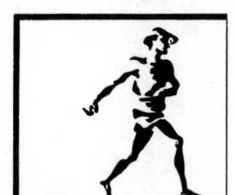

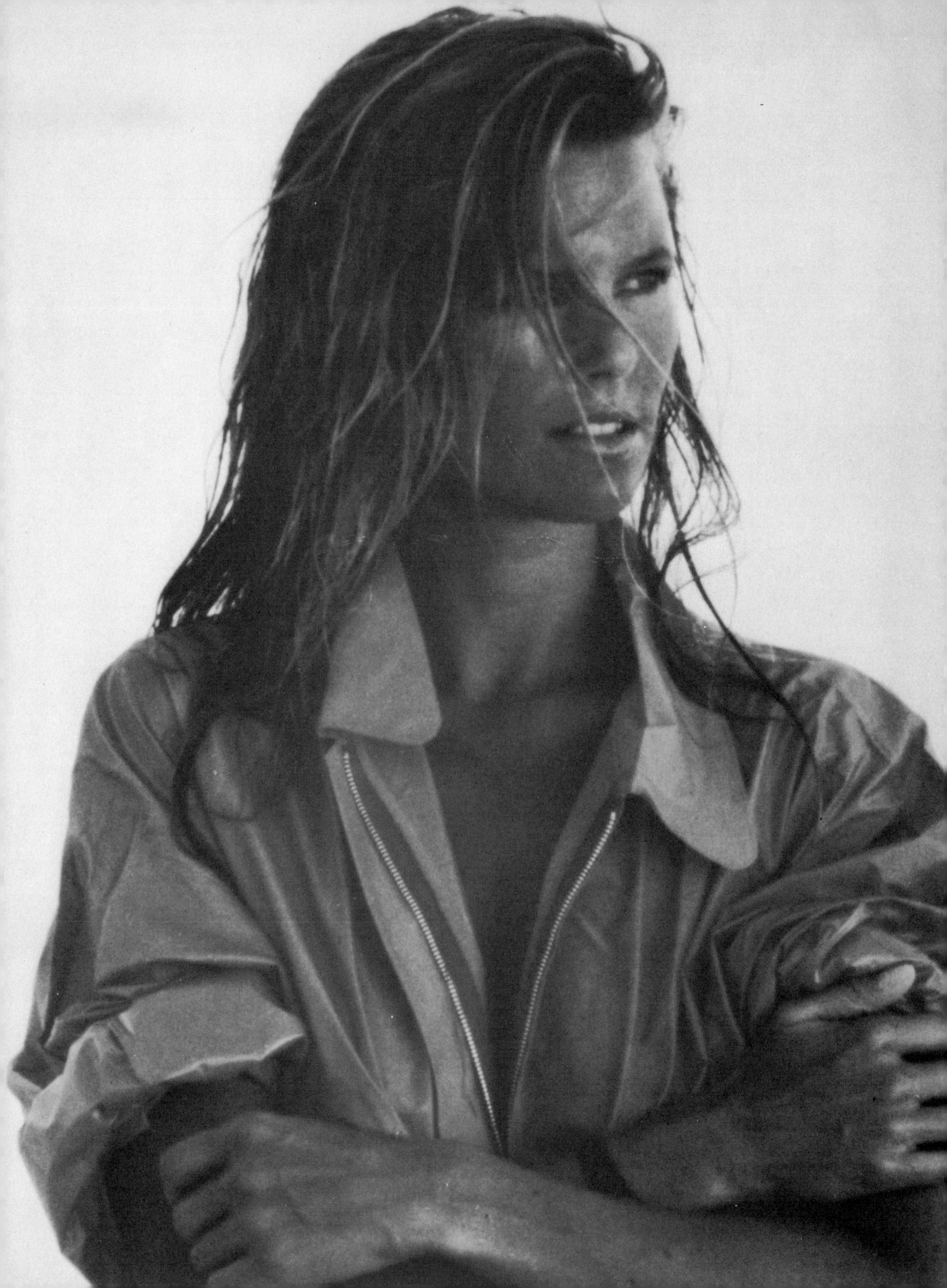

Christie Brinkley's Outdoor Beauty & Fitness Book

Photography by Alex Chatelain
Illustrations by Christie Brinkley
Research by Kathy Matthews

SIMON AND SCHUSTER • New York

Published by Simon and Schuster
A Division of Gulf & Western Corporation
Simon & Schuster Building
Rockefeller Center
1230 Avenue of the Americas
New York, New York 10020
SIMON AND SCHUSTER and colophon are registered trademarks of Simon & Schuster
Designed by Christie Brinkley/C. Linda Dingler
Manufactured in the United States of America

10 9 8 7 6 5 4 3 2 1

Library of Congress Cataloging in Publication Data
Brinkley, Christie.
    Christie Brinkley's Outdoor Beauty Book

    1. Beauty, Personal.   2. Women—Health and hygiene.
3. Physical fitness of women.   I. Title.
RA778.B84   1983   613'.04244   83-454
ISBN 0-671-46190-7

FOR OLIVIER CHANDON

ACKNOWLEDGMENTS

Thank you, *grazie, merci mille fois* to the fantastic photographers who have contributed their beautiful photographs for use in this book—Les Goldberg, Walter Ioos, Jr., Jacques Malignon, Mike Rhinehart, Jean-Claude Sauer/*Paris Match,* Albert Watson, Bruce Weber, John Zimmerman/*Sports Illustrated*— and a very special thanks to Alex Chatelain and Patrick Demarchelier for their generous contributions of time and talent.

I would also like to extend my thanks and gratitude to Liza Bruce, Norma Kamali, Julio, Danskin, Fieldcrest Towels, Keesha Keeval, and Arthur Kleinman . . . and a very special note of thanks to Francesca Casciaro for her continued interest, support and endless energy . . . and of course, thanks, Mom and Dad!

FOR EVERYONE WHO LOVES AND PROTECTS THE SEA

CONTENTS

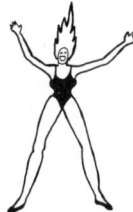

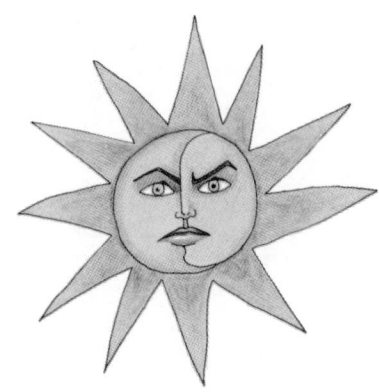

THE SUN

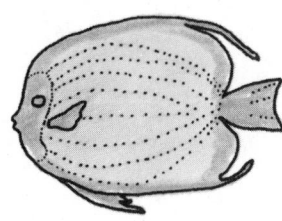

THE SEA   **155**

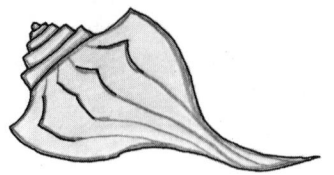

THE SAND 181

Christie Brinkley's Outdoor Beauty & Fitness Book

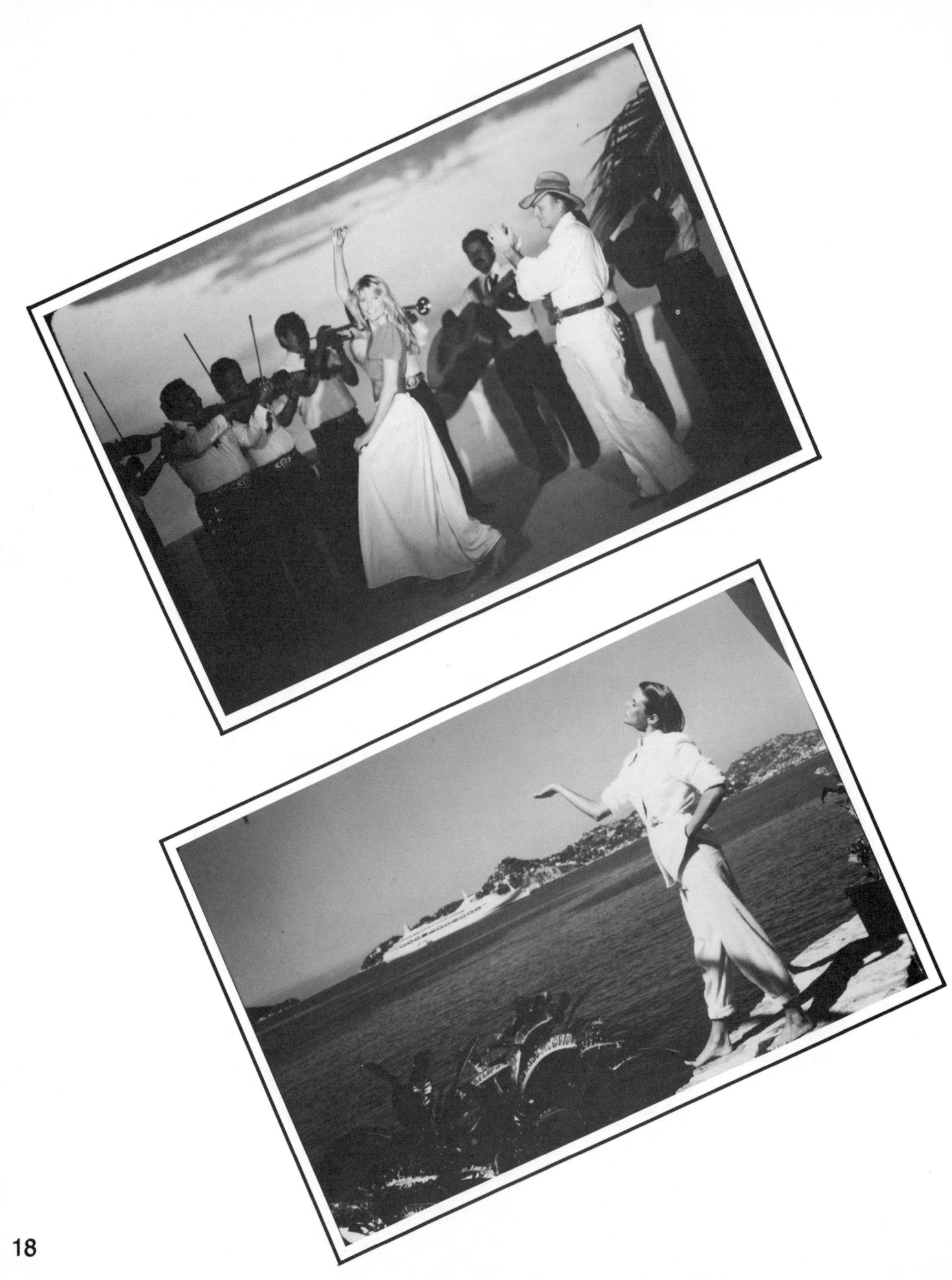

I grew up on the beach in Malibu, California, with a blob of zinc oxide on my nose. I was the only surfer on the beach with a fake French accent, for as much as I cherished being a suntanned tomboy by the sea, I dreamed of becoming an artist in France. So, zats *exactement* what I did.

At 18, I moved to Paris. I studied art, became fluent in French, worked as an illustrator, stopped wearing zinc oxide *sur mon nez,* had the time of my life, got a dog, got "discovered" and ended up right back on the beach!

Modeling by the sea may sound glamorous, and in many ways it *is,* but it also means:

teeny bikinis—they must fit!

makeup in the water—it must not smudge!

humid weather—try curling your hair!

dry heat—try not to peel!

exotic food—I must not eat it!

exotic bugs—they must not eat *me!*

and sunburns—you can't wear zinc oxide on your burning nose when you're selling the makeup that covers it!

I learned a lot of beauty tricks as a matter of survival, and now I'm sharing all my tricks and tips with you!

Bonnes vacances!

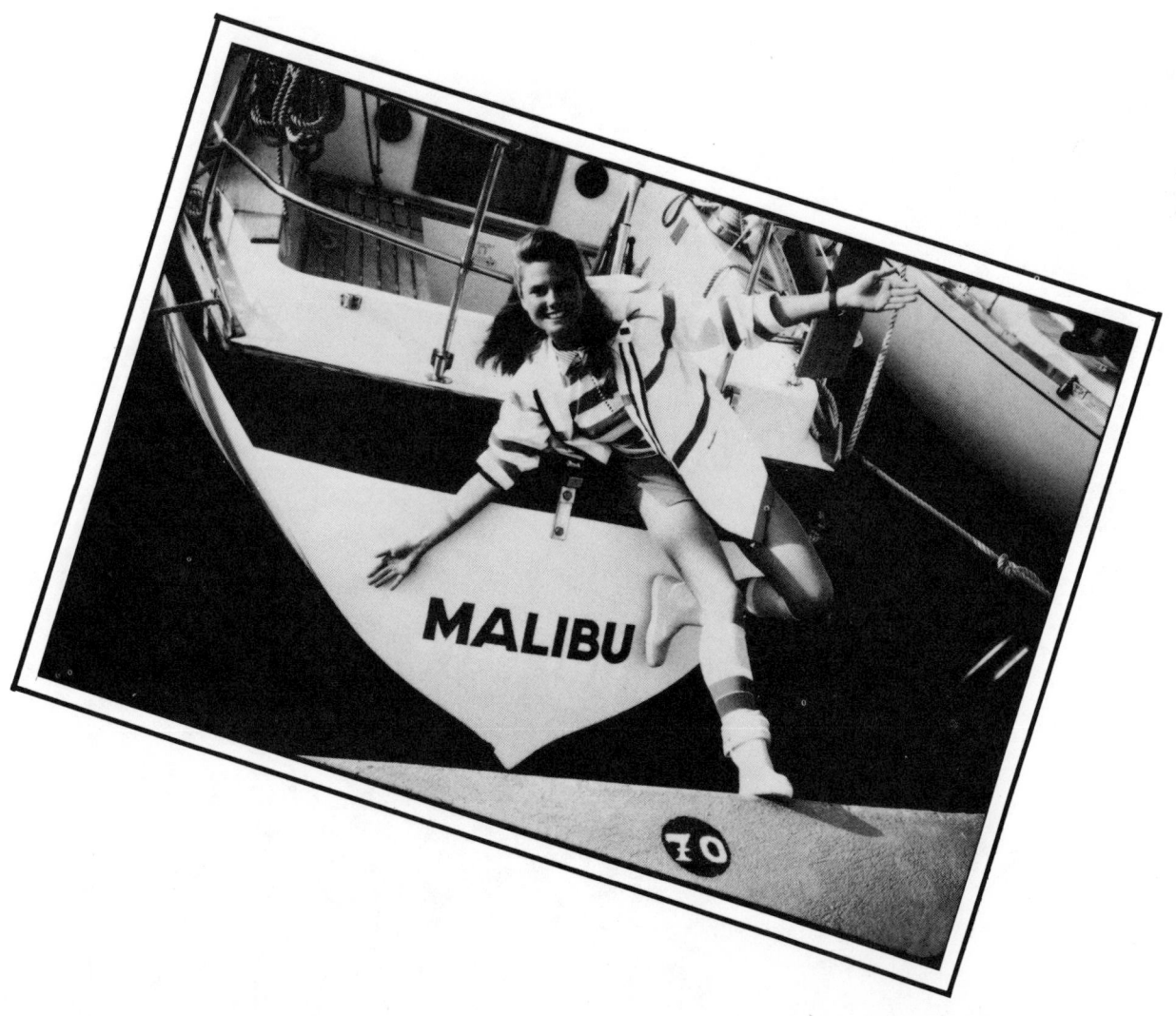

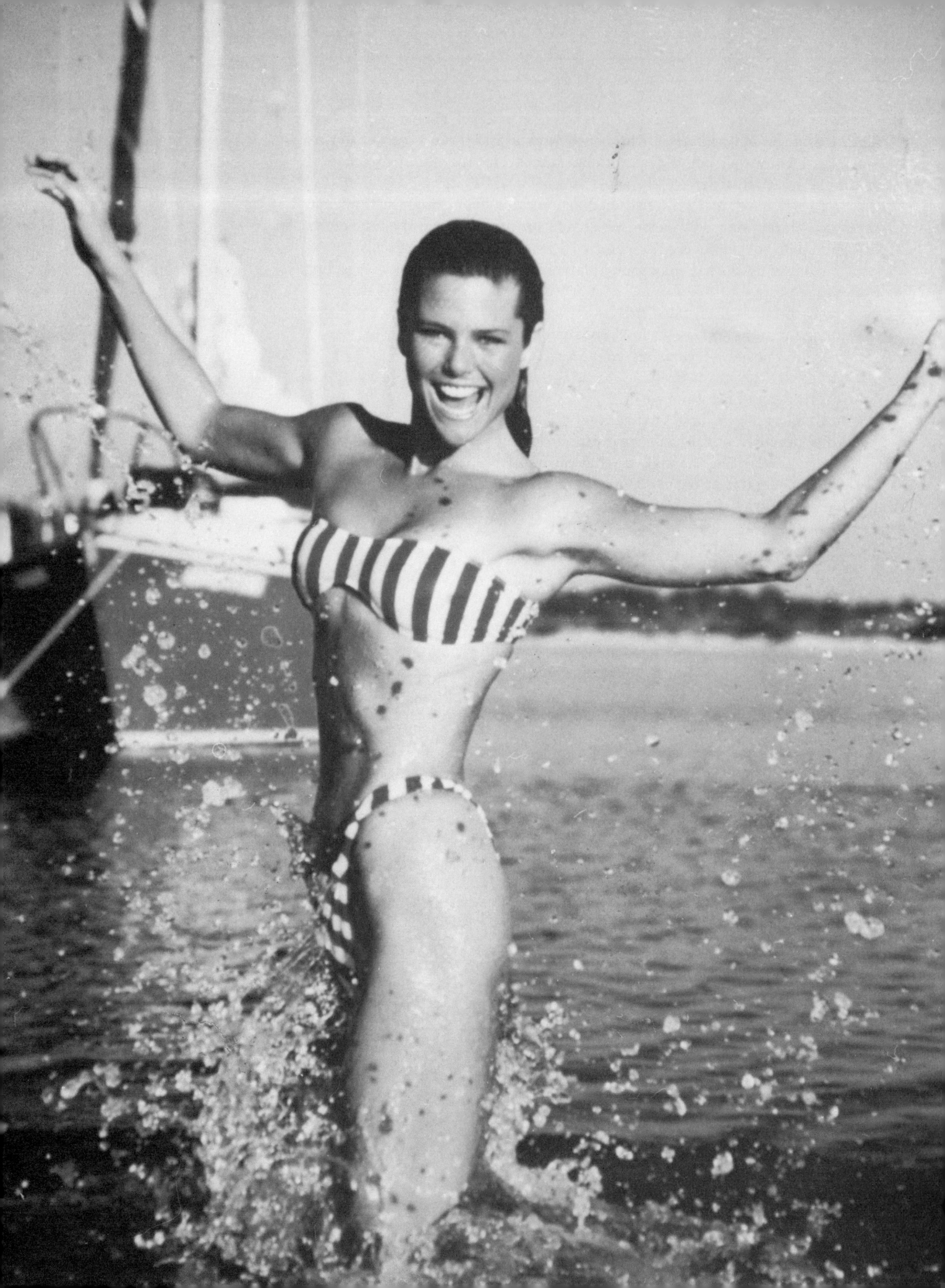

GETTING READY TO BARE IT!

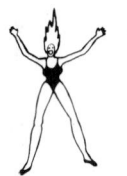

Me, fat??? You should have seen me in Mexico!

There I was, immersed in a few simple margaritas, tostarilas, etceterita, etceterita, etceterita . . . And suddenly, it was the Battle of El Bulgo!

What is it about Mexican food that seems to shrink bikinis? Okay, I'll tell you.

The main ingredient in Mexican food is *not*, as you may have thought, beans—it's *calories!*

Yes, I've fallen prey to temptation many times, and discovered, to my regret, that there are no simple diet tricks.

I've tried the watermelon diet,
> the no-fats diet,
> the juice diet,
> the fish-only diet,
> the lonely apple diet,
> the grapefruit diet.

I've dieted from the suburbs of Beverly Hills to the outskirts of Cambridge!

But, let's face it, the only one that really works is a low-calorie, well-balanced diet.

THE REMOVABLE FEAST

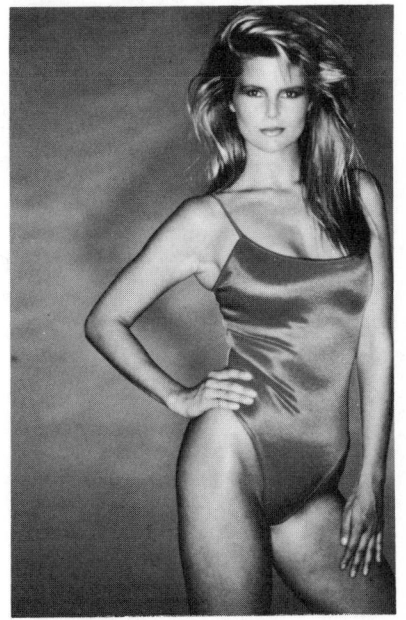

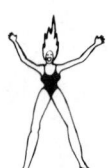

Is that your stomach growling? Just the mere mention of the word "diet" makes *me* hungry! But with *this* diet you don't have to be hungry! If you choose the right foods that are low in calories, you'd be amazed at the enormous quantity you're allowed!

Being calorie-conscious has taught me to compare foods in a vivid, visual way. I think about some foods as being friendly, harmless, healthful, big-quantity foods. Others as concentrated, heavy-calorie, small-portion foods. And I choose accordingly. Once your doctor has told you how many calories you can eat to lose weight, you can eat your calorie quota in ice cream and cake and *still* lose weight—but you'll end up with dull, lifeless hair, bad skin and teeth, and other serious health problems. You want to not only look better but feel better, too! You have to eat balanced meals in order to keep your energy up, your hair shiny, your complexion glowing, and your body functioning at its very best.

When I was first asked to model in Paris, I immediately assumed I had to be as skinny as the other models. My first assignment? A magazine cover—in a bikini. Panic! I stopped eating everything except yogurt. I had always heard that yogurt is healthy, and it is. One week later the bikini fit, and I shot the cover. I was thrilled, so I continued my yogurt-only regimen another week. My diet ended when I passed out in a café and woke up in the doctor's office—with, of all things, a calcium deficiency. Although yogurt is full of calcium, my body was unable to assimilate it because it lacked the proper nutrients needed in order to do so.

THE LOW-CALORIE, WELL-BALANCED DIET
(or How to Keep Your Bikini from Shrinking)

Another case of learning the hard way. Now I make a point of eating vegetables, fruits, fish, and grains every day. (I've been a vegetarian since I was 14 years old so I skip the meat entirely.)

Become calorie smart! Get yourself one of those little calorie books and study it. Use your book to make a food diary. List everything that passes your lips. Choose foods from each food group every day and tally up your calories. With the facts in front of you it's hard to cheat!

Remember, if you want to lose weight, you have to stick to your diet—and you can with this diet that offers such a wide variety of food and even an occasional splurge!

Now my mind is trained. I know how to choose the low-calorie alternatives automatically. And I can eat a full and balanced diet. Here are some suggestions from the five major food groups that you might find interesting and that will help you get started on your calorie-wise education.

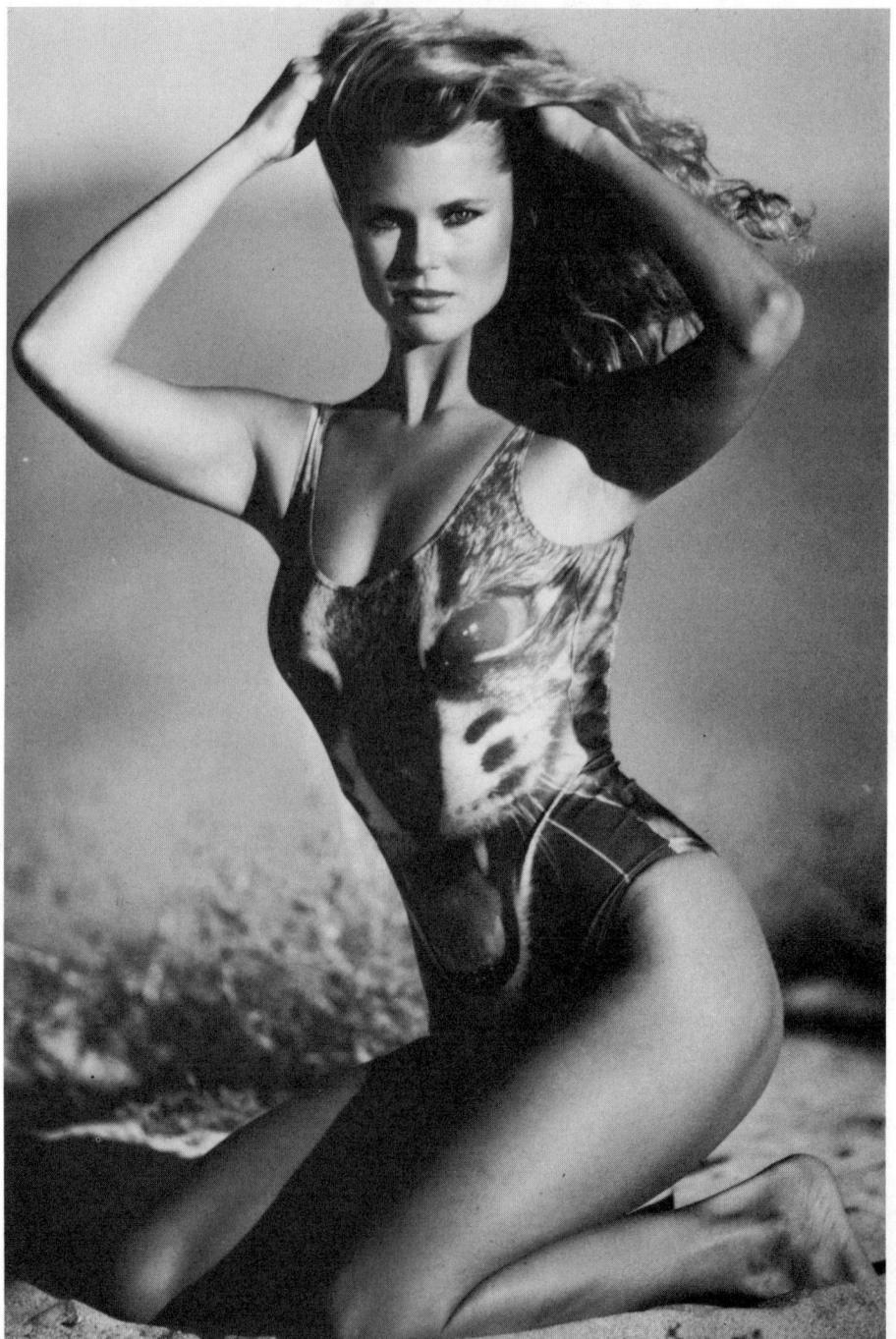

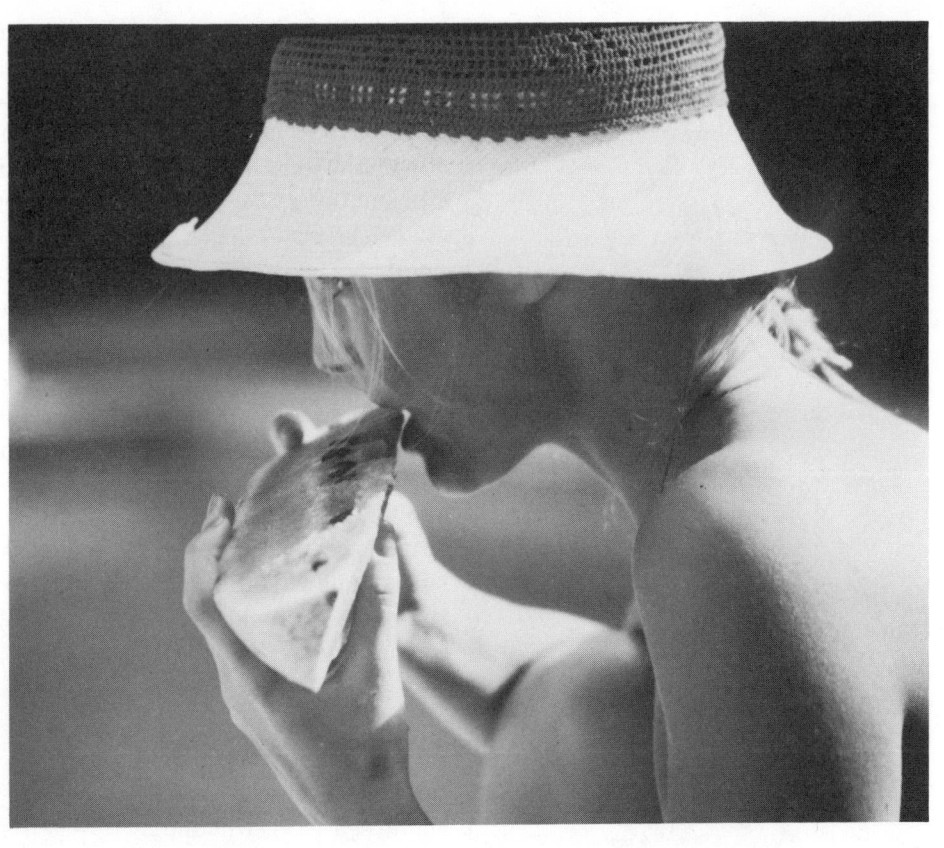

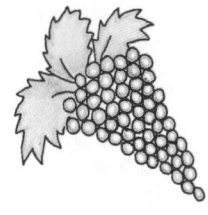

Fruit/calories

1 medium orange	60
2 tangerines	78
1 banana	101
½ cup strawberries	26
½ cantaloupe	60
1 medium apple	80
½ papaya	60
½ grapefruit	48

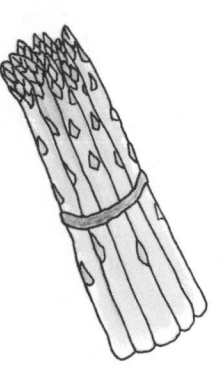

Vegetables/calories

1 cup cooked, sliced zucchini	18
½ cup green beans	16
1 average artichoke	53
4 spears asparagus	8
1 medium cucumber (no skin)	21
3 leaves (8″ long) romaine lettuce	5
1 stalk broccoli	18
1 ear corn	74

THE MAIN FOOD GROUPS

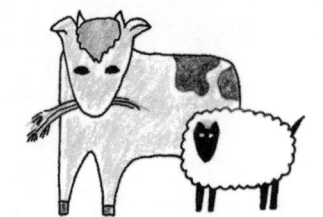

Meat and Poultry/Calories

3 ounces lean pot roast	183
3 ounces sliced ham	198
1 chicken drumstick	78
½ chicken breast	156
3 ounces broiled burger	243
1 hot dog	134
4 ounces turkey (with skin)	250
4 ounces loin veal chop	265

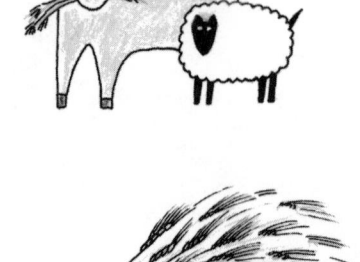

Bread and Cereal/Calories

½ cup cooked brown rice	89
¾ cup toasted, puffed millet	50
1 ounce wheat germ	93
1 slice whole wheat bread	66
1 cup oatmeal, cooked	132
1 corn muffin	129

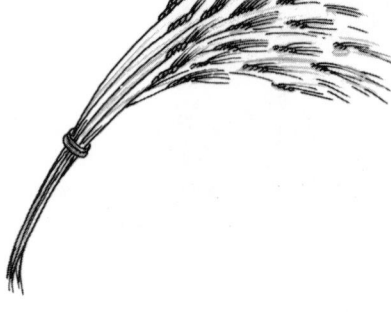

Fish/Calories

1 can tuna in water (7 ounces)	234
1 whole sea bass (1 pound)	165
3 ounces scallops	96
1 whole lobster	107
4 raw clams	65
1 fish cake	153
4 ounces baked flounder	230

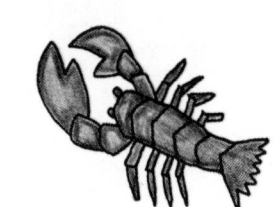

Dairy/Calories

1 cup skim milk	88
1 cup yogurt (plain)	150
1 ounce cottage cheese	30
1 ounce Camembert	85
1 ounce mozzarella	79
1 ounce cheddar cheese	113

COUNTING CALORIES

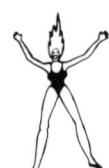

How many calories does it take to keep you going each day? Nutritionists estimate that someone who is moderately active burns 12 to 15 calories per pound of body weight per day. So a 120-pound woman would burn about 1560 calories a day (at the rate of 13 per pound) just to maintain her weight.

But what if she wanted to lose weight? How many calories should she consume?

Well, first imagine that your body is a machine that runs on two possible fuels: food and/or stored fat. As you go through your day, you're drawing on these energy sources. To compare the energy sources, we know that 1 pound of fat equals 3500 calories. If our 120-pound woman burned all the 1560 calories we said she needed to keep going but still kept going, she'd be using the stored fat in her body for energy. She'd be burning up fat and losing weight. If, in a week, she burned an extra 3500 calories, she'd lose a pound.

Here's how to figure how many calories you should be eating to lose 2 pounds a week. Grab your calculator; it's easy:

1. Your current weight × 13 = M (M is how many calories you need a day to maintain your weight.)

2. If you want to lose 2 pounds per week, you've got to eliminate a total of 7000 calories (3500 for each pound) per week or 1000 calories each day,

so

3. M − 1000 = your daily calorie intake, which will make you lose 2 pounds per week!

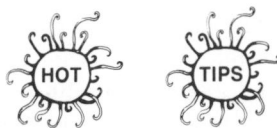

Your Ideal Weight: Want a quick rule of thumb for figuring your ideal weight? If you're 5 feet tall, you should weigh 100 pounds. For every additional inch, add 5 pounds. So if you're 5 feet 4 inches, you should weigh 120 pounds.

Of course, this applies to an average frame. If you have a small or a large frame, your ideal weight would vary accordingly.

Chew slowly!

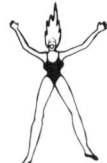

WAIT! Before you put that chocolate into your mouth—let me entice you with a list of healthy low-cal fantastic figure foods:

FANTASTIC FIGURE FOODS

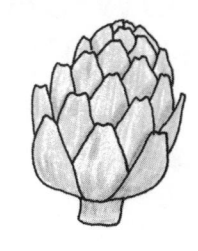

Artichokes! What tastes great, takes forever to eat, and makes you feel full? Artichokes! I eat them all the time. I always keep them around the house, especially when I'm trying to lose weight. I use just a tiny bit of olive oil as a dip. You could also mix up a yogurt dip which is tasty and low in calories.

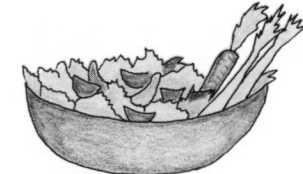

Salads! Salads as "diet" food can seem bland and boring. So liven them up with unusual ingredients or combinations. My very favorite salad is *insalata Caprese,* which is fresh tomatoes, fresh basil, and pieces of mozzarella cheese. With just the slightest bit of olive oil drizzled over, there's nothing like it! Don't forget fresh herbs—they can make a *huge* difference in an otherwise ordinary salad.

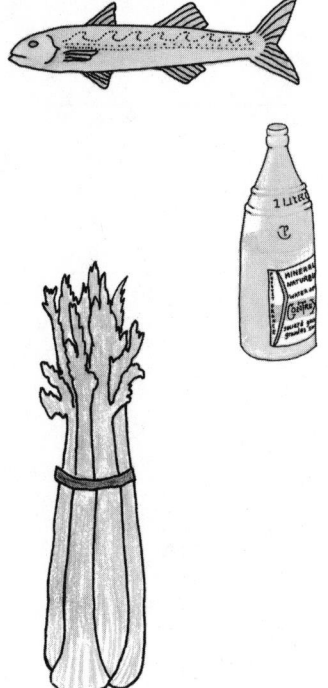

Seafood! I love seafood! It's best at the beach where it's fresh and delicious, but even dining in midtown Manhattan I make a point of ordering it (without sauces, please)! It fills me up for the day. Fish is low in calories, high in protein, and can be easily prepared in a variety of ways.

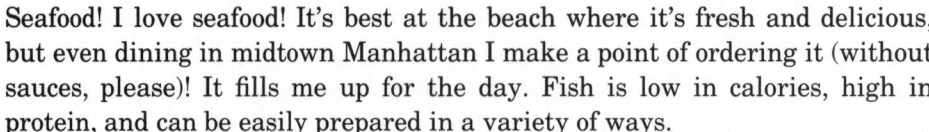

Water! You're not hungry, you're thirsty! So don't have a cookie, have a tall glass of club soda or mineral water. Add a slice of lemon, lime, or even orange. Or add some fresh fruit juice. Sip it slowly. It works! Drink eight glasses a day, every day. (But don't drink it within a half hour before or after eating meals, as it dilutes your digestive juices.)

Vegetables! Vegetables! They're really the backbone of my diet. I love them. They're filling, satisfying, and they give you lots of valuable vitamins and minerals. They are also complex carbohydrates which take a while to digest and give you a gradual energy supply that holds up throughout the day. How about fresh steamed broccoli with a wedge of lemon? Or steamed carrots with some yogurt/dill sauce? Be imaginative! Yumm, this is making me hungry!

Snacks! Snacks are an important part of losing weight—because as soon as you decide to go on a diet, you're hungry all the time. All you think about is food. So be prepared! When you steam vegetables for dinner, steam extra to snack on the next day. Freeze a banana (yum!). It tastes like ice cream and takes a long time to eat. (Peel it first—have you ever tried to peel a frozen banana?) Keep treats like uncoated frozen yogurt bars around. They have only 70 calories and make you feel as if you're having ice cream. Put the fattening foods in the back of the fridge. When you open the door you want to see a beautiful bowl of vegetables and perhaps a yogurt/curry or yogurt/scallion dip.

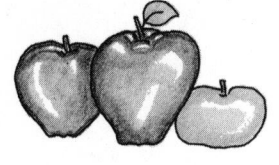

SOME EASY LOW-CAL RECIPES

Guacamole

This makes a great dip for raw vegetables. Mash together the flesh of 1 avocado, 1 clove of minced garlic, 1 small chopped tomato, the juice of ½ lemon, 2 chopped green onions, 1 small chopped green chili pepper, ½ teaspoon of chili powder, and 1 tablespoon of minced fresh coriander (cilantro). Each tablespoon is only about 28 calories, so you can dip freely!

Yogurt Sauce

Sometimes plain steamed vegetables can be a bore. So whip up some yogurt sauce to liven things up. Simmer about ¼ cup of white wine in a saucepan for a few minutes till it reduces. Then swirl in about ¼ cup of plain yogurt and some fresh herbs, such as dill or basil. Don't let the yogurt boil; just heat it through, then pour over veggies. It's only about 35 calories.

Lite Russian Dressing

Whenever you're in the mood for a creamy-style dressing, here's one that's low in calories. Mix 3 tablespoons of imitation or diet mayonnaise with 2 teaspoons each of ketchup and chili sauce. Add Worcestershire sauce to taste.

Beaten Banana

Whenever you've got a banana that's overripe, use it for a low-cal breakfast or snack. Toss it in the blender with about ½ cup of plain yogurt, 1 teaspoon of lemon juice, a dash of vanilla or almond extract, and 2 or 3 ice cubes. Blend till foamy. It's only about 150 calories for the whole drink.

Mock Caramels

Desperate for some candy? Satisfy yourself with frozen raisins. Let them thaw just a bit and they'll taste like caramels. At 30 calories a tablespoon you can really satisfy your sweet tooth!

Hot Melon

Here's a great alternative to your usual breakfast fruit. It also makes a filling snack. Take a half a cantaloupe, drizzle it with a teaspoon of honey and about ½ cup of strong herb tea (like Red Zinger). Put it in a 350-degree oven for about 15 minutes and enjoy warm. About 55 calories.

Super Slim Soup

Want a quick cool soup for a hot afternoon? Take a seeded, chopped cucumber, 1 cup yogurt, 2 teaspoons fresh, chopped dill and 2 chopped green onions. Into the blender and presto! Cool-as-a-cucumber soup at only about 50 calories.

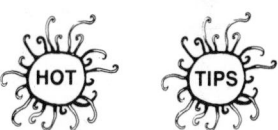

A minute on the lips, a lifetime on your hips.

Dieting? Weigh yourself at the same time of day *once a week!* Those daily weigh-ins are too confusing and discouraging, as they reflect natural water fluctuations.

Low-fat yogurt makes a great low-cal replacement for mayonnaise!

Do you find that whenever you try to diet you wind up obsessed with food and snacking all day? Then why don't you try "snack dieting." Eat lots of tiny meals all day long; this will help eliminate hunger pangs and keep your energy level up all day long. As long as the total calorie intake is within your diet limit and all your nutritional needs are being met, you'll be losing weight.

Carry healthy, natural food with you to work or to the beach so you won't be tempted by all the fast junk food around you!

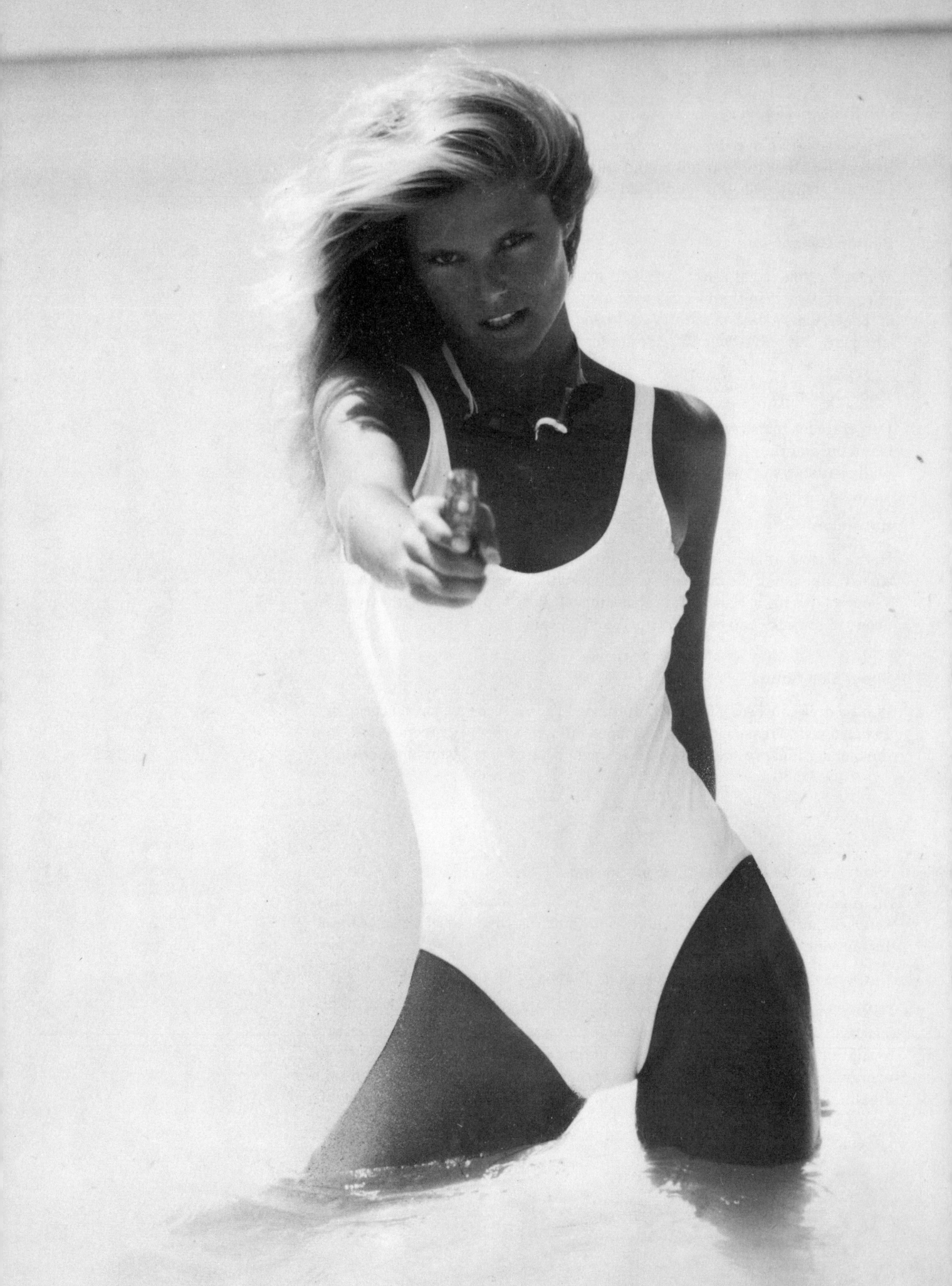

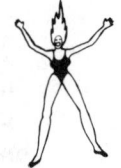 **HOLD IT! HANDS UP!** Move away from that cookie jar! I know it's tough. *Temptation* is everywhere. It's not easy to change your eating habits. You need to fight the battle of "El Bulgo" on every front. To give yourself every weapon and advantage, arm yourself with these helpful plans of action.

Exercise! It's your best friend. It firms you, burns calories, and suppresses your appetite. And if you exercise vigorously, you'll still be burning calories even after you stop. Besides, it's hard to eat while you're standing on your head! Instead of having a snack, do 10 sit-ups and then . . . do 10 more!

Sleep hungry! I try never to eat after 6 P.M. or 7 P.M. I may be hungry but it doesn't hurt to *dream* about hot fudge sundaes! This way your stomach growls while you're sleeping and you don't even feel it. It's given up growling by morning. When I wake up, I'm ready for a decent breakfast: some fruit, maybe a small piece of cheese, and a cup of herbal tea.

Adjust for the big night out! If I know I'm going to splurge with friends in a fancy restaurant, I prepare for it all day. I eat a small breakfast of perhaps half a papaya, and just an apple and a bit of cheese for lunch. My stomach growls its loudest at 5 P.M. or 6 P.M., so I'll have a small snack then—maybe a glass of fruit juice. By the time I get to the restaurant, I'm ready for a great meal, and I deserve it!

Fill your fridge with fruits and vegetables!

Fool your stomach! Did you know that it takes your stomach 20 minutes to realize you've eaten something? When you go on a binge, by the time your stomach knows it's full, it's too late. So fool your stomach with before-meal snacks. Do what your mother always warned against: Spoil your appetite! Have a carrot, a cup of broth, a few sticks of celery 20 minutes before dinner. By the time you sit down to eat, you'll be less hungry.

Eliminate salt! Especially at the beginning of a diet. Salt makes you retain water (and weight) and gives you a puffy feeling. If you eliminate it at the beginning of your diet, you'll lose pounds and inches more quickly and that'll give you the psychological boost to stick with it.

The more you eat, the hungrier you are! I find if I splurge on a big meal at dinner, the next morning I'm ravenous. But if I stick with light meals my stomach somehow adjusts and I'm not tempted to binge.

Alcohol is the downfall of many dieters! The trick here is to know yourself. If you *must* have a drink in the evening, make it a dry white-wine spritzer. Sip slowly. Add more ice when you're halfway through instead of refilling sooner. I love margaritas, but when I order one I order water, too. I alternate sips from both and make it last all night. And remember that the calories in alcohol have no nutritional benefit. Adjust your daily calorie count accordingly.

Avoid processed foods! Most of them are high in calories and laden with preservatives and salt. Make it yourself from scratch, or better yet, whenever possible eat it raw.

Never, never let yourself get ravenous! It'll be your downfall. If you're going to have to go a long stretch between lunch and dinner, plan on a healthy snack: an apple, some steamed vegetables, some cottage cheese with chives on melba toast. That way you won't go nuts when you finally get to your meal. (But the *best* way to avoid extra snack calories is to keep yourself so busy you don't have time to even think about snacking!)

Ban junk food from your home! This may be difficult if you live with a crowd but, after all, it benefits them, too. I never keep junk food at home. How can you resist salted peanuts if they're on the coffee table or chocolate cake if it's calling to you from the refrigerator? Make it easy on yourself.

Wallpaper your refrigerator with photos of thin thighs!

Buy yourself a wonderful dress two sizes too small! Then plan a party for the end of the month where you'll slip on your gorgeous gown and show off your new figure.

Or go bathing-suit shopping—it always takes away my appetite!

And, must I say it? Leave the sugar to the birds.

DIETING— À LA CARTE

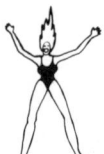

I'm always eating in restaurants. Often I'm working on location where the meal is whatever is brought in. Other times I'm in transit and eating on the run. And when I finally do get home and get a chance to see my friends, we often meet in a restaurant. This requires some special techniques for staying slim. Restaurants are getting better these days—they often offer light meals—but still, it helps to have some tried and true strategies.

Order appetizers only! Of course you can't expect to sit in a busy coffee shop and nibble for an hour on a fruit cocktail. But in a more relaxed restaurant you can order, say, a shrimp cocktail, a salad, and a tomato juice. Or how about two appetizers and a vegetable? Most restaurants will be happy to oblige and the presentation will often be pretty and appetizing. You won't miss that fattening casserole after all.

No bread! But don't try to resist once it's there; tell the waiter not to put it down in the first place.

Head for the salad bar! But skip the croutons, bacon bits, olives, and heavy dressings and stick with lemon juice and a bit of oil.

If you're traveling by plane, remember when making your reservation to ask for a special fruit or vegetable plate. Not only will it keep you on your diet, it will taste a lot better than what everyone around you will eat!

Be fearless! Don't be afraid in a restaurant, on an airplane, or at someone's home (within reason) to ask for something special. If you explain that you're on a special diet, most people are happy to help out. Ask for the entrée without the sauce. Ask for the fish broiled without butter. Ask for the salad to be served without dressing. And don't ask for dessert!

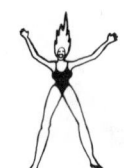

As I write this, over a million women in the United States are suffering from anorexia nervosa. As you probably know, this is a disorder connected with obsessive dieting. Its consequences are tragic.

Though I think it's important for your body to be in good condition, I believe that many women use the wrong guidelines for their ideal figures. They measure themselves by an unreasonably small clothing size or a picture in a magazine of a woman with a tiny bone structure or the weight and height statistics of a fashion model.

Good health and good nutrition are the only sensible foundations for dieting. I am constantly aware of my figure but I am very active. I exercise constantly and I need to eat healthy meals to maintain my energy level and my appearance. I think that the terribly thin body that results from excessive dieting is unattractive. But worse, it's unhealthy.

If you are dieting and you find yourself obsessed with dieting to an unreasonable degree, even though you are quite thin, you may need help. Talk to your doctor or write to the American Anorexia Nervosa Association, 101 Cedar Lane, Teaneck, N.J. 07666 for advice.

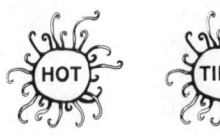

Good health is good business.
—slogan, President's Council for Physical Education

As you get older your body needs fewer calories to stay the same weight. So every birthday you should drop 10 calories off your daily total intake.

NAVEL

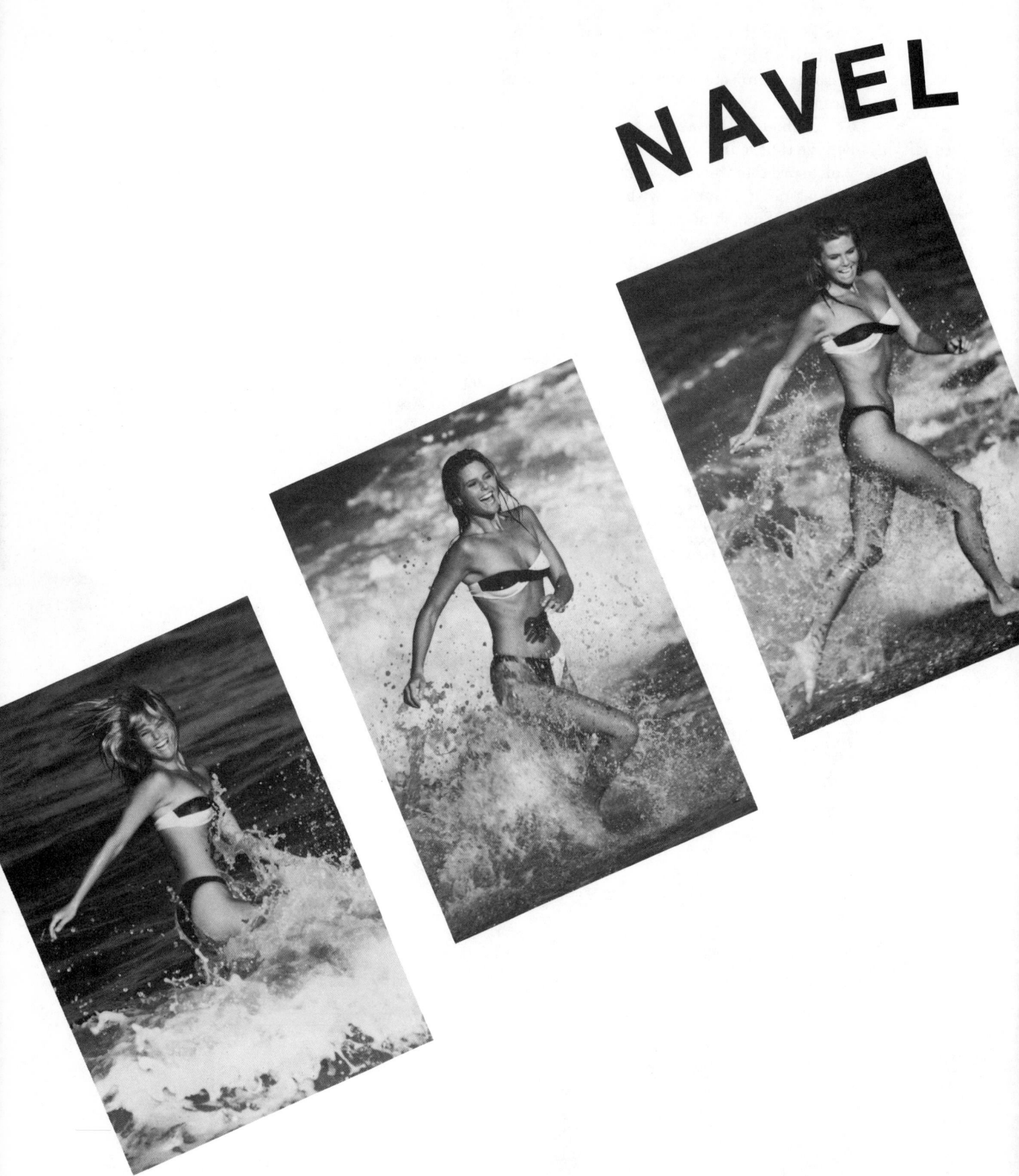

MANEUVERS

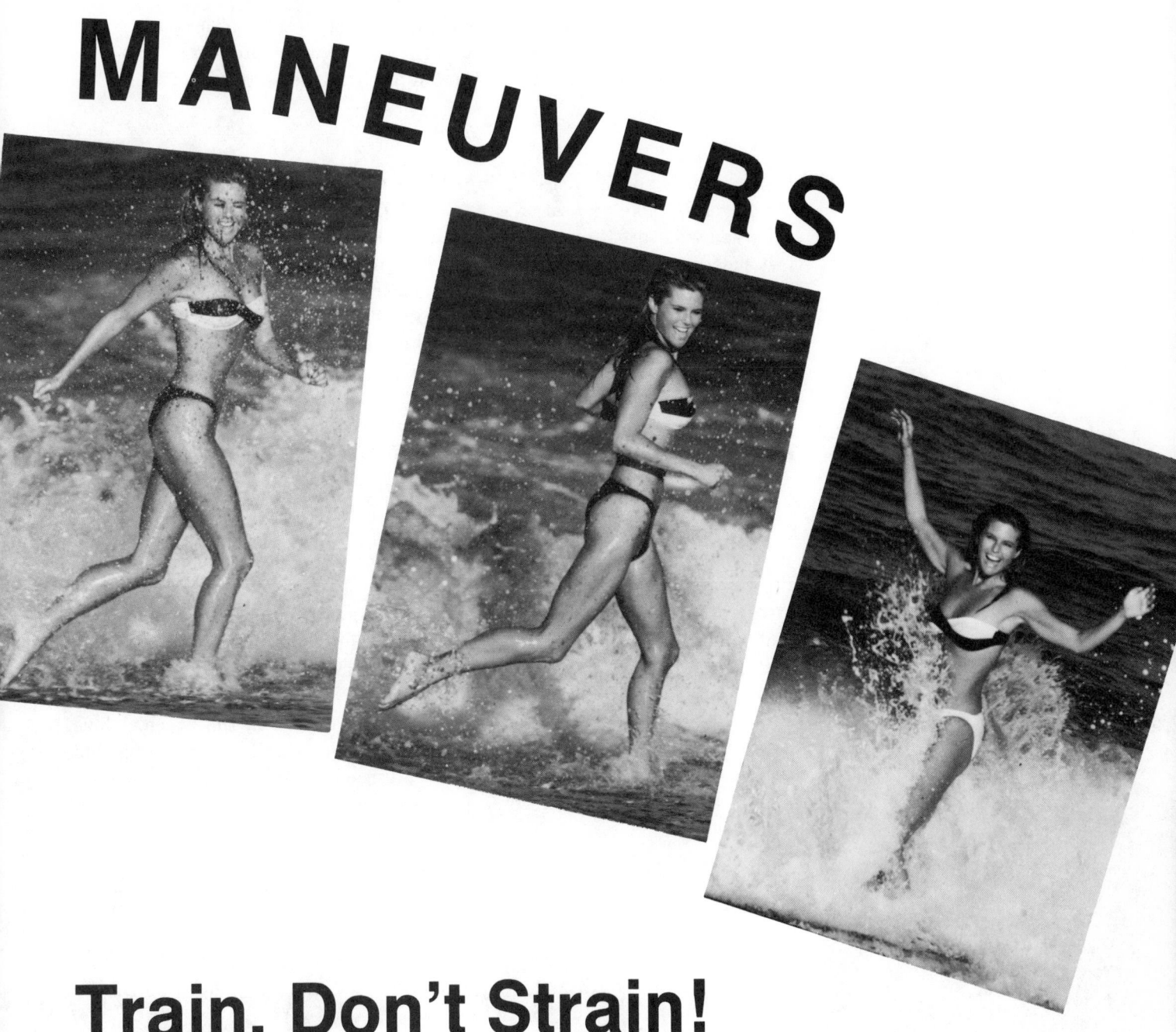

Train, Don't Strain!

Exercise routines are boring and difficult to stick to. But that doesn't mean I don't exercise. I do—every day! To look and feel fantastic, your body needs a daily workout. The best way to ensure that you will do it is to make it fun. I've discovered the key word that makes exercise something I look forward to: it's *variety!* This helps to eliminate boredom and keeps you going when the going gets tough.

BE ACTIVE!

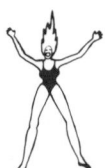

Start by spicing up your life with active sports. There are other places to lose weight besides your living-room floor. And you'll enjoy sports so much you'll forget that it's exercise too!

Winter

Last winter I added cross-country skiing to my downhill skiing trips and discovered a whole new set of sore muscles. While working on my ice-skating I learned what great exercise falling down is! A friend introduced me to the fast indoor game of racquetball, and it's great for getting that cold winter blood pumping. I bought rollers for my bicycle so that I could keep pedaling while I was looking out the window and waiting for the thaw. Take a horseback ride across a snowy field. Go sledding. How about disco roller-skating? Or why not learn a martial art? I now study Tae Kwon Do under the great Master Lee Kwon Young and I've included his warm-ups in my exercise chapter. Tae Kwon Do not only keeps me fit but it gives me confidence when I'm alone at night! Winter is also a great time to join a gym.

Summer

As things warm up it becomes easier and easier to incorporate sports into your life. I practically live outdoors in the summer. My bicycle goes back out to the streets (the calm ones, that is!). I start losing tennis games to my mom and dad again (they're too good!). Friends start organizing hiking trips and baseball games in the park. I manage to have at least one sore muscle all summer long!

But my favorite way to spend a summer day is on the beach. I love anything happening in, on, or near the water. Volleyball, scuba diving (I'm certified), water-skiing (with one ski), falling off windsurfs (just learning), racing sailboats with my brother, Greg (he's an expert sailor), or just riding the waves.

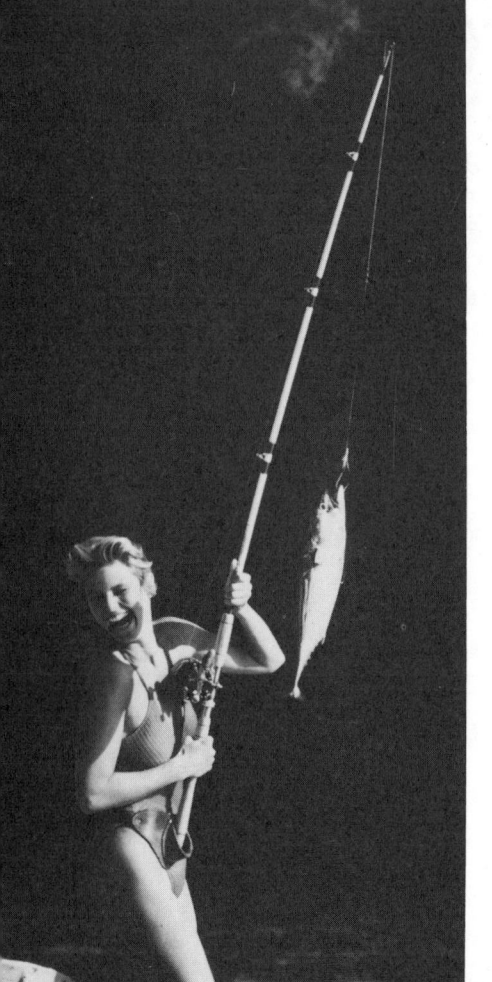

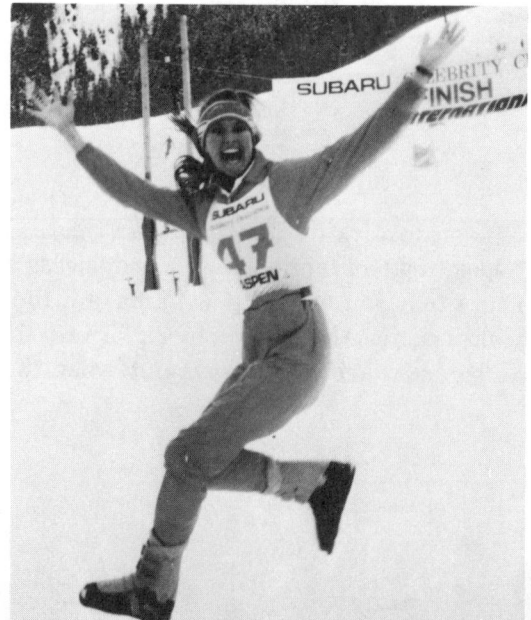

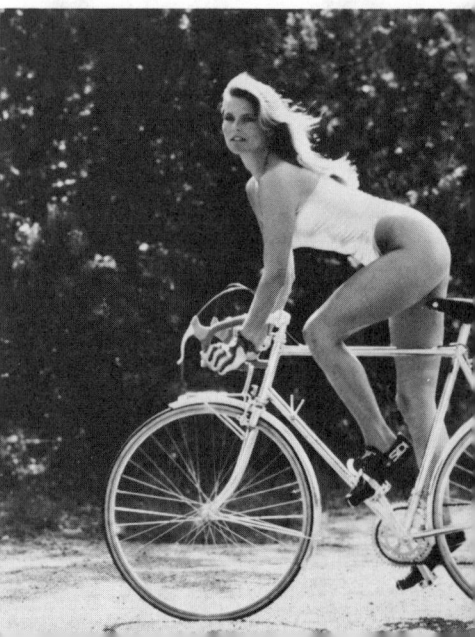

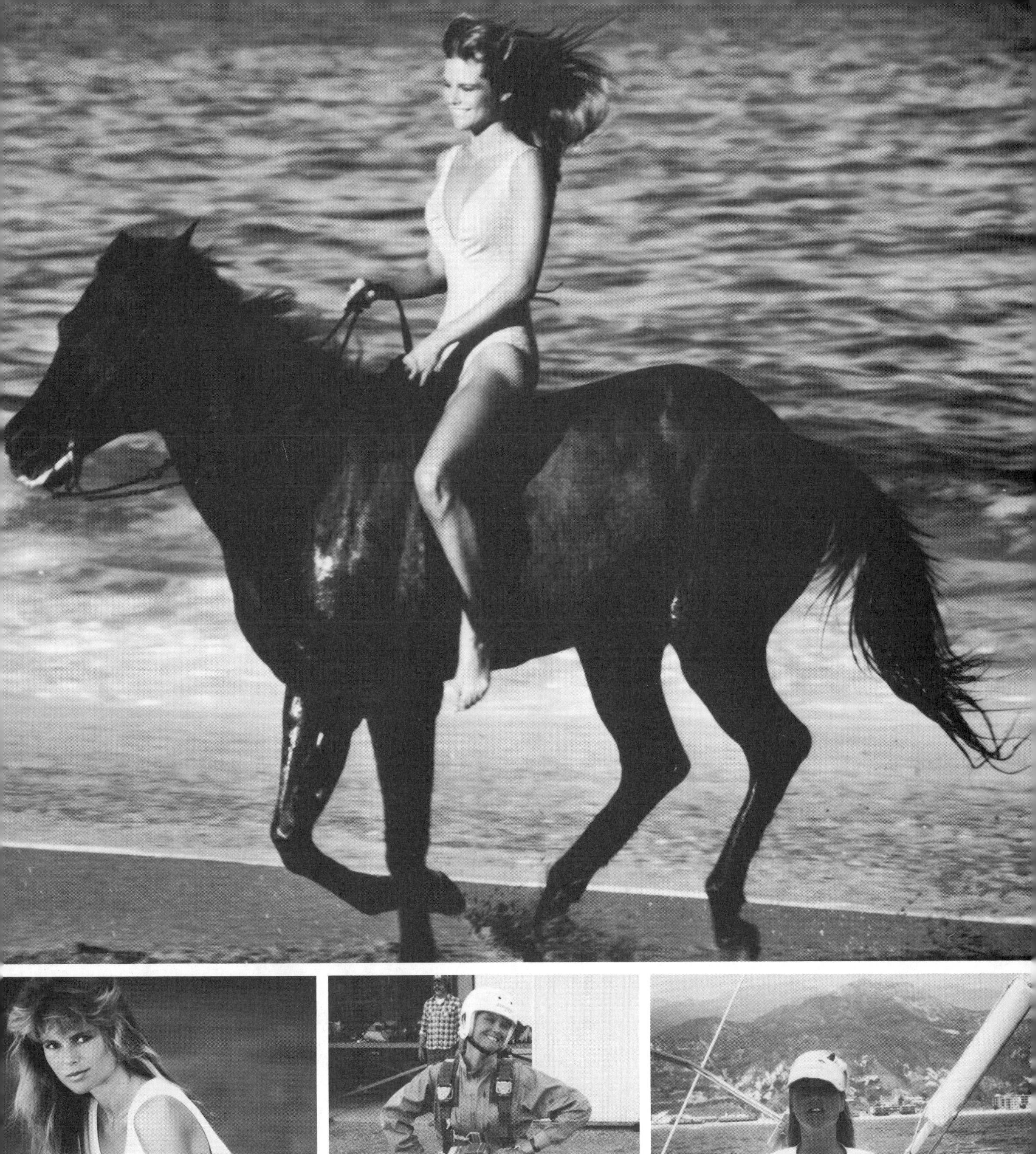

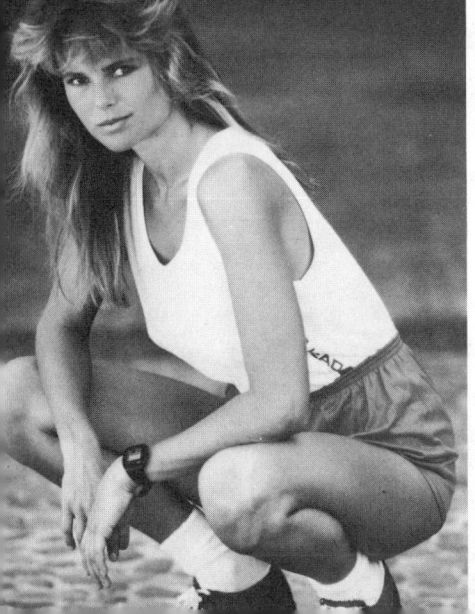
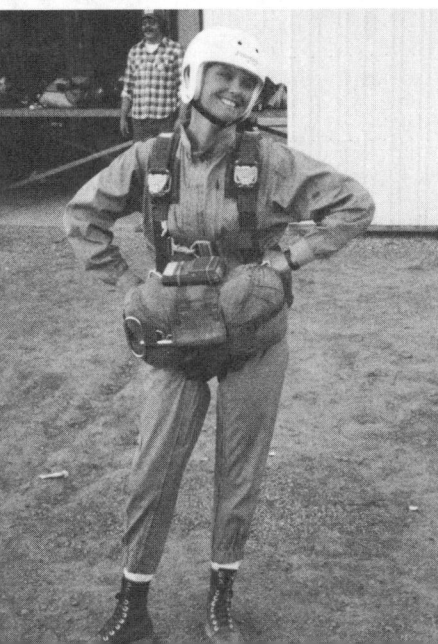
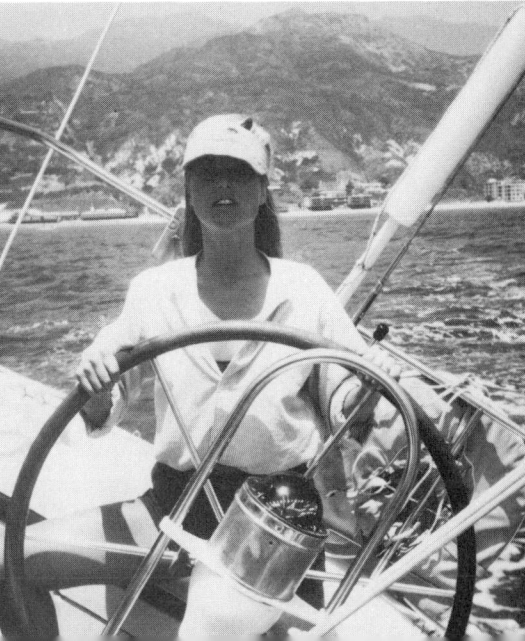

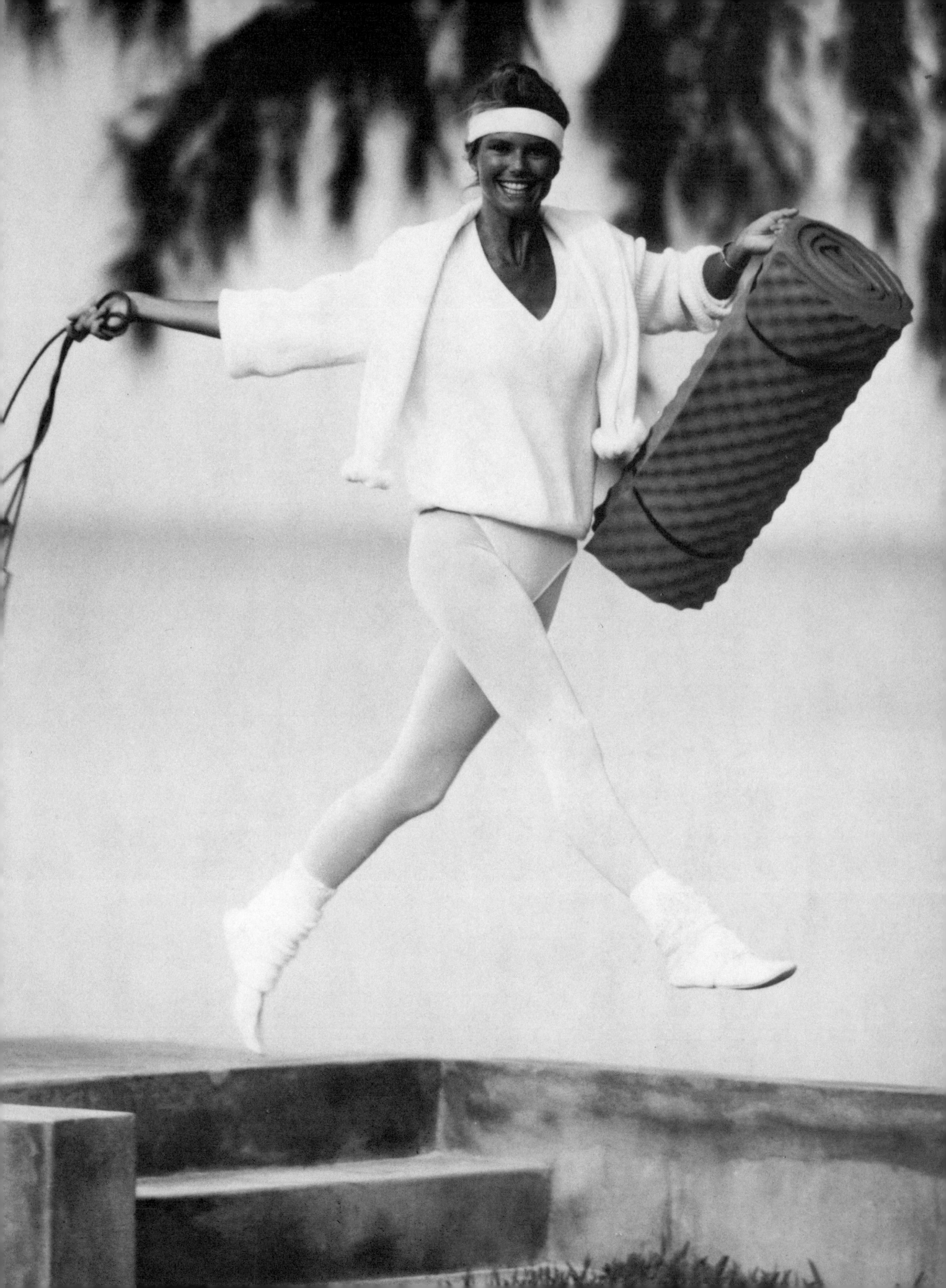

MOTIVATION
(Tips to Keep You in Motion!)

1. Become an exercise collector. Start your exercise notebook *today!*

2. Keep your weight and tape measurements up to date in your exercise notebook.

3. Buy some new exercise clothes so you feel good when you put them on.

4. Step out of bed and into your exercise clothes. That way you'll have no excuses: You'll be ready to go.

5. Keep the rest of your equipment in full view as a reminder that you should be using it! Hang a jump rope on the doorknob, keep your exercise mat *on the floor*.

6. Put on your favorite happy "up" music. That will get you going!

7. Try posting a photo of a body you admire on your refrigerator door to remind you of your goal.

8. Be flexible with your time. Just because you missed your morning exercises doesn't mean you've blown it for the day. Do them at lunchtime or before dinner.

9. And forget about making excuses. *They* won't slim down thighs!!!

EXERCISE STRATEGY

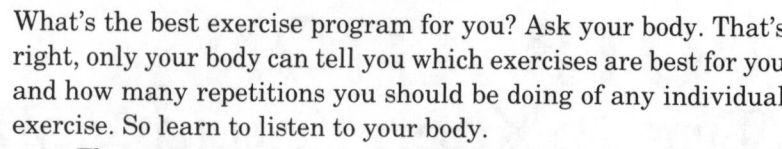

What's the best exercise program for you? Ask your body. That's right, only your body can tell you which exercises are best for you and how many repetitions you should be doing of any individual exercise. So learn to listen to your body.

The exercises in this book are ones that I do all the time and the repetitions given are the number of reps that I do. But I've been doing these exercises every day for a long time. If you're a beginner, you have to let your body dictate how many reps you should be doing and at what speed.

Here are some important keys to effective exercise:

Whether you're starting fresh or an old hand at daily exercises, be sure to warm up first. A warm, relaxed muscle has more potential power than a cold, tense one. It's also less liable to injury.

If an exercise hurts, stop! No exercise should hurt you. You may feel tired and your muscles may twitch with effort but you shouldn't hurt. If you do, you may be doing the exercise wrong. Check the instructions again and if it still hurts you should check with a professional—a doctor or a trained exercise expert.

Start slowly. If you push yourself unmercifully the first day, you may get so knocked out that you'll want to quit forever. It's okay to feel that pleasant ache that tells you your muscles worked out yesterday. But anything more than that is counterproductive. If I say you should touch your toes in a certain exercise and you can't, don't skip the exercise. Instead, go for your ankles or your knees. You'll be working the same set of muscles and that's what counts. If 20 reps are recommended and you can't do more than 5, fine. Make your goal 6 and work toward that. Remember, you're not competing, you're improving.

Go for subtlety. Most people think of exercise as all action; they can't wait to kick and jump and bend. But often the effectiveness of an exercise comes from doing it less flamboyantly but perfectly. Sometimes it's easy to kick high if you let your stomach muscles go. Don't fall into this trap. Do every exercise perfectly. Think of your body as a sculpture. Work every muscle, keep the correct alignment, breathe deeply. The results will be more dramatic and satisfying.

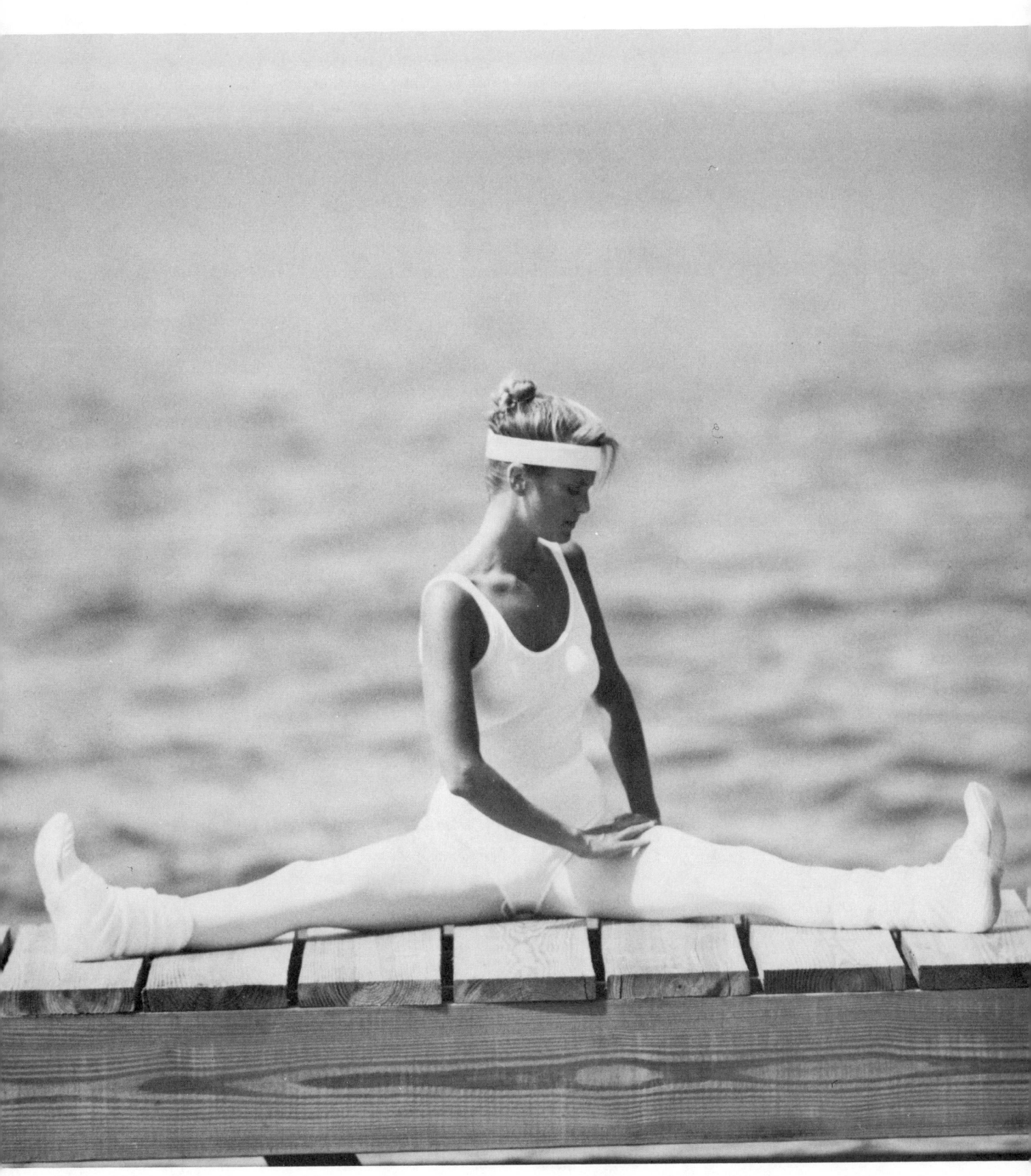

EXERCISE NOTEBOOK

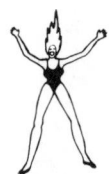

Spot exercises are the mainstay of your exercise system. They're the links between tennis and skiing. They're the exercises you do on a rainy day or a busy day that doesn't allow time for a scuba dive. They will firm you up and keep you in shape for all your active sports!

These are the exercises you will face on a regular basis, so it's up to you to be imaginative so you don't slip into a boring routine! Each day I make a point of varying my workout. I'm always on the lookout for new exercises, which I record in an exercise notebook so I have hundreds to choose from.

I own exercise books, tapes, and video cassettes. At work I exchange exercises with models from around the world. I have had modeling assignments that had me demonstrating exercises from top experts. Ballerinas Melinda Roy and Antonia Francesci of the New York City Ballet have taught me some real killers. I've even picked up some fancy jump-rope footwork from boxing champions like Roberto Duran and Sugar Ray Leonard.

I'm not an exercise expert able to name every muscle in my body, but as a model part of my job is staying in shape. So now I want to share with you some of my favorite exercises. Remember, this is not a routine. It's up to you to develop a new awareness about exercising. Try these out and see which ones work for you, and then add them to *your* exercise notebook.

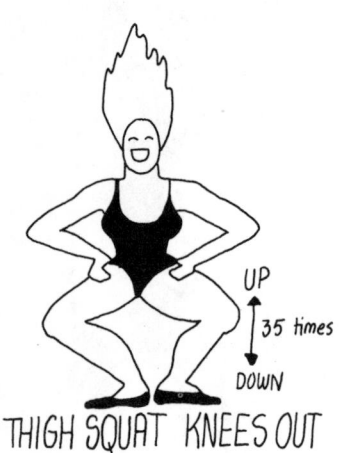

UP
35 times
DOWN

THIGH SQUAT KNEES OUT

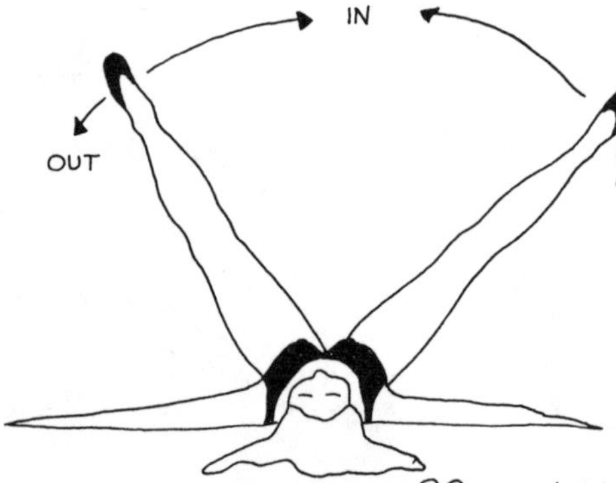

IN
OUT
OUT

WIDE-LEG SCISSORS _ count 40

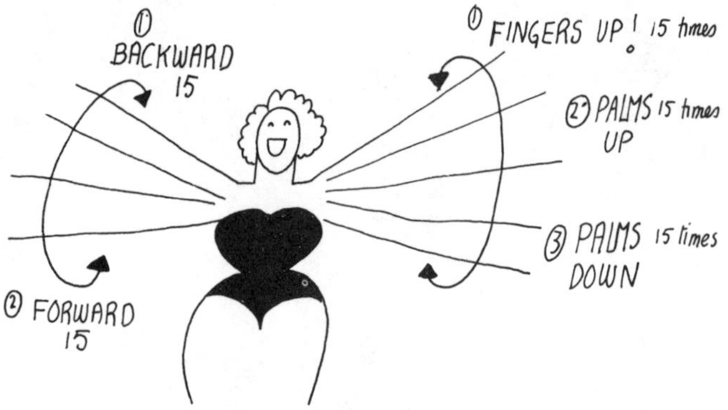

① BACKWARD 15
② FORWARD 15
① FINGERS UP! 15 times
② PALMS 15 times UP
③ PALMS 15 times DOWN

ARM PROPELLERS
a great warm-up exercise

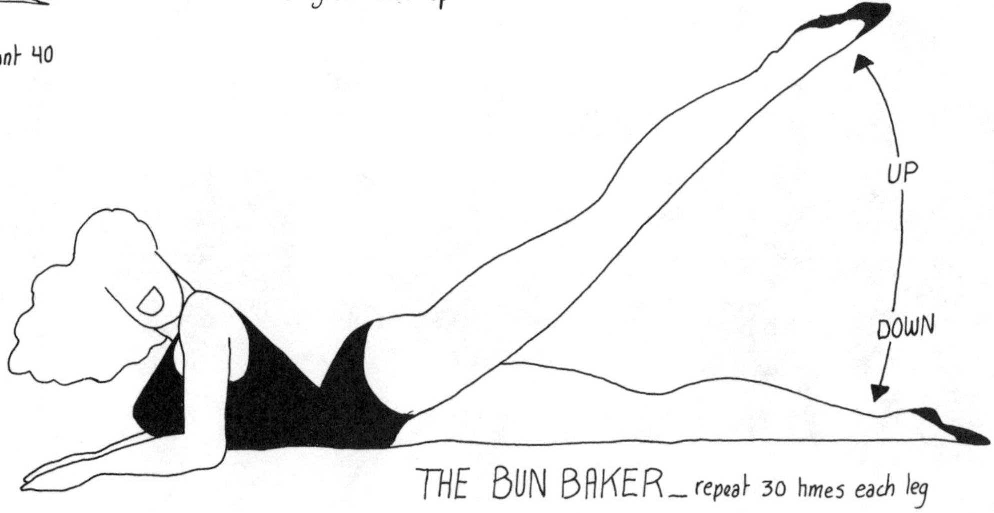

UP
DOWN

THE BUN BAKER _ repeat 30 times each leg

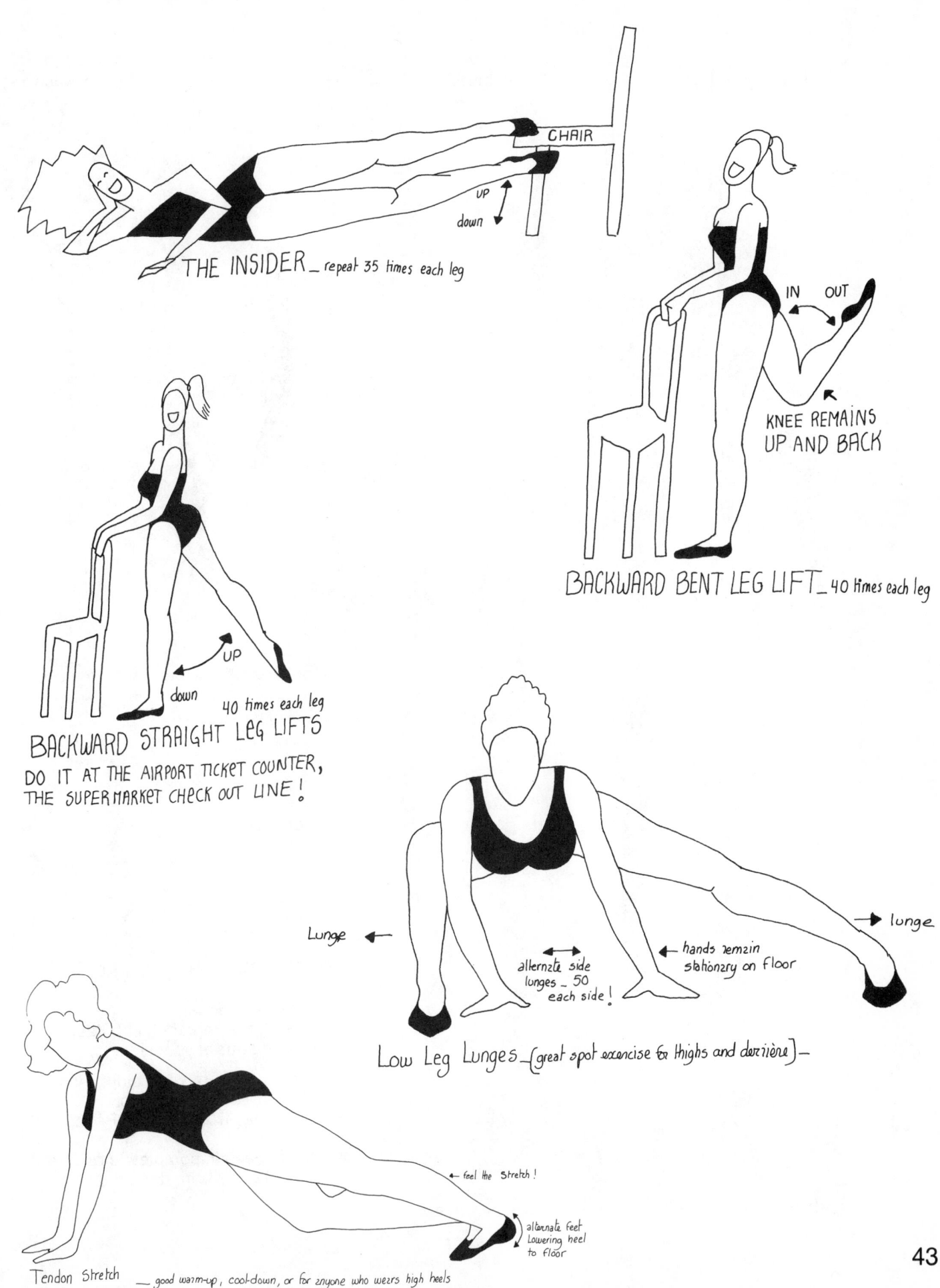

THE INSIDER — repeat 35 times each leg

UP
down

CHAIR

IN   OUT

KNEE REMAINS
UP AND BACK

BACKWARD BENT LEG LIFT — 40 times each leg

UP
down
40 times each leg

BACKWARD STRAIGHT LEG LIFTS
DO IT AT THE AIRPORT TICKET COUNTER,
THE SUPERMARKET CHECK OUT LINE!

Lunge

lunge

alternate side
lunges — 50
each side!

hands remain
stationary on floor

Low Leg Lunges — (great spot exercise for thighs and derrière) —

← feel the stretch!

alternate feet
lowering heel
to floor

Tendon Stretch — good warm-up, cool-down, or for anyone who wears high heels

43

WARM UP!

Cold muscles can be easily injured regardless of what you've planned for the day. Protect yourself by always doing a few stretches and aerobics to really get you going.

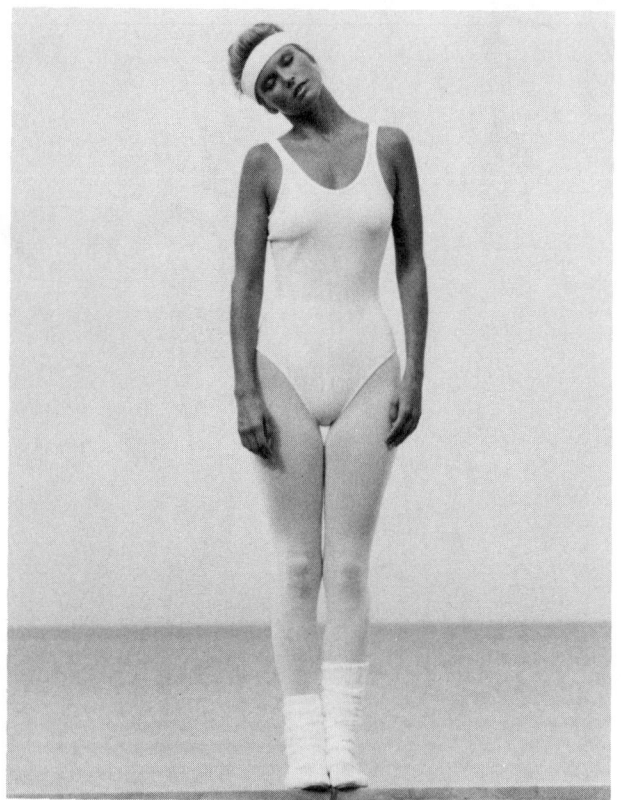

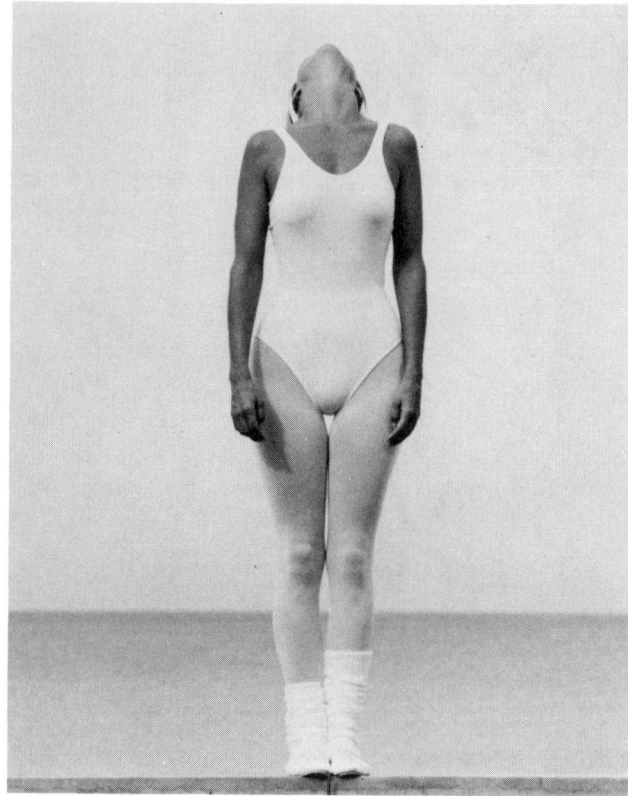

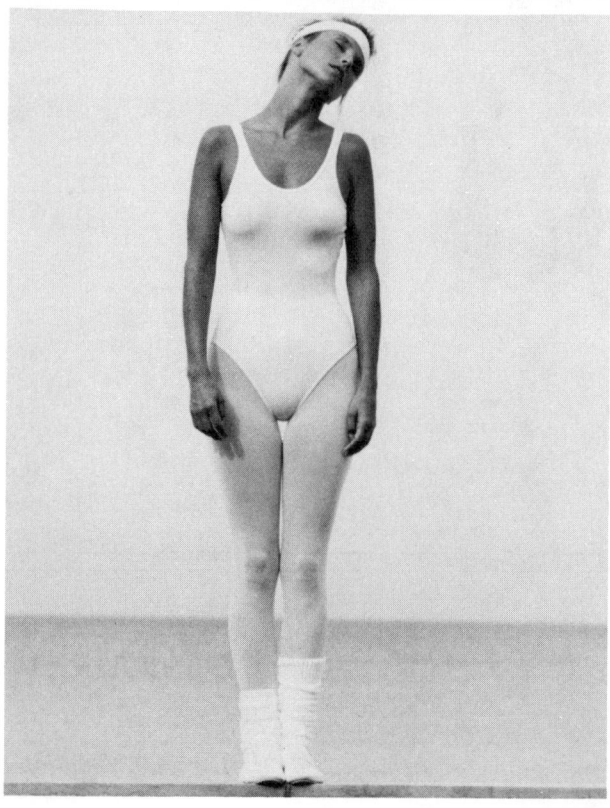

DO ALL STRETCHES VERY SLOWLY.

The Rubber Neck
Stand with feet together, shoulders relaxed, and arms at your side.

1. Stretch head to right side, then to left side. Repeat 10 times.
2. Move head front to back. Repeat 10 times.
3. Rotate head in complete circle. Repeat 10 times both directions.

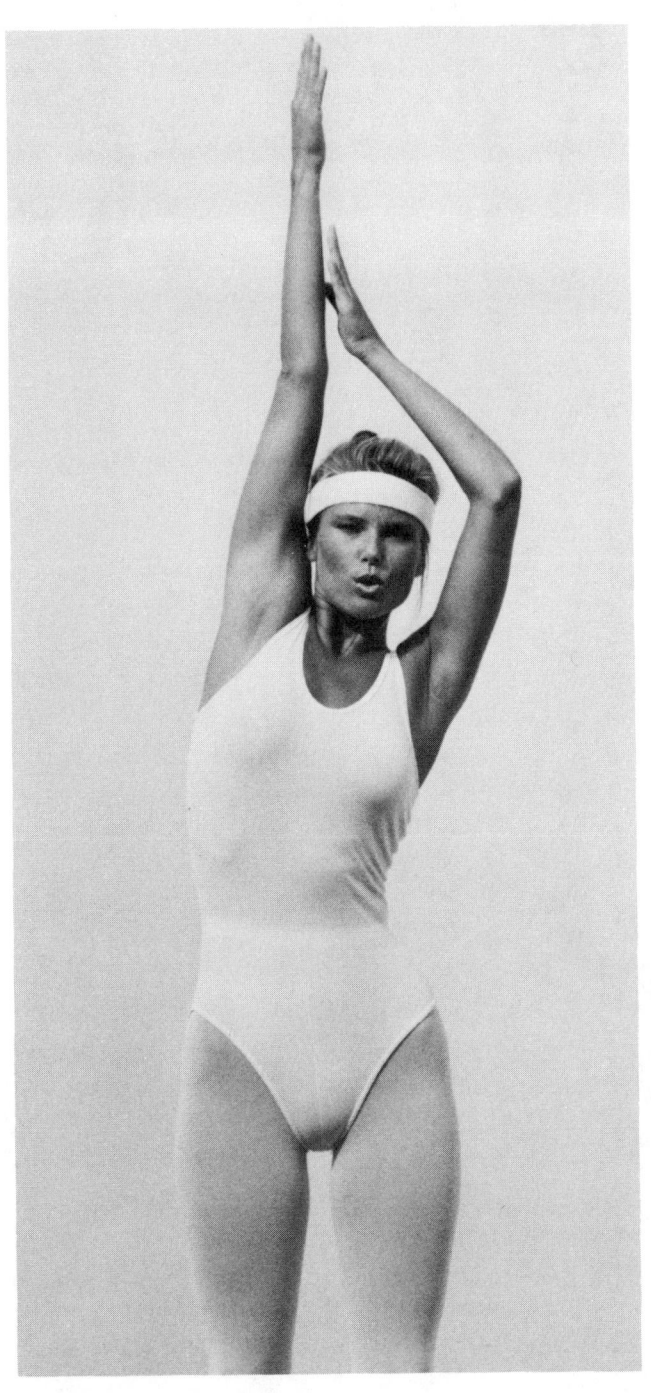

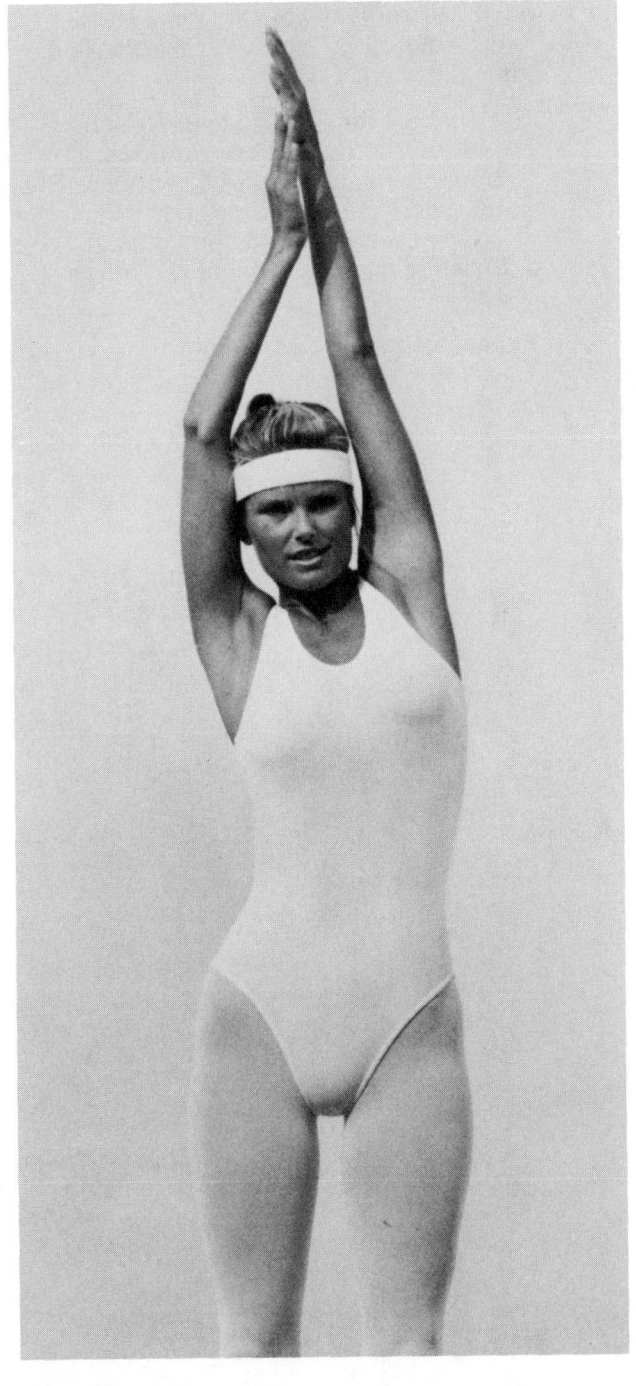

Rope Reach
Stand with feet shoulder-distance apart.

1. As if you were climbing a rope with your hands, reach with the right hand, stretching all the muscles along the side of your upper torso.
2. Then reach with the left hand.

Repeat steps 1 and 2 fifteen or twenty times.

And remember, TRAIN, DON'T STRAIN!

45

WARM UP!

Oblique Stretch
This stretches the oblique muscles and works the waist.

Stand with your arms at your sides, feet shoulder-distance apart. Raise one arm over your head and drop the other in front of you at waist level. Keep your body straight, shoulders right above your hips.

1. Bounce 4 times to the left, stretching out a little more with each bounce. Remember, when "bouncing" don't strain—take it easy until you're sure you won't hurt yourself.
2. Reverse and bounce 4 times to the right.

Repeat steps 1 and 2 ten times.

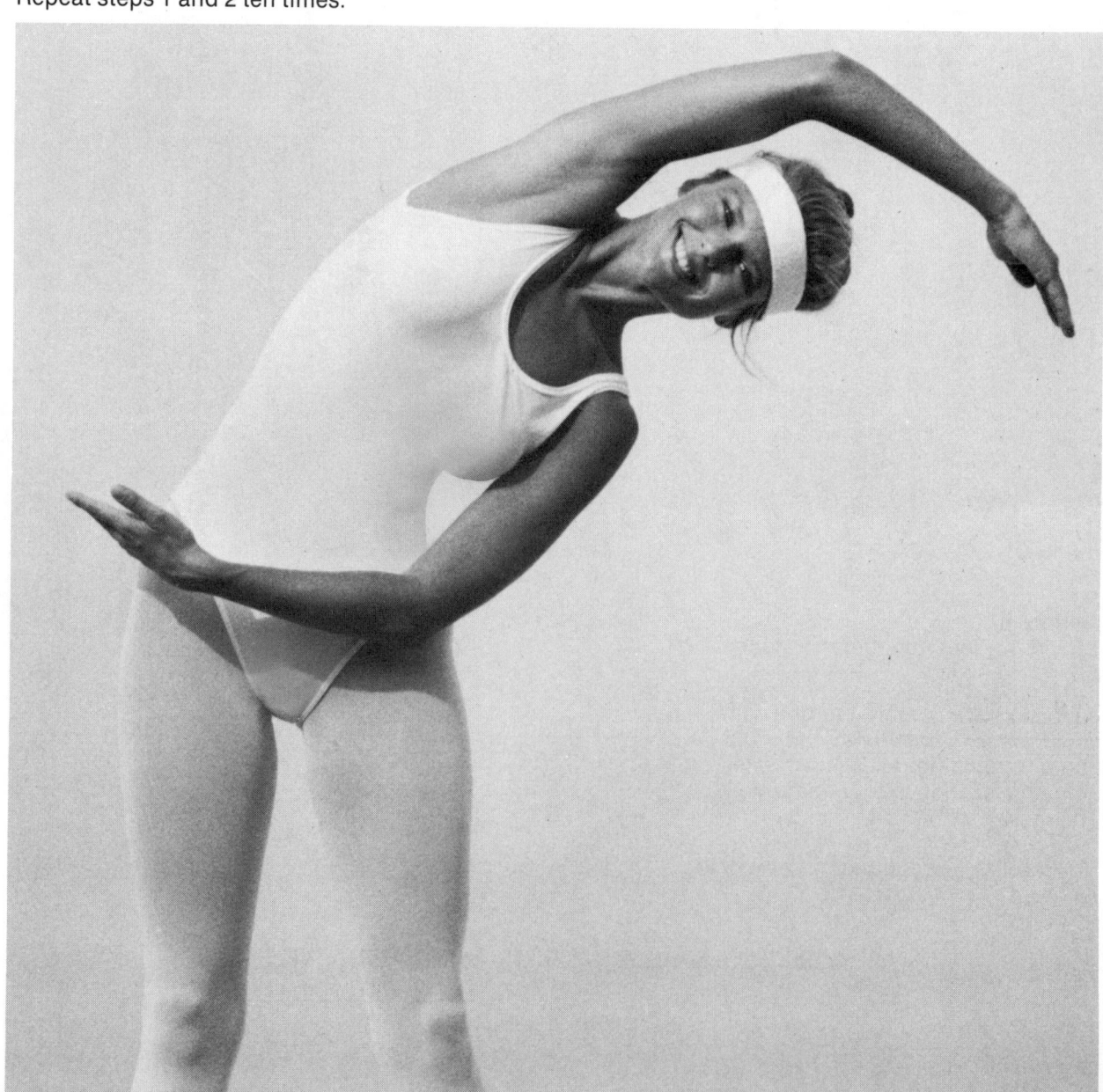

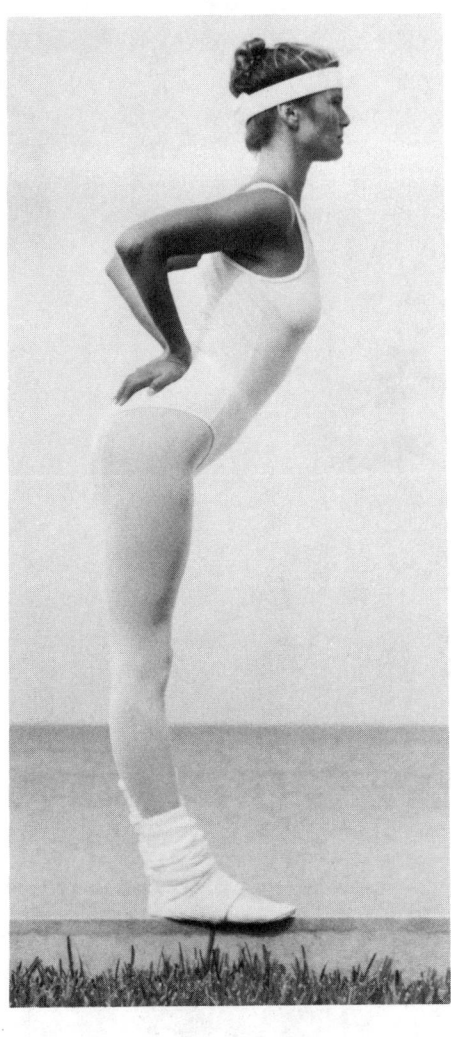

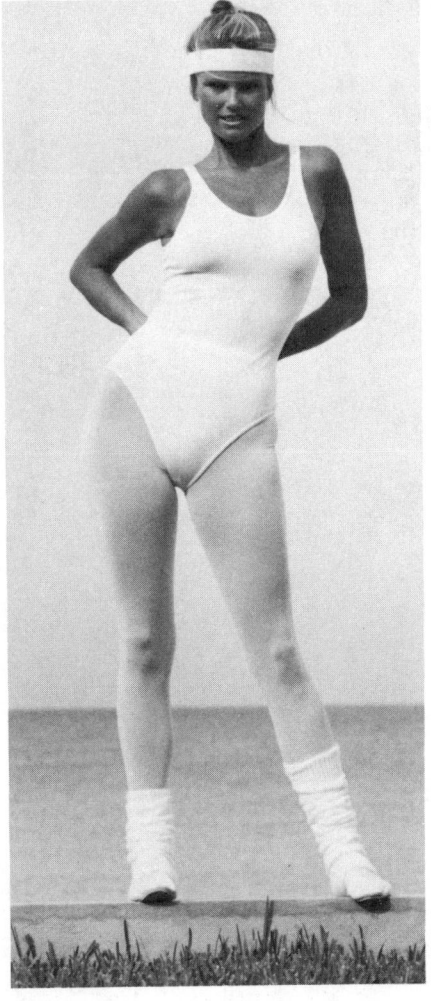

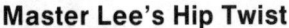

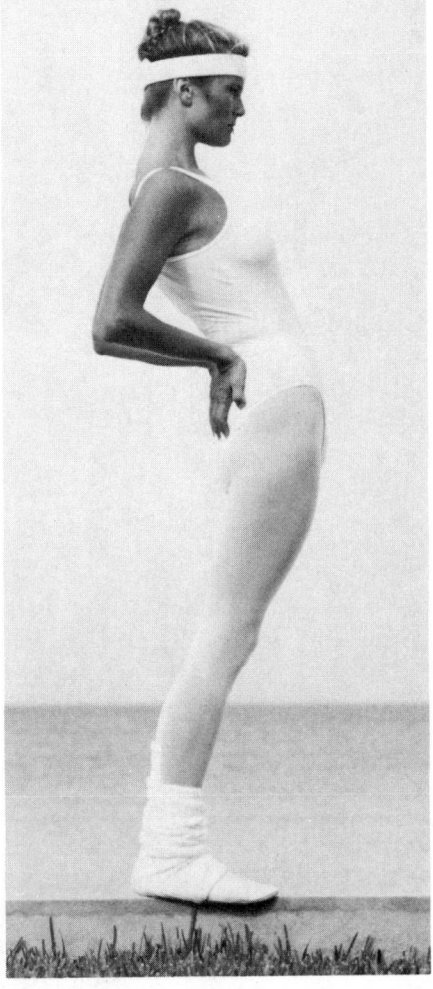

Master Lee's Hip Twist
This exercise limbers up the joints at the hips.

Stand with feet shoulder-width apart and hands on hips. In a giant circular motion:

1. Swing hips to the back.
2. Swing hips to the right.
3. Swing hips to the front.
4. Swing hips to the left.

Repeat steps 1 to 4 ten times.

WARM UP!

Master Lee's Knee and Ankle Twist
This will really loosen up your knees and ankles.

Stand with feet together, hands resting on thighs or knees with knees bent. Keep your heels on the floor throughout.

1. Swing knees in a circle to the left and end with knees straight. Repeat 5 times in this direction.
2. Bend knees and move in a circle to the right and end with knees straight. Repeat 5 times in this direction.

Repeat steps 1 and 2 ten times.

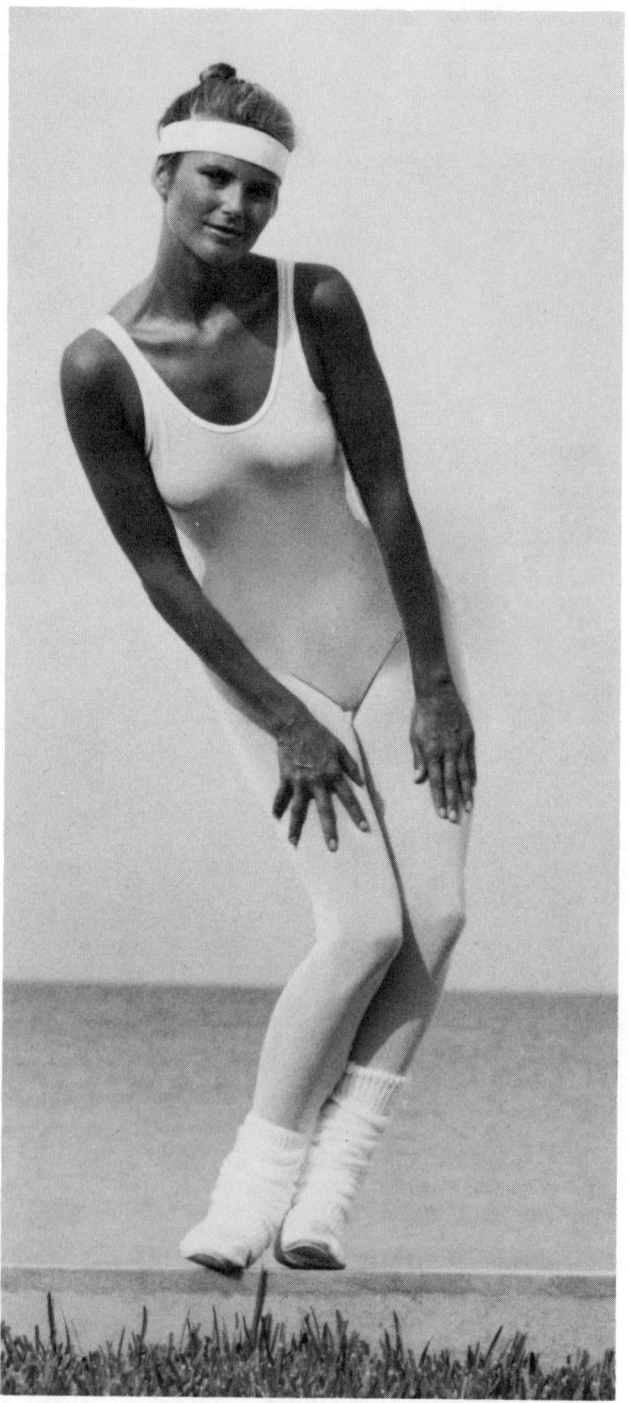

48

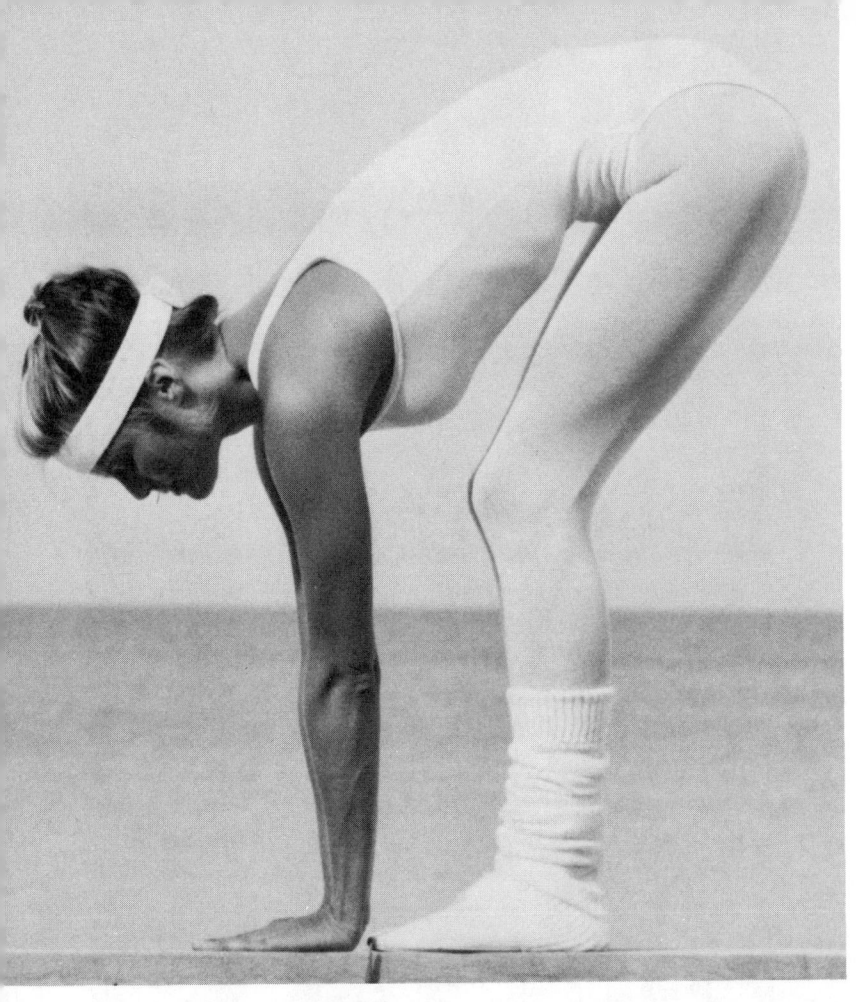

Hamstring Stretch

This gives the tendons (hamstrings) in the back of the knees a real stretch. But remember not to stretch more than you can do without straining.

Stand with feet together, knees bent. Bend at the waist. Rest your palms on the floor in front of your feet (or fingertips if you're a beginner).

1. Slowly straighten your legs, leaving hands on the floor. Feel the stretch in your hamstrings.
2. Return to starting position.

Repeat steps 1 and 2 ten times.

As you become more advanced, you wind up this exercise by walking your hands behind you on the floor, pulling your chest to your knees. The farther back you go, the greater the stretch.

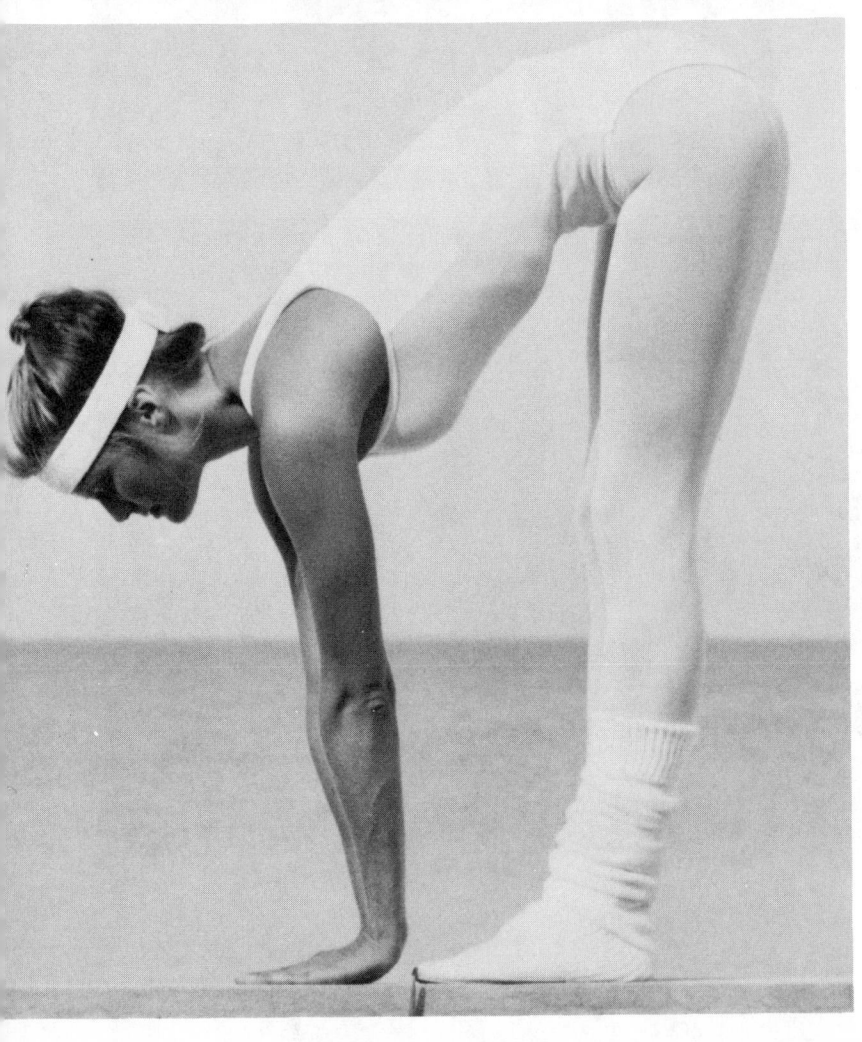

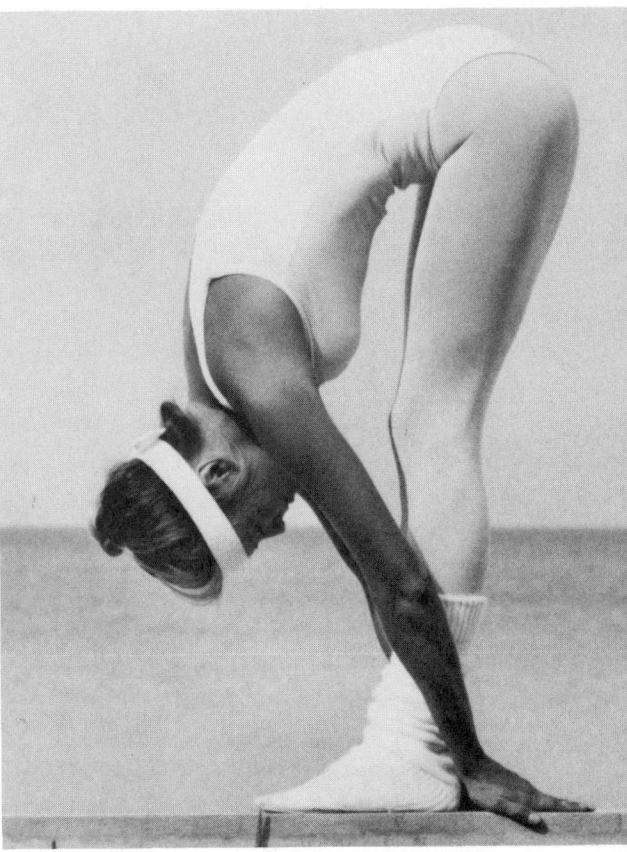

49

WARM UP!

Banana Splits
This exercise will give the legs a complete stretch.

Sit on the floor with your legs extended to either side.

1. With toes flexed and arms relaxed, stretch toward your right knee, trying to touch your chest to the knee. Bounce *gently* about 5 times, keeping your back flat.
2. Bounce gently to the middle 5 times.
3. Bounce gently to your left knee 5 times.

Repeat steps 1 to 3 ten times.
Then . . .
Repeat the entire exercise with your toes pointed to work a different set of muscles.

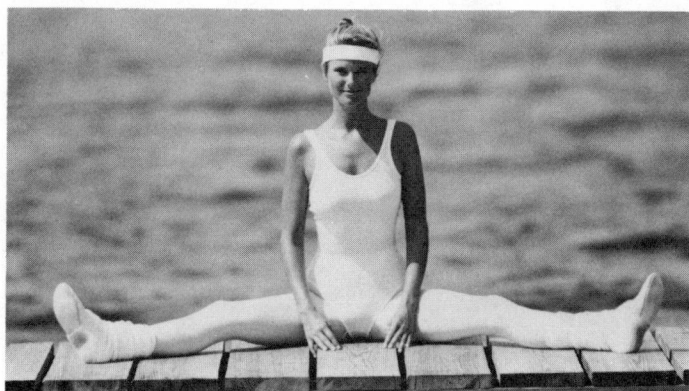
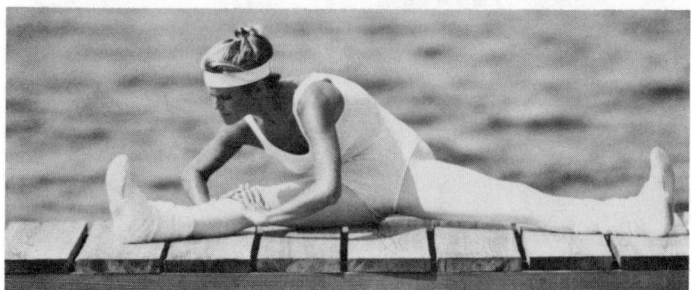
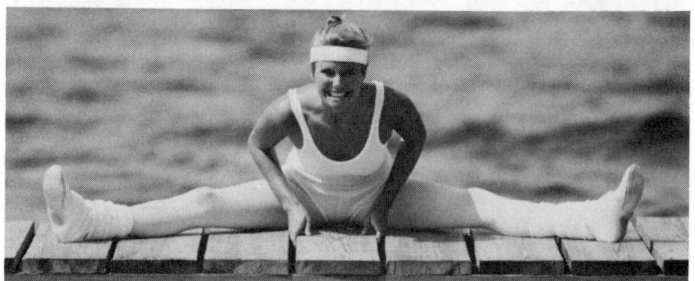

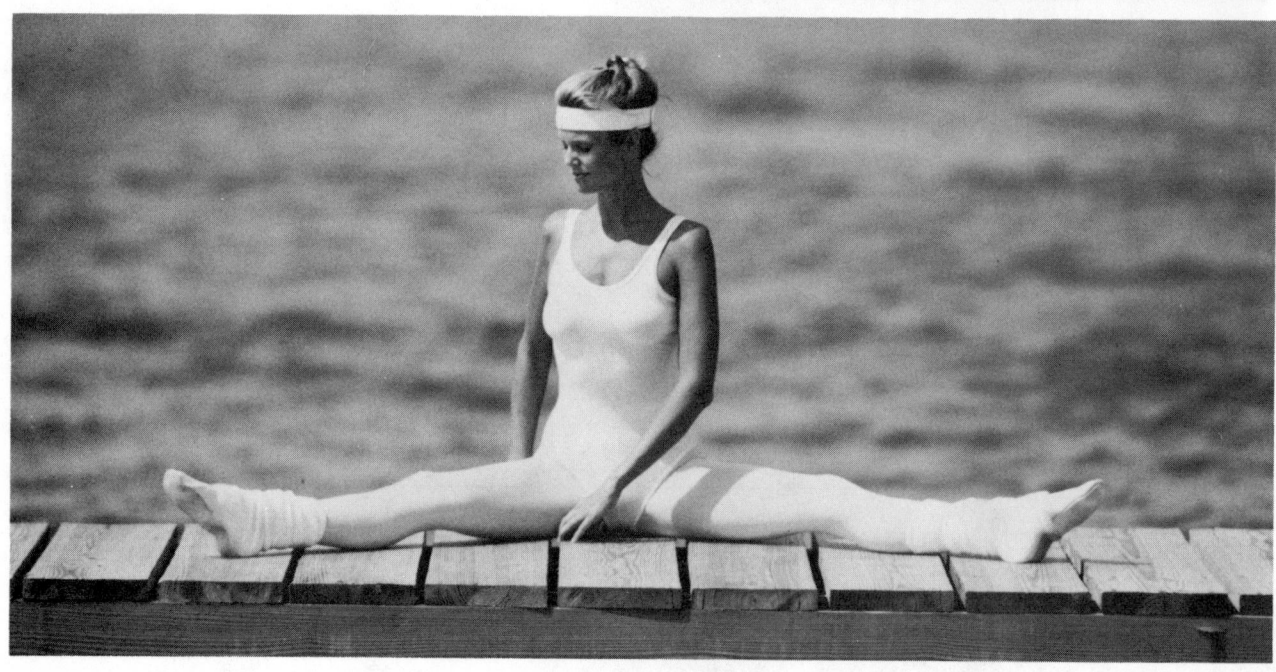

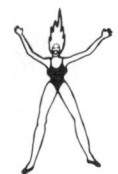 Aerobics should be an important part of your general exercise program. Calisthenics work on your muscles but aerobics work on your life. That's because aerobic exercise—exercise that, depending on age and duration of activity, increases your heartbeat to 130 to 150 beats per minute for a sustained time—has lots of hidden benefits that dramatically affect your health (and figure!).

Aerobic exercise burns calories and helps you lose weight.

Regular aerobic exercise helps you avoid heart, circulatory, respiratory, and metabolic diseases.

Aerobic exercise decreases your appetite.

Aerobic exercise works for you not only while you're doing it but afterwards as well. It increases your metabolism and burns calories more rapidly than usual even after you've stopped working.

Aerobic exercise is fun.

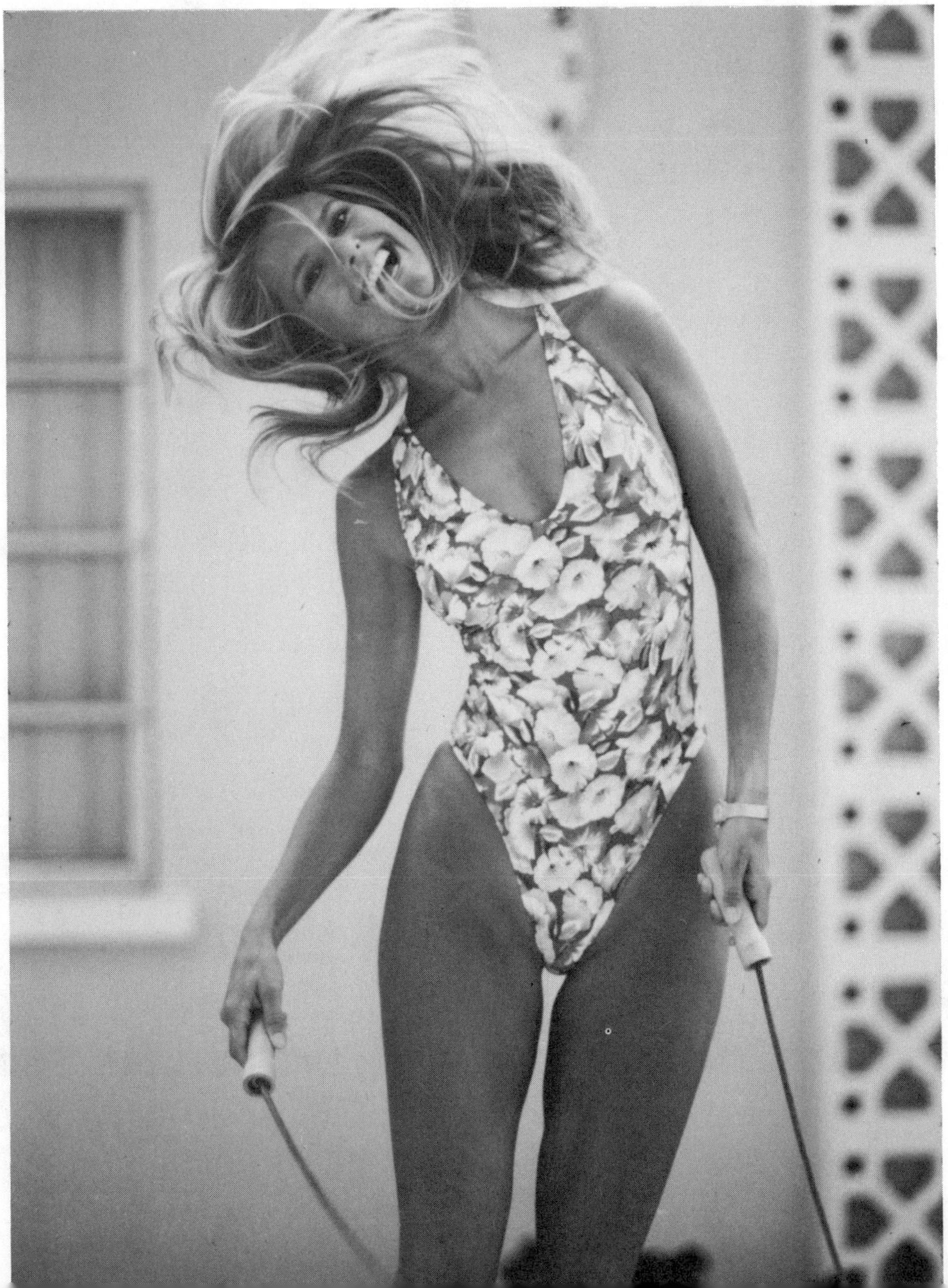

AEROBICS

AEROBICS

Aerobic Dance
My favorite aerobic exercise is simply to put on some terrific music and keep moving! Hop, skip, jump, twist, lunge, use your imagination to keep your muscles limber and heart pumping!

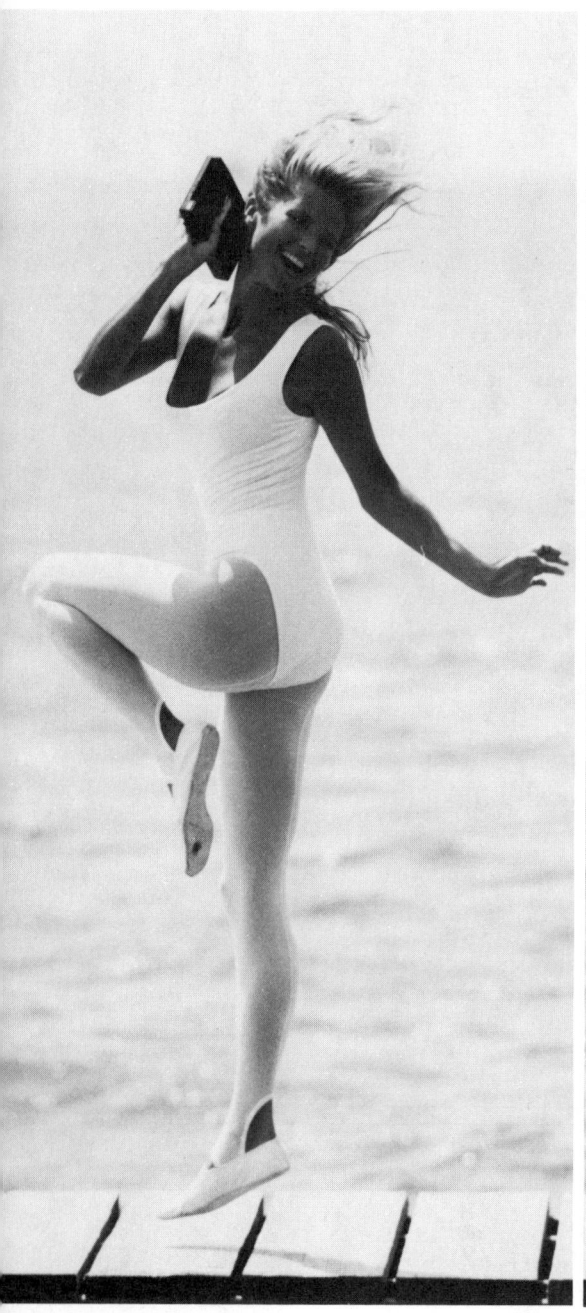
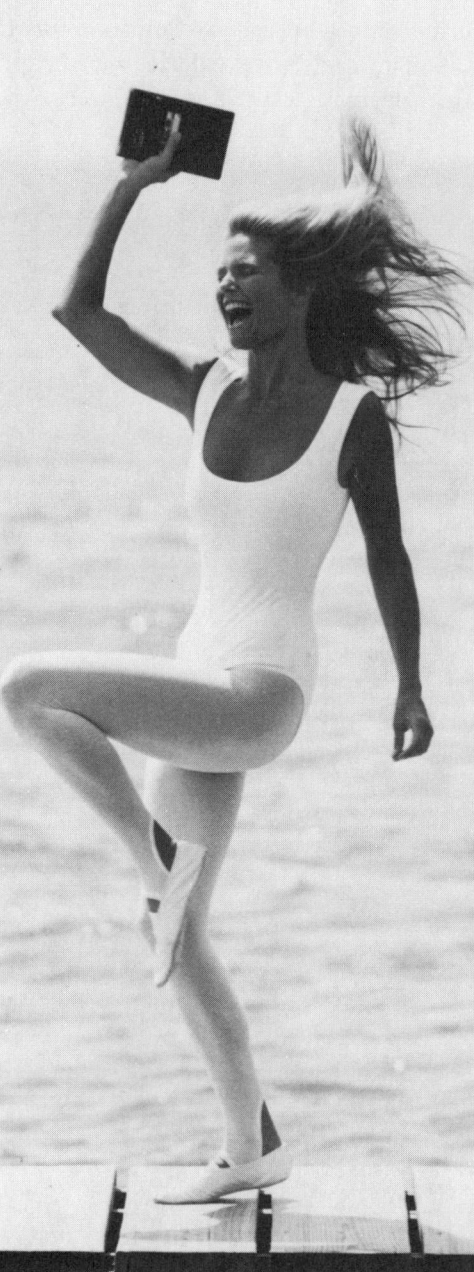
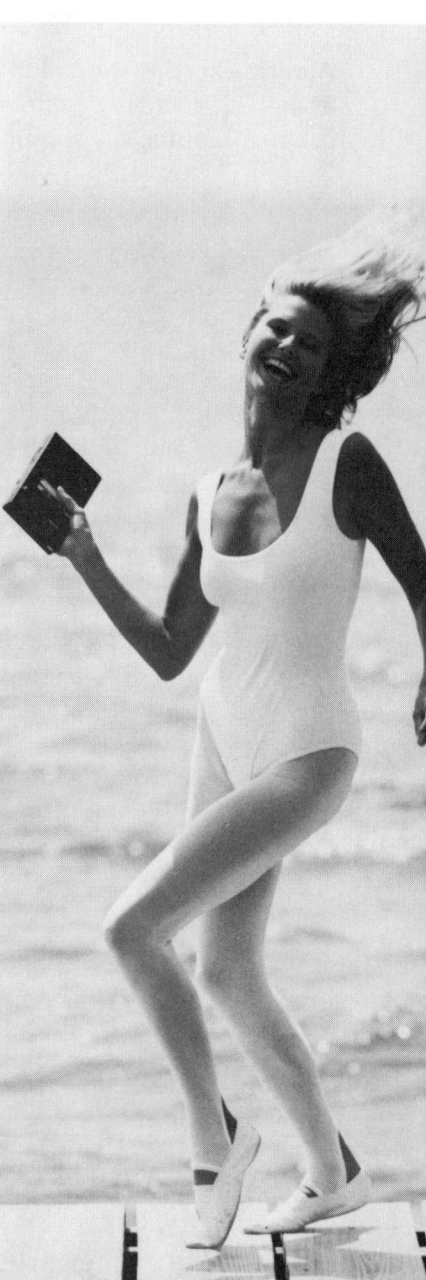

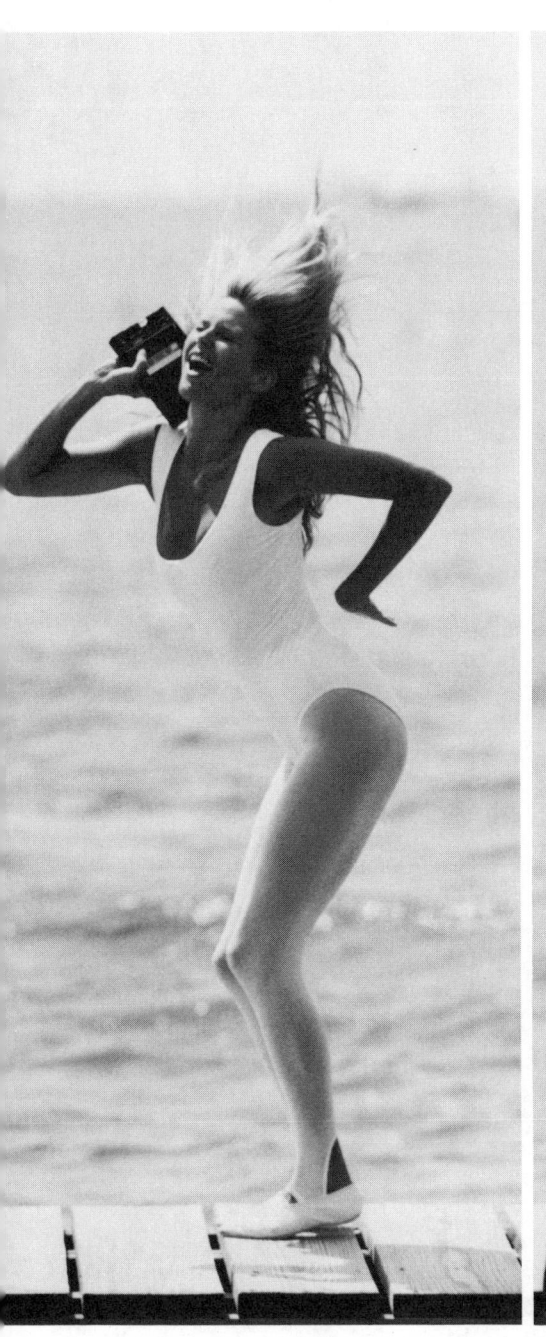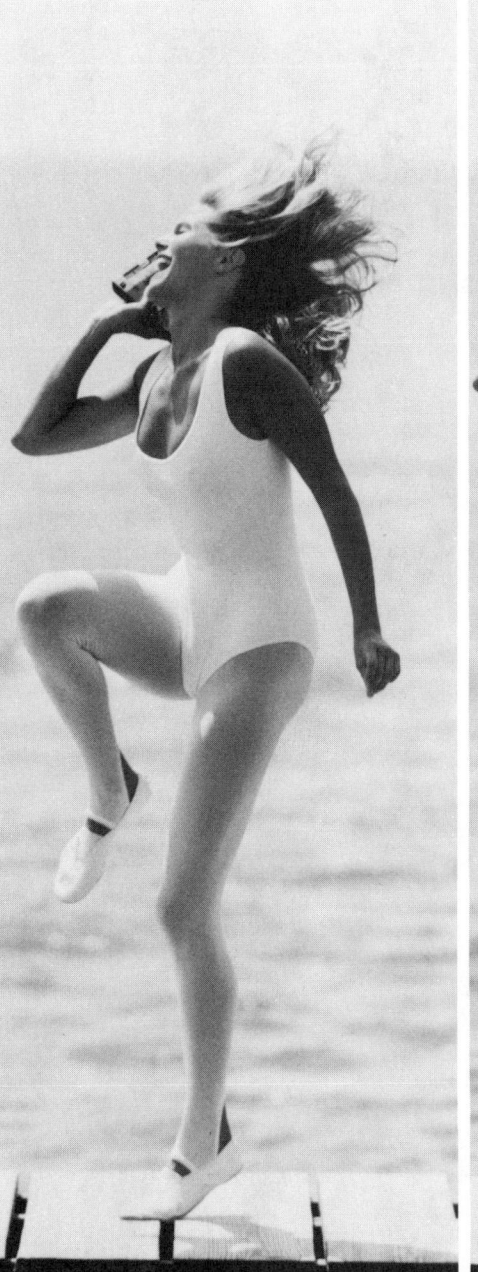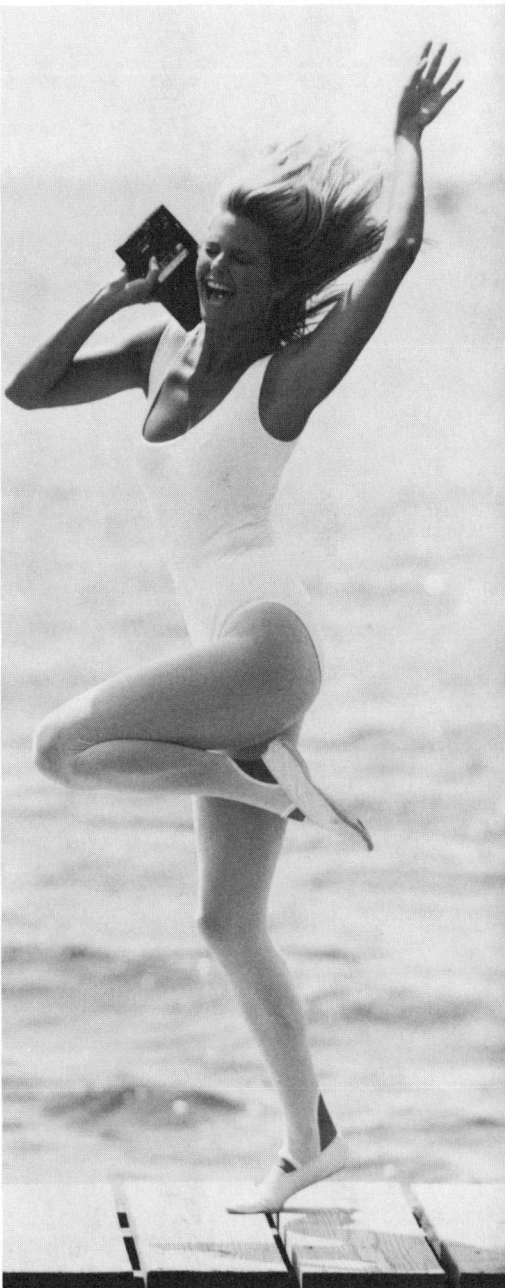

AEROBICS

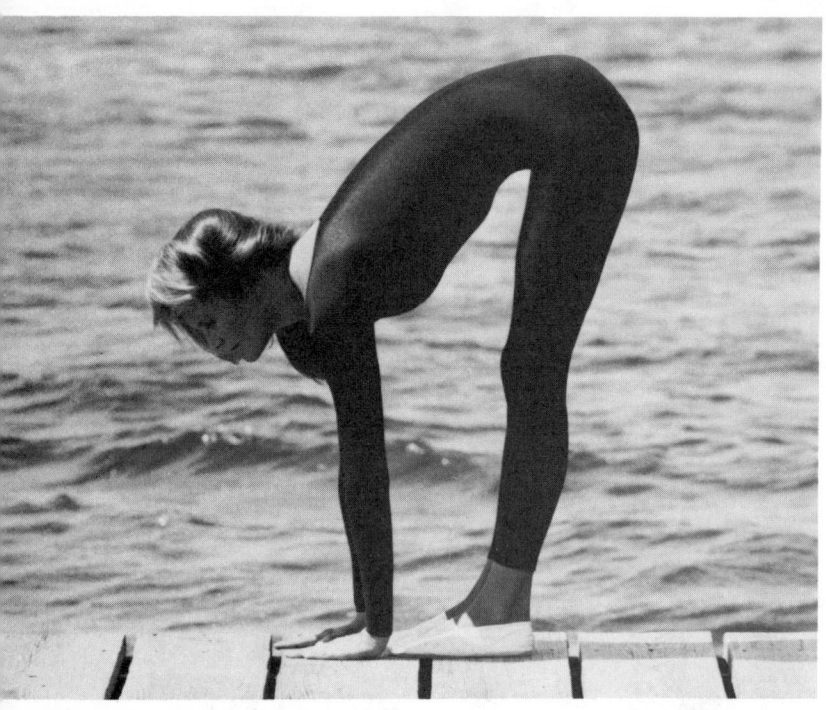

Aerobic Bounce

Stand with feet together. Bend forward at the waist, keeping your knees straight, and put palms (or fingertips) on the floor. Remember to breathe deeply.

1. Bend knees and move into a crouch, extending arms in front of you for balance.
2. Return to starting position.

Repeat steps 1 and 2 fifteen times.

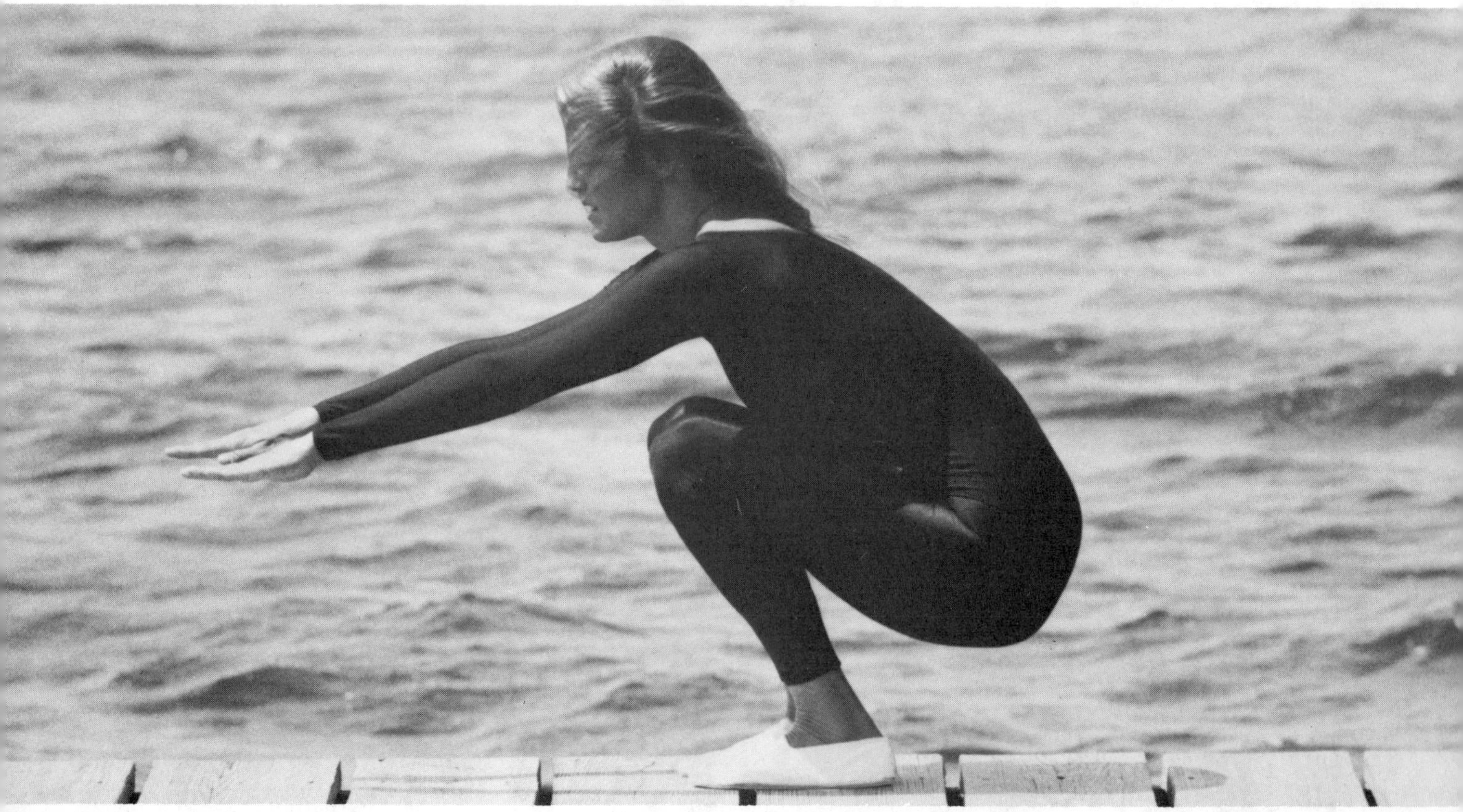

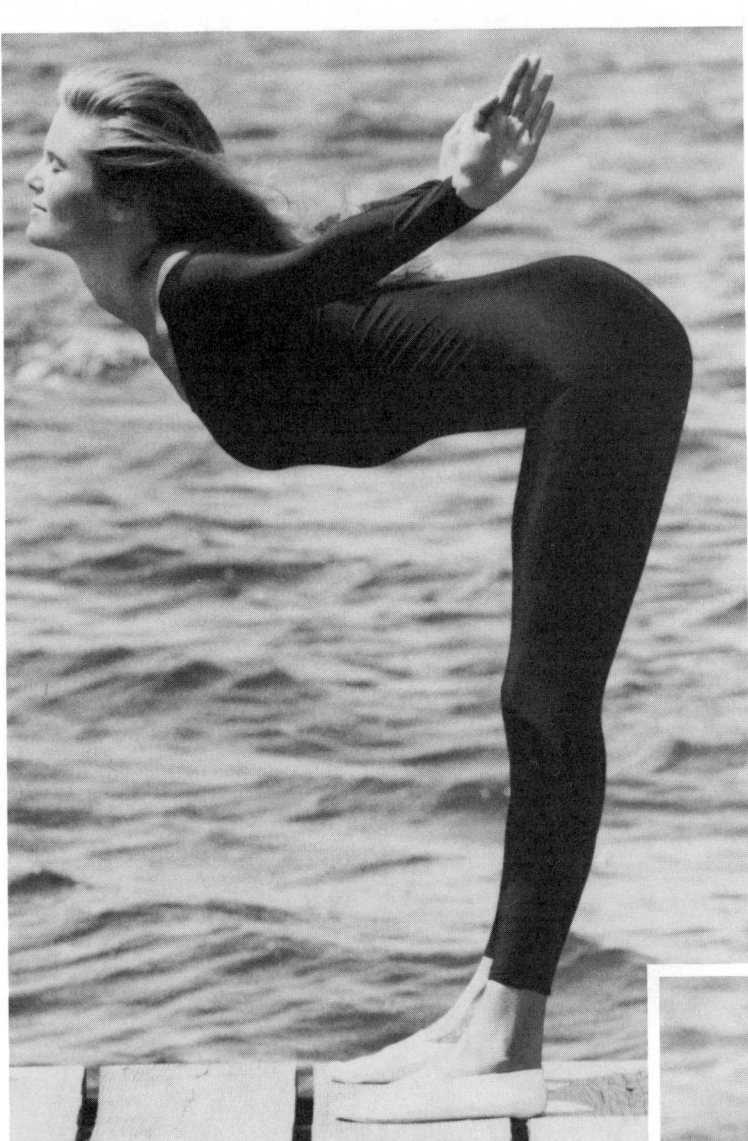

Aerobic Reach

Stand with feet one foot apart, bend forward until body is parallel to the floor, keeping back straight and arms extended out to sides.

1. Bend all the way down, putting hands between legs—reaching as far behind as you can.
2. Return to starting position.

Repeat steps 1 and 2 fifteen times.

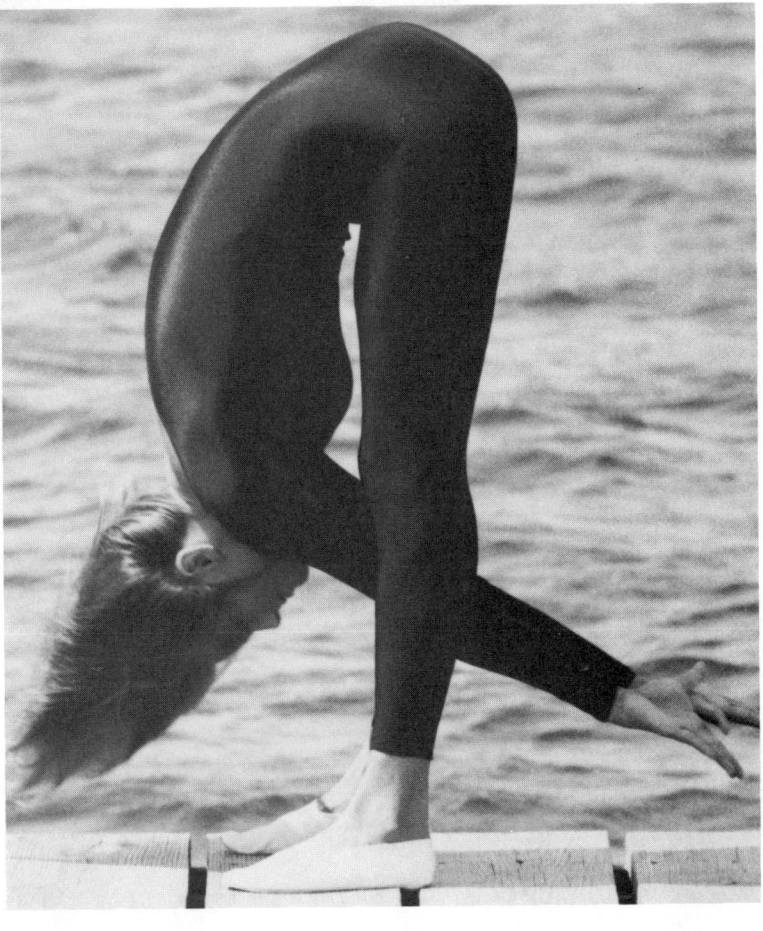

AEROBICS

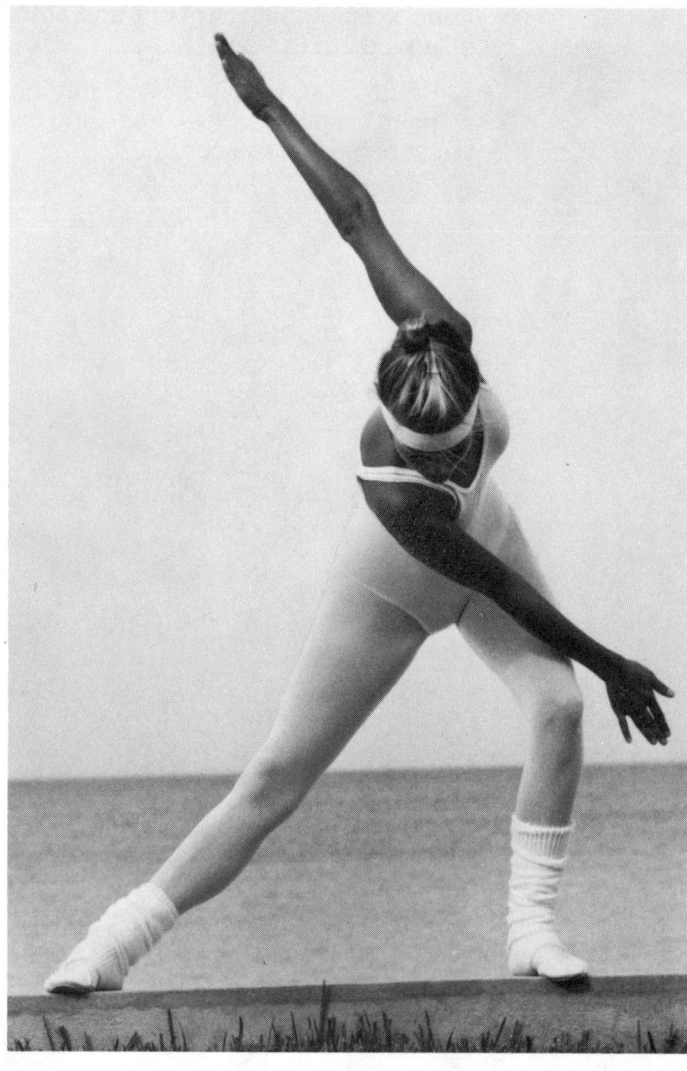

Aerobic Leg Lunge

I do this to the beat of music (not too fast). It works your thighs and your waist and is a super warm-up. Remember to breathe deeply.

Stand with legs apart two times the width of your shoulders, arms outstretched.

1. Lunge forward with the full weight of your body over the left knee, touching your left knee with your right hand, extending your left hand behind you.
2. Lunge to the right touching your right knee with your left hand, extending your right hand behind you.
3. Return to starting position.

Repeat steps 1 to 3 ten times.

Then repeat the exercise touching the opposite *foot* instead of the knee. Repeat this variation ten times, alternating right and left.

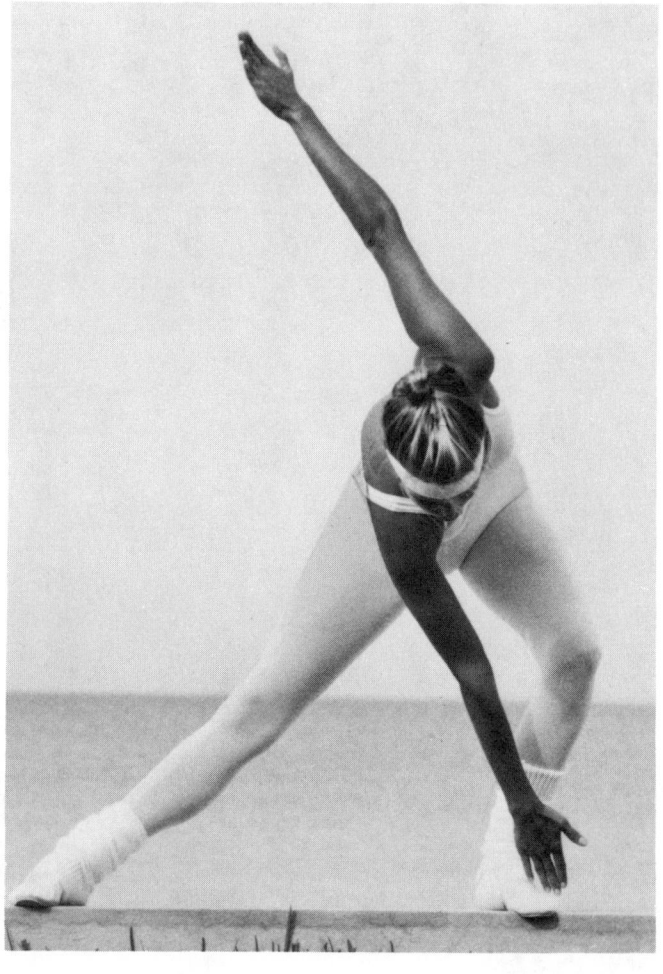

SPOT EXERCISES

Arms and Bust

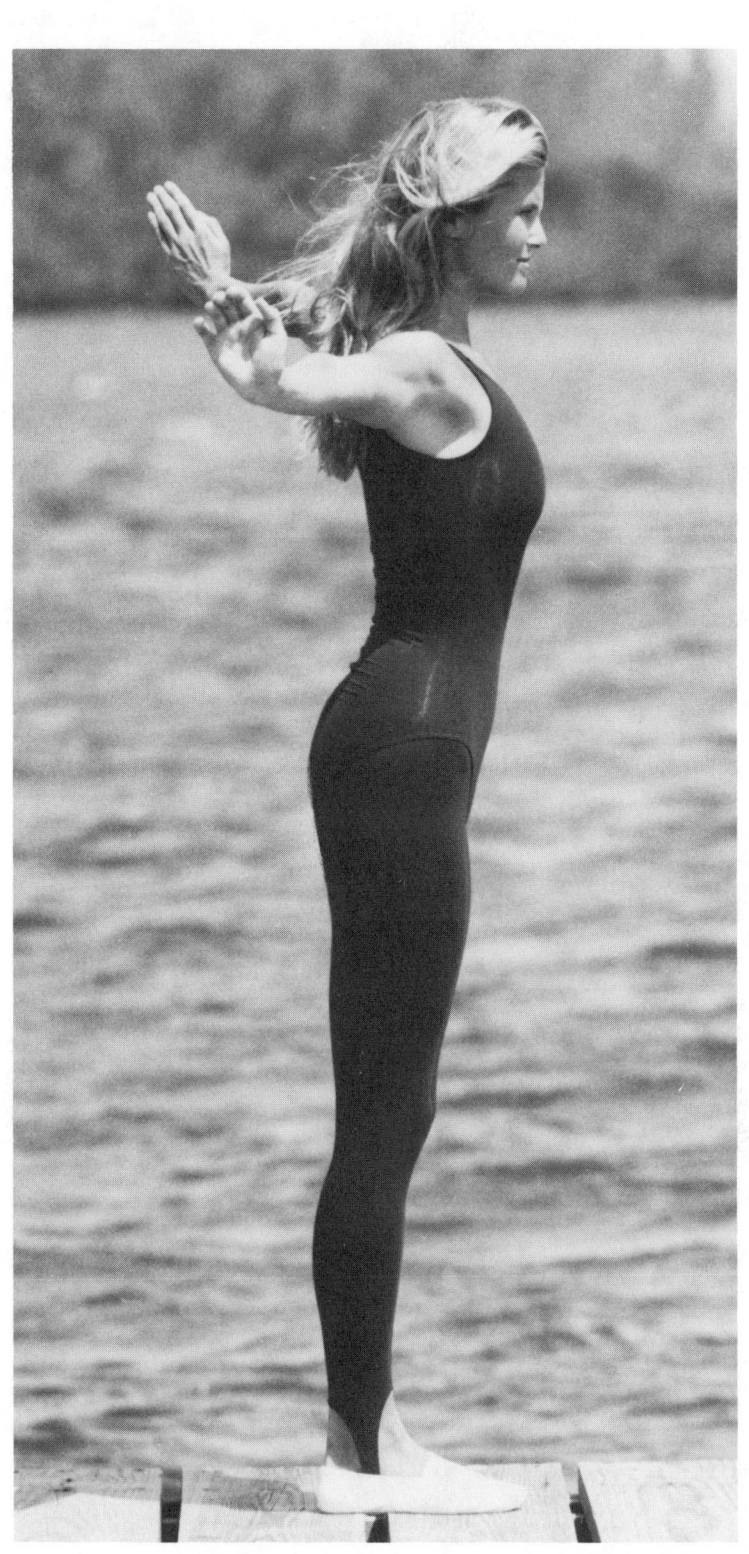

Propellers

This will firm your upper arm muscles.

Stand with feet together and arms stretched out to the side, your fingers pointing upward.

1. Rotate your arms in small circles forward 15 times.
2. Rotate your arms in small circles backward 15 times.

Repeat exercise making large circles 15 times forward and 15 times back.

Arms and Bust

Arm Tightener

This is terrific for firming backs of upper arms.

Stand with feet together; bend over at the waist, keeping your back flat; bend your arms up, keeping elbows close to sides and hands against your chest.

1. Staying in bent position, unfold your arms up behind you as high as you can. Feel it work the backs of your arms.
2. Return to starting position.

Start with 20 repetitions and go for 100!

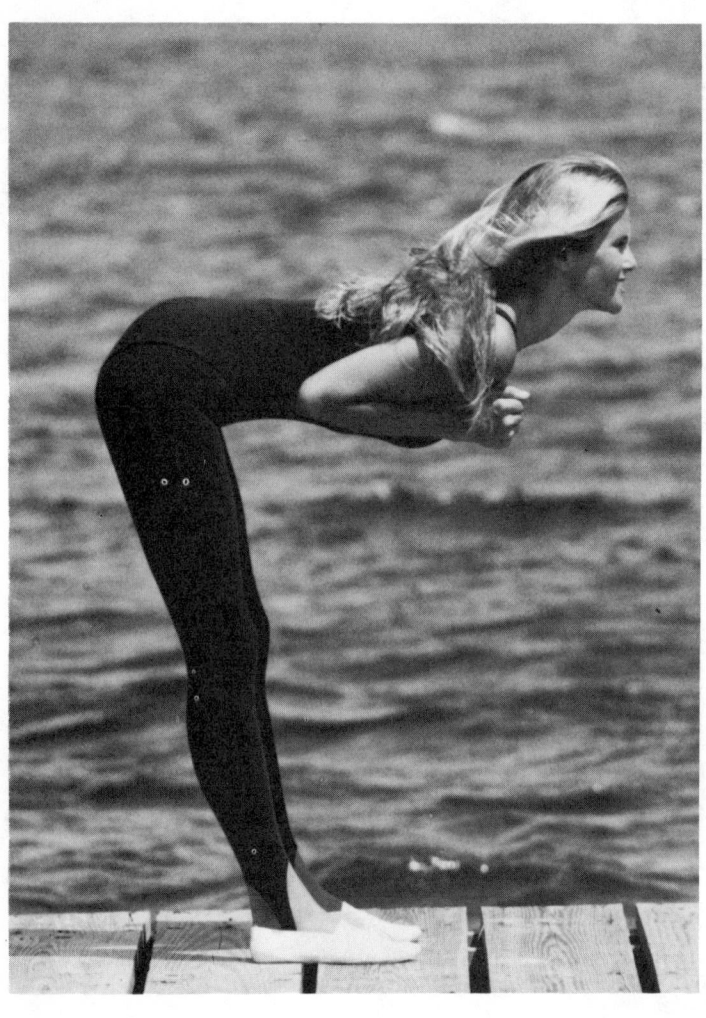
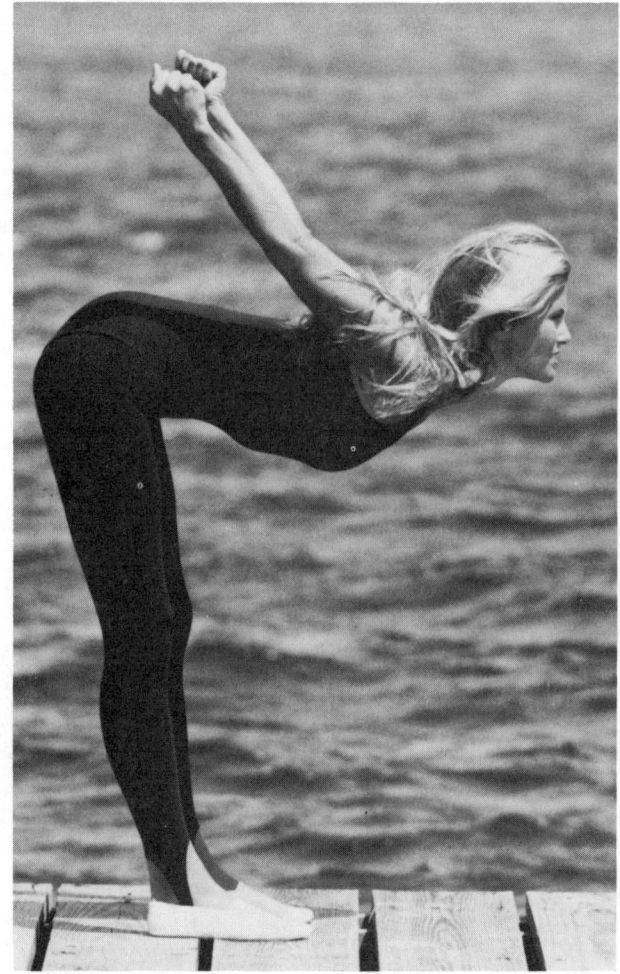

The Butterfly
This is great for the pectorals!

Stand with feet together, arms in a "prayer" position above your head.

1. Keeping your hands above your head, press elbows together in front.
2. Return to starting position.

Repeat steps 1 and 2 twenty-five times.

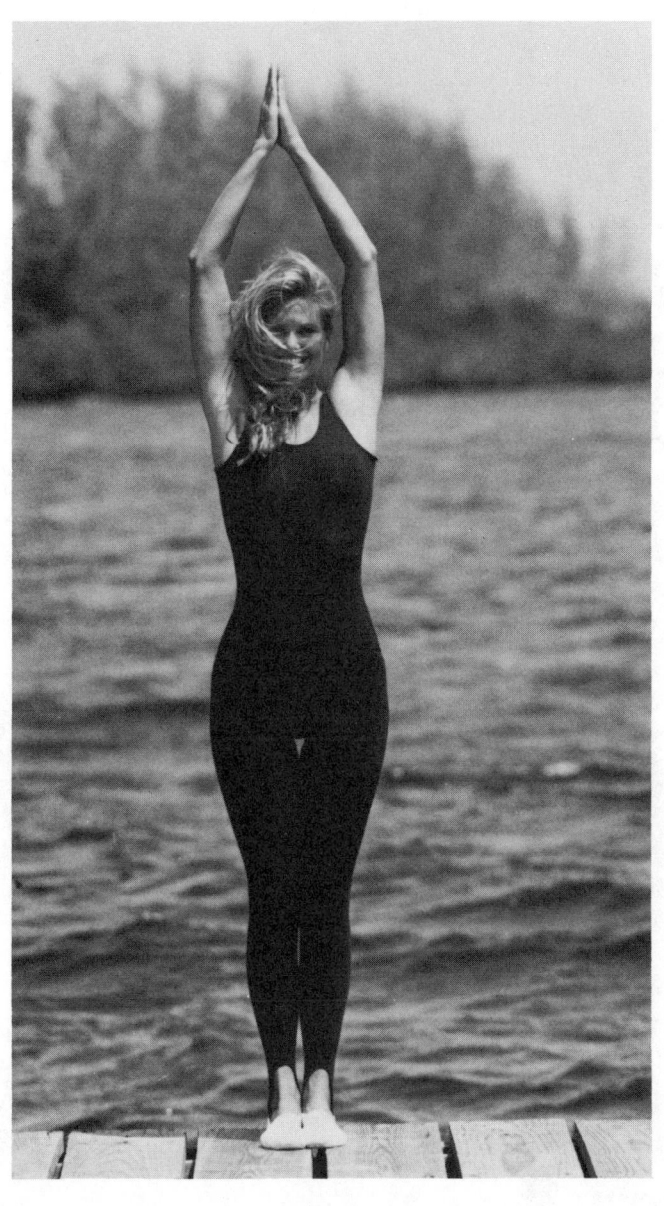

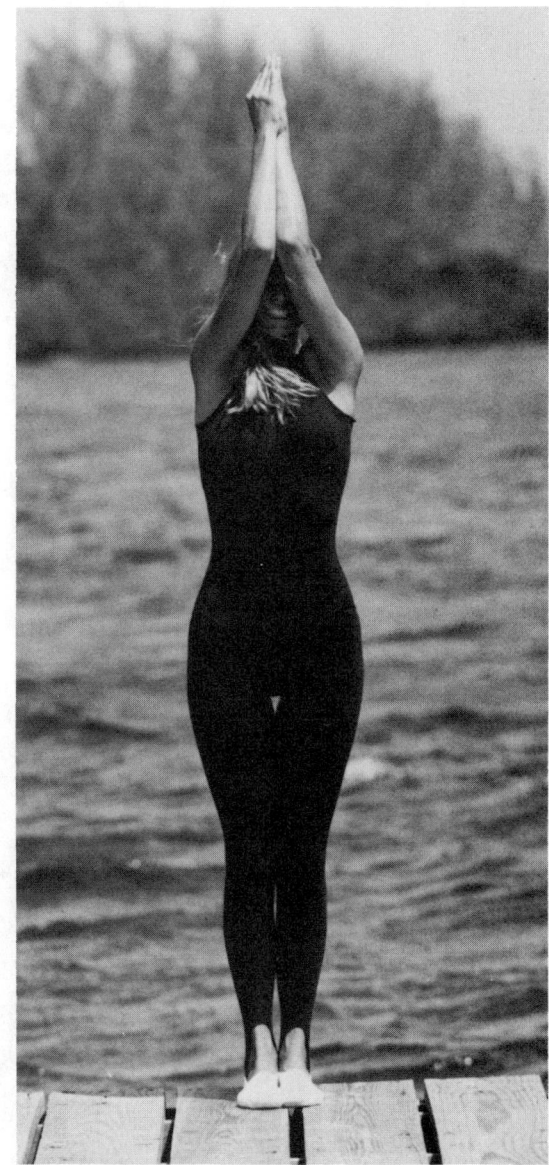

Waist

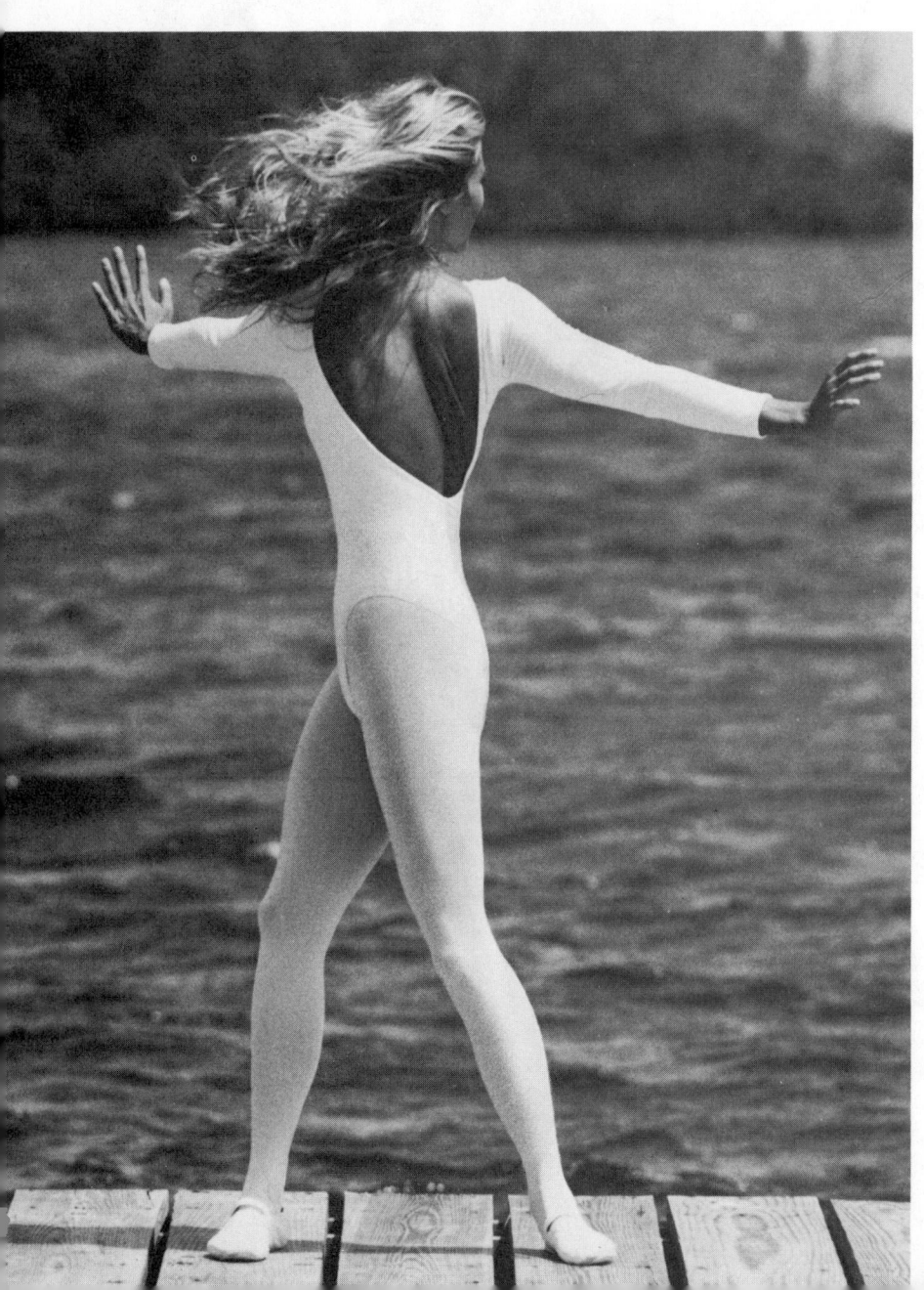

The Dizzy Dame (Three Variations)
This is perfect for trimming your waist. Stand with feet apart at shoulder width, arms extended to the sides at shoulder height.

1. Twist upper body and head to the right as far as you can without straining.
2. Then twist to the left as far as possible.

Repeat steps 1 and 2 twenty-five times.

The Dizzy Dame II
Done this way, the Dizzy Dame is good for the waist, but works the stomach muscles as well.

Stand with feet apart at shoulder width. Clasp arms on top or behind head.

1. Twist to right, turning as far as possible.
2. Twist to left, turning as far as you can.

Repeat steps 1 and 2 twenty-five times.

The Dizzy Dame III
Stand with feet apart at shoulder width. Now reach up as high as you can, clasp hands over your head, and twist.

1. Twist upper body and head to the right, turning as far as possible.
2. Then twist to the left, turning as far as you can.

Repeat steps 1 and 2 fifteen times.

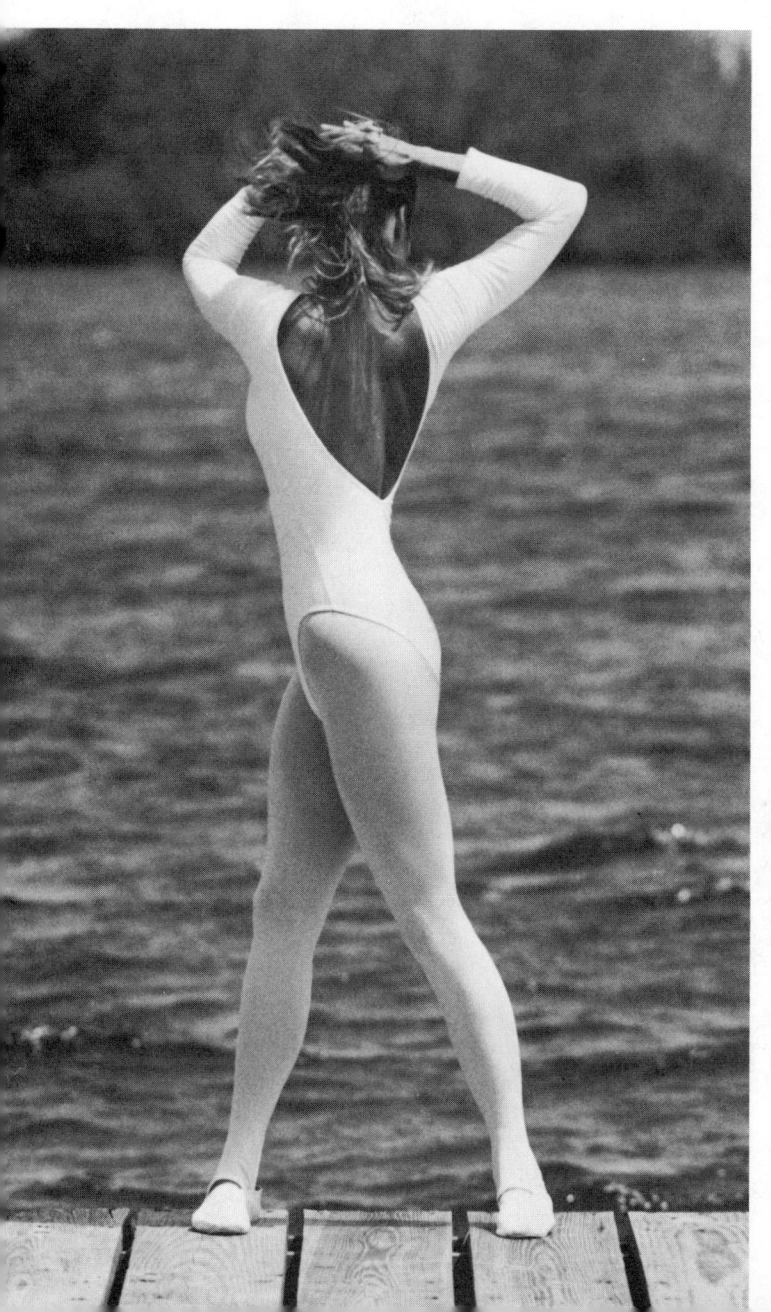

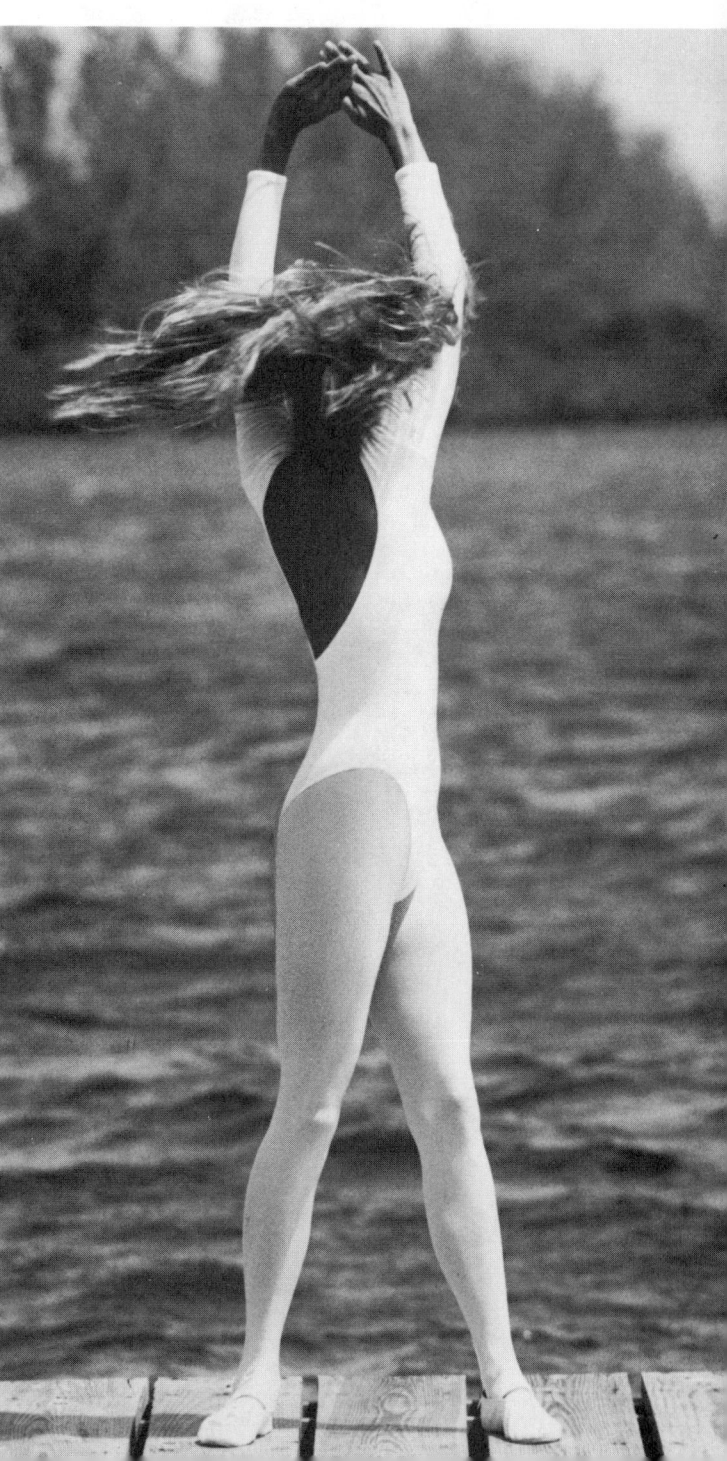

Stomach

Lindy's Stomachache

Lie on back with knees bent and feet flat on floor. Keep the feet close together for beginners, far apart for advanced. Exhale when you come up; inhale going down.

1. Sit up slowly, keeping hips straight, reach under left knee with left hand to touch inside of right foot. Lie back down slowly.

2. Repeat using right hand to touch left foot.

Repeat steps 1 and 2 twenty times.

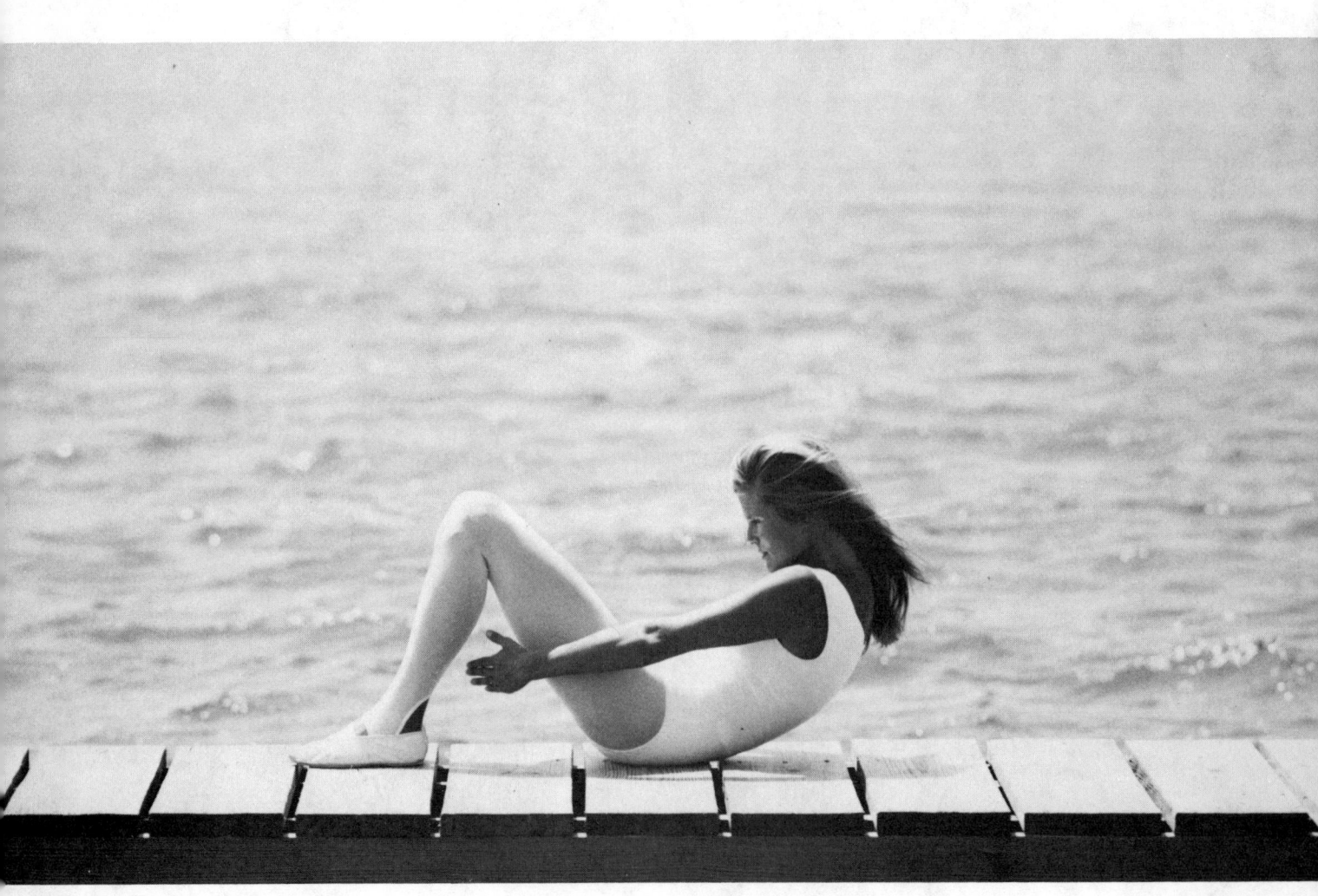

Lindy's Bicycle

Lying on back with legs straight, toes pointed and head up, lift your legs slightly. Keep your legs and head off the floor throughout the exercise.

1. Bend your right knee and try to touch your chest with it while you clap hands under your knee.
2. Reverse and do same with left leg.

Repeat steps 1 and 2 twenty times.

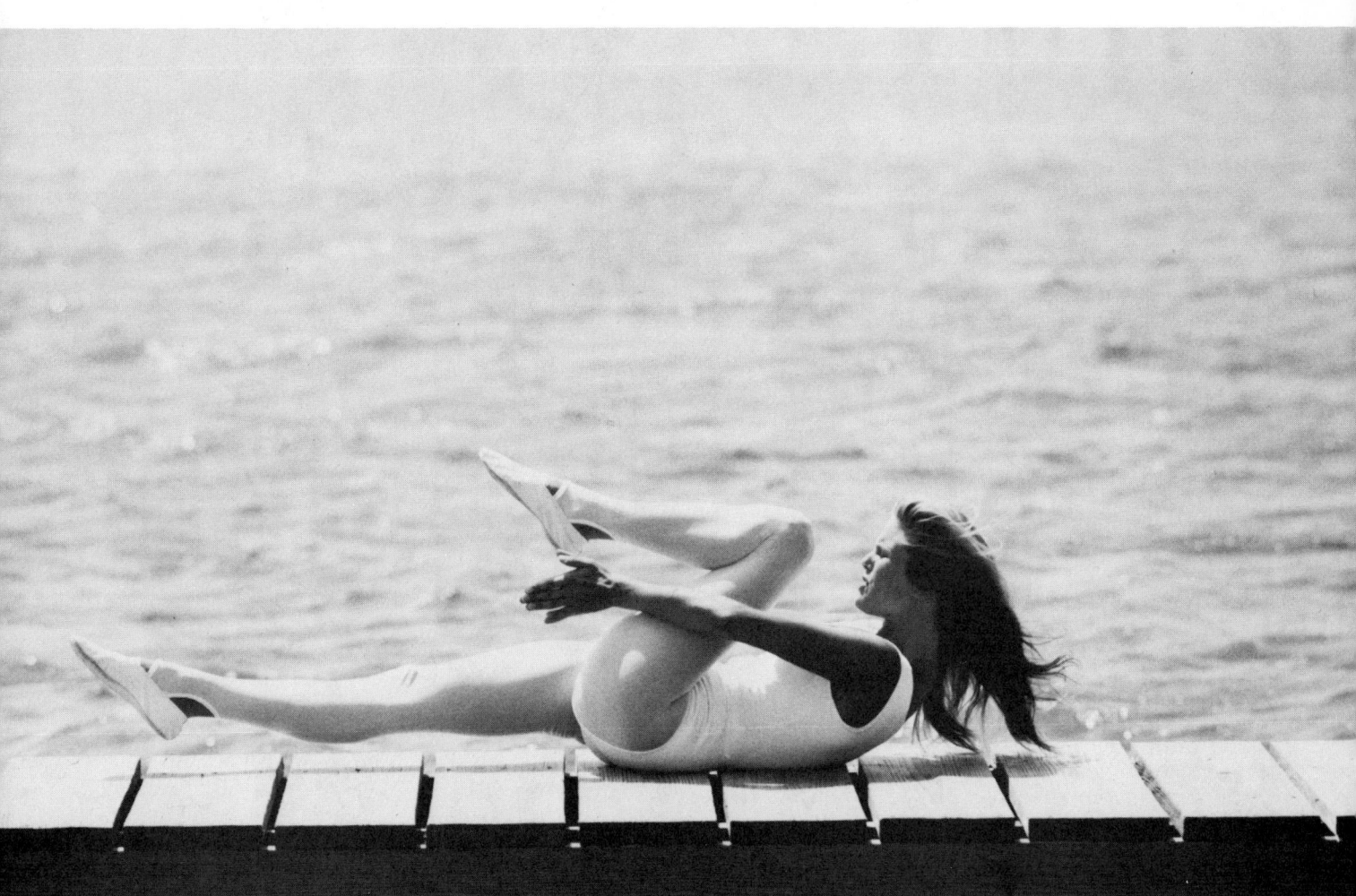

Stomach

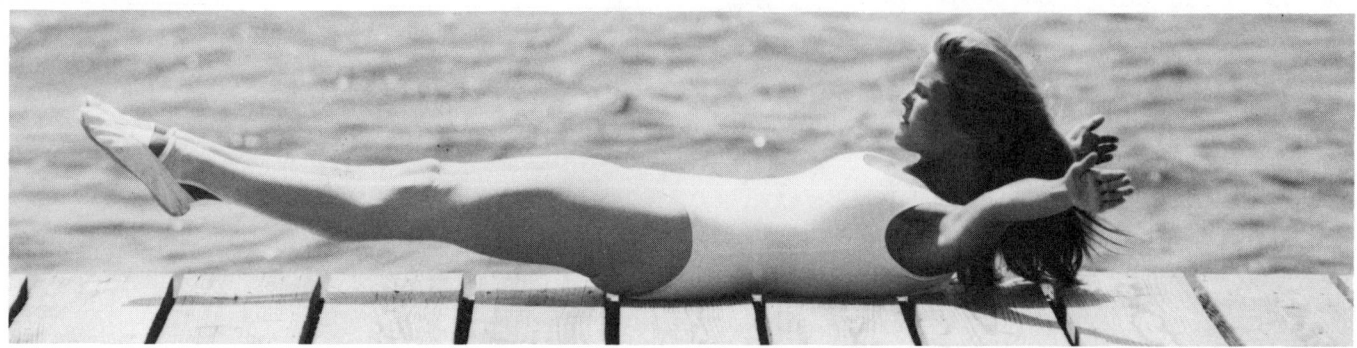

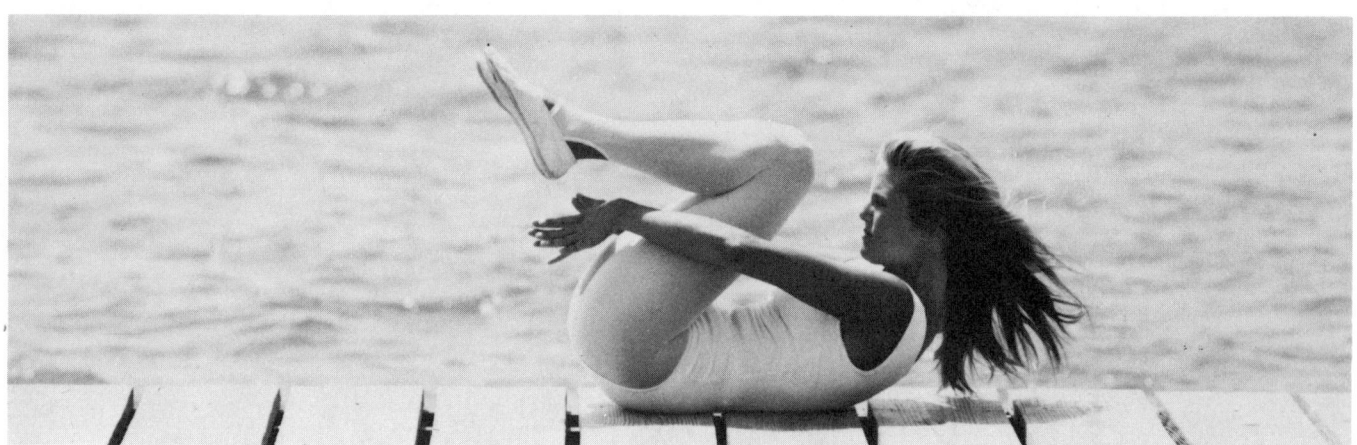

Antonia's Toner
This works the stomach (as well as the legs and buttocks).

Lie on back, legs extended, toes pointed, head raised and arms stretched out to sides. Head, arms, and legs must not touch the floor during the exercise.

1. Bend both knees and bring them toward the chest while clapping hands under your knees.
2. Extend legs and arms to starting position.

Repeat steps 1 and 2 twenty times.

Lindy's Leg Killer

Great for stretching backs of legs, but works stomach muscles, too.

Lie on back with arms at sides, feet together, toes pointed.

1. Lift left knee to chest with knee bent.
2. Straighten knee until leg is perpendicular to body with foot flexed.
3. Lower foot to starting position.
4. Repeat with other leg.

Repeat steps 1 to 4 twenty times.

Legs

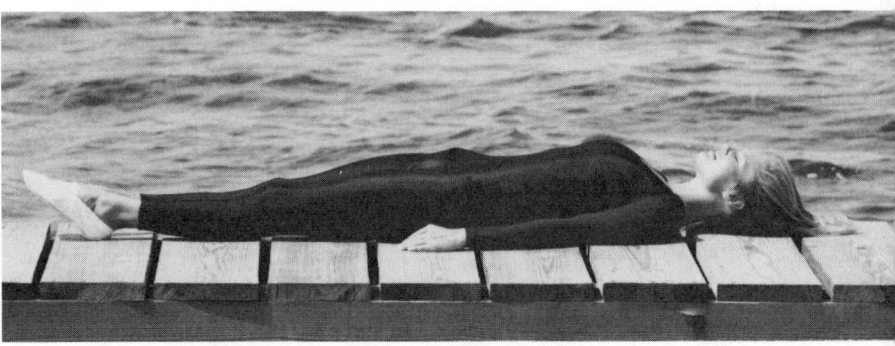

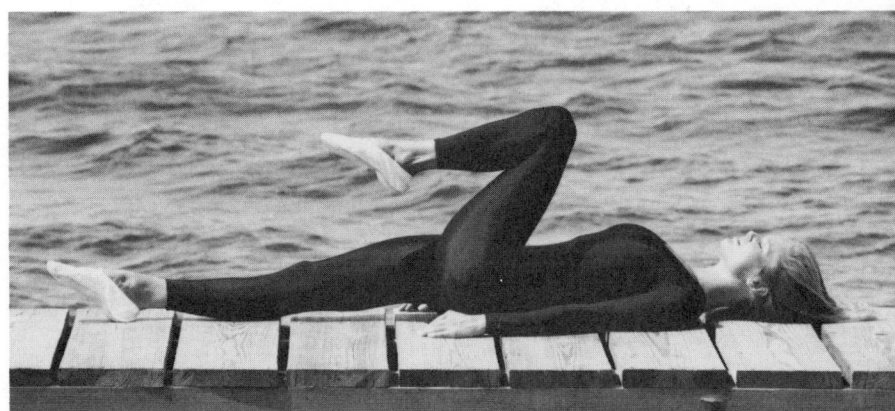

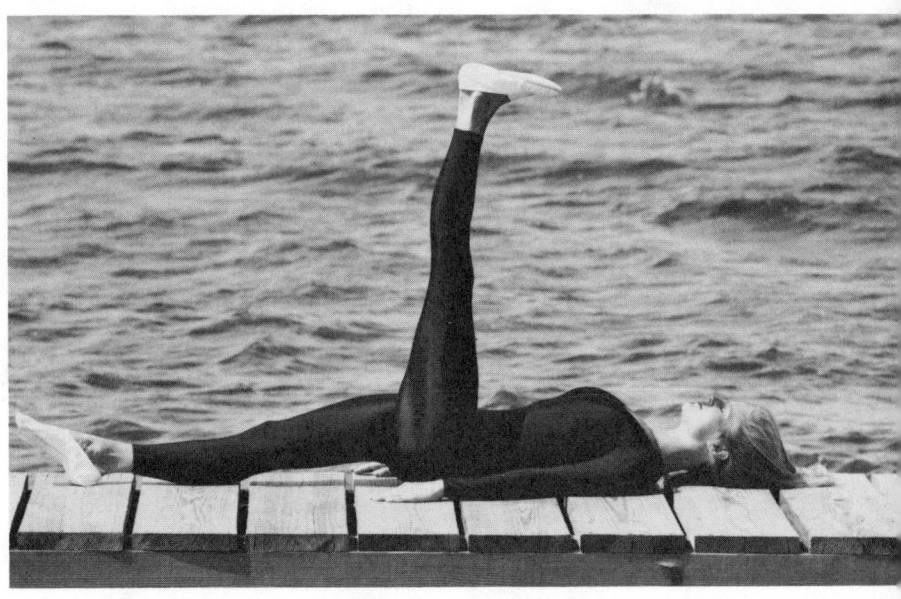

Legs

Roy's Revolver

Lie on back, arms at sides and feet together, with toes pointed.

1. Lift left leg, flexing foot.
2. Hold leg perpendicular to body with foot flexed.
3. Lower left leg to floor on left side, keeping foot flexed.
4. Return leg to starting position.

Repeat steps 1 to 4 ten times.

Repeat with opposite leg.

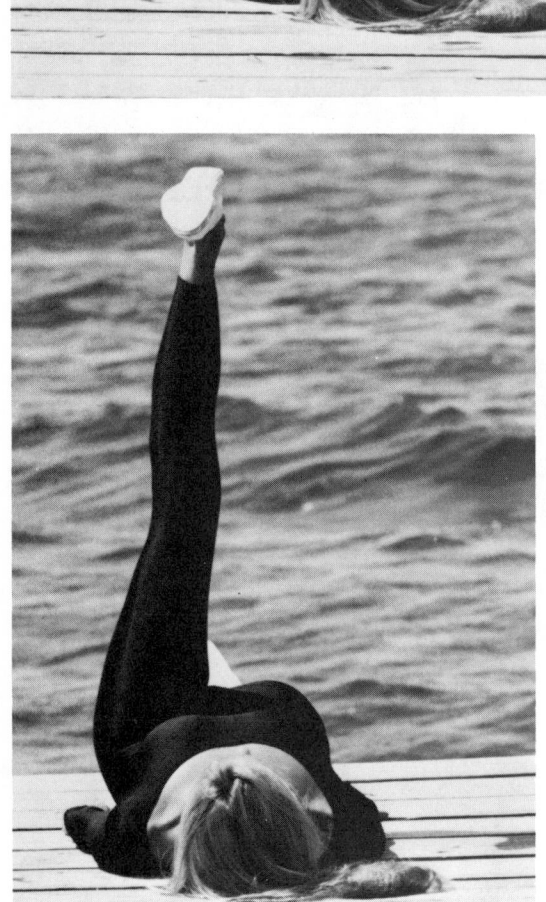

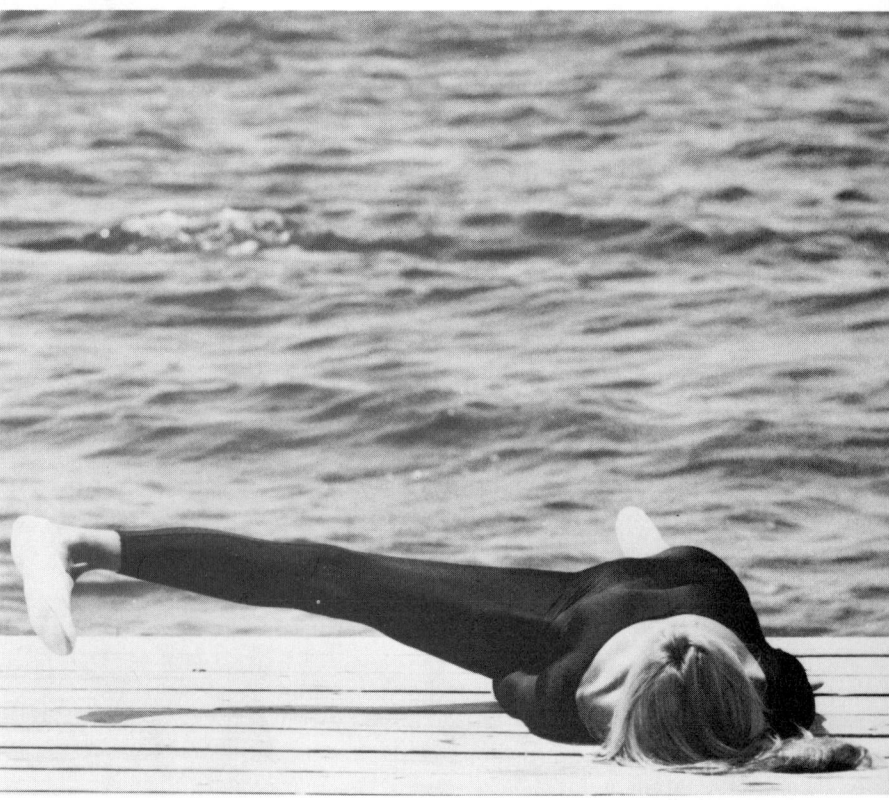

Flexed Foot Leg Lift

Lie on side, head resting on raised hand, other arm relaxed in front of body.

1. Flex foot and raise leg straight up as high as you can.
2. Return to starting position.

Repeat 20 times.
Then . . .
Turn to other side and repeat steps 1 and 2 with opposite leg 20 times.

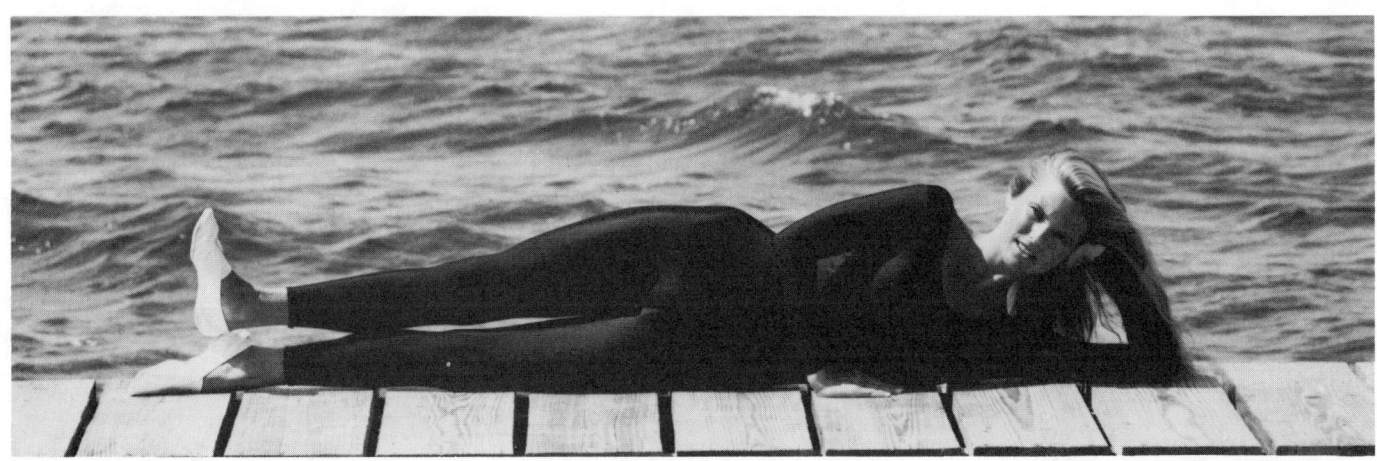

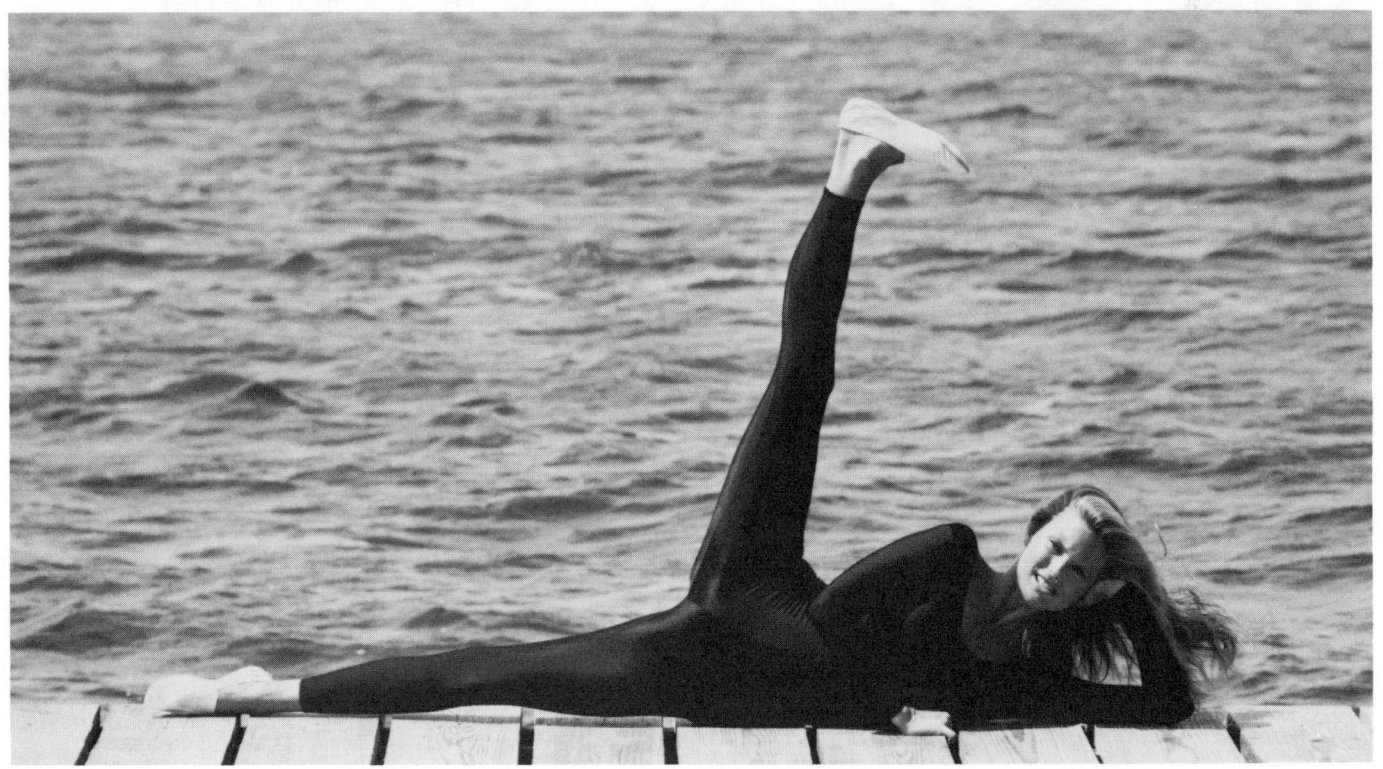

Legs

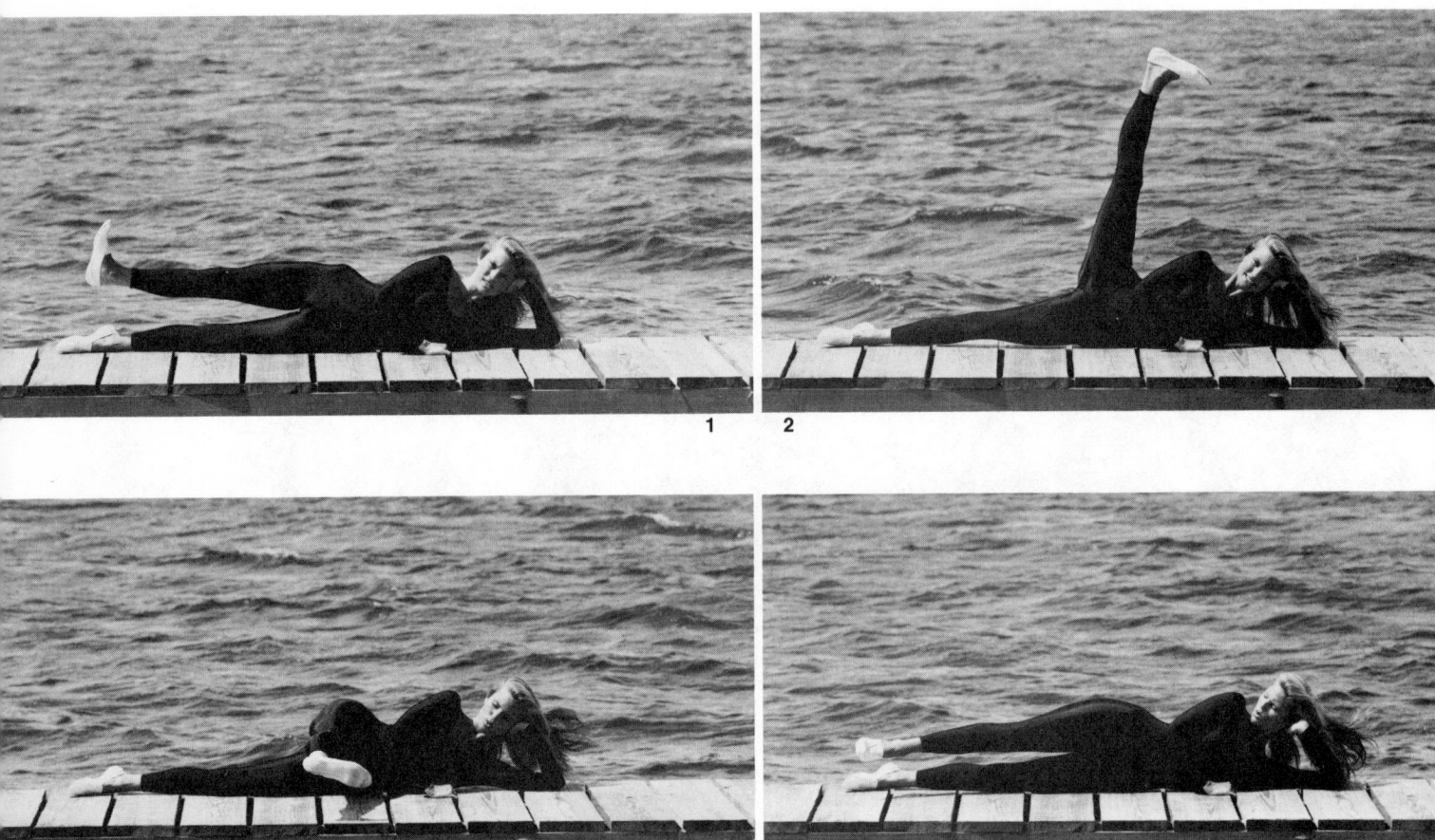

1 2

3 4

Ballet Circles
Lie on side with head resting on raised hand and other arm relaxed in front of body.

1. Raise top leg slightly and flex foot.
2. Then lift leg as high as you can.
3. Lower leg so it's extended in front of you.
4. Bring leg back to starting position (completing circle).

Repeat steps 1 to 4 fifteen times.
Then . . .
Turn to other side and repeat steps 1 to 4 with opposite leg 15 times.

Fran's Slant

You'll feel this in the muscles in the front of the thighs as well as in the buttocks.

Kneel on ground with legs together and arms extended straight in front of you, palms facing downward.

1. Keeping your upper body straight, lower yourself backward as far as possible and hold position for 1 minute.
2. Slowly return to starting position.

Repeat steps 1 and 2 ten times.

Thighs and Buttocks

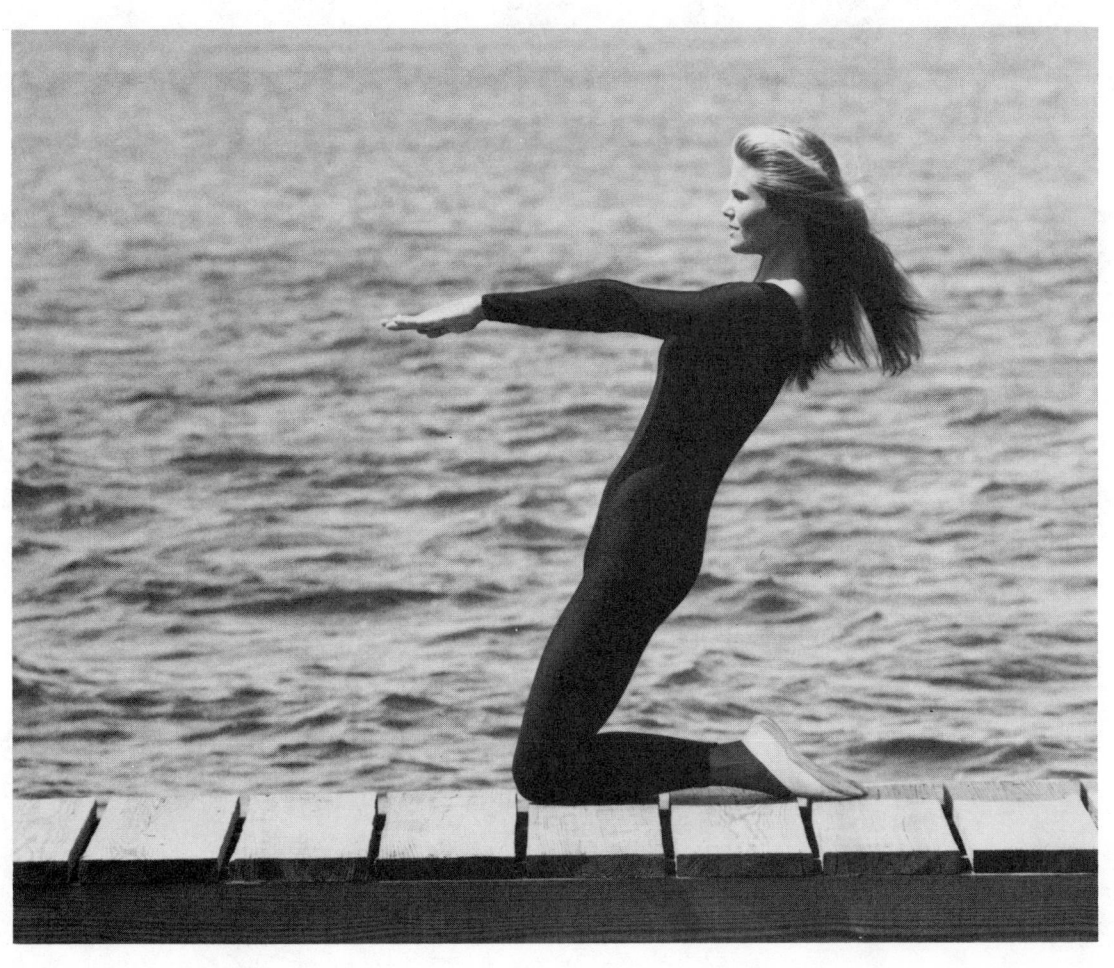

Thighs and Buttocks

Pelvic Squeeze
Lie on your back, arms at sides, palms down. Bend knees, keeping feet flat on floor. Raise pelvis slightly.

1. Then lift pelvis as high as you can. Holding the position for a moment, squeeze buttocks *hard!*
2. Slowly lower pelvis into starting position. Pelvis should not touch the floor at any time during exercise.

Repeat steps 1 and 2 thirty times.

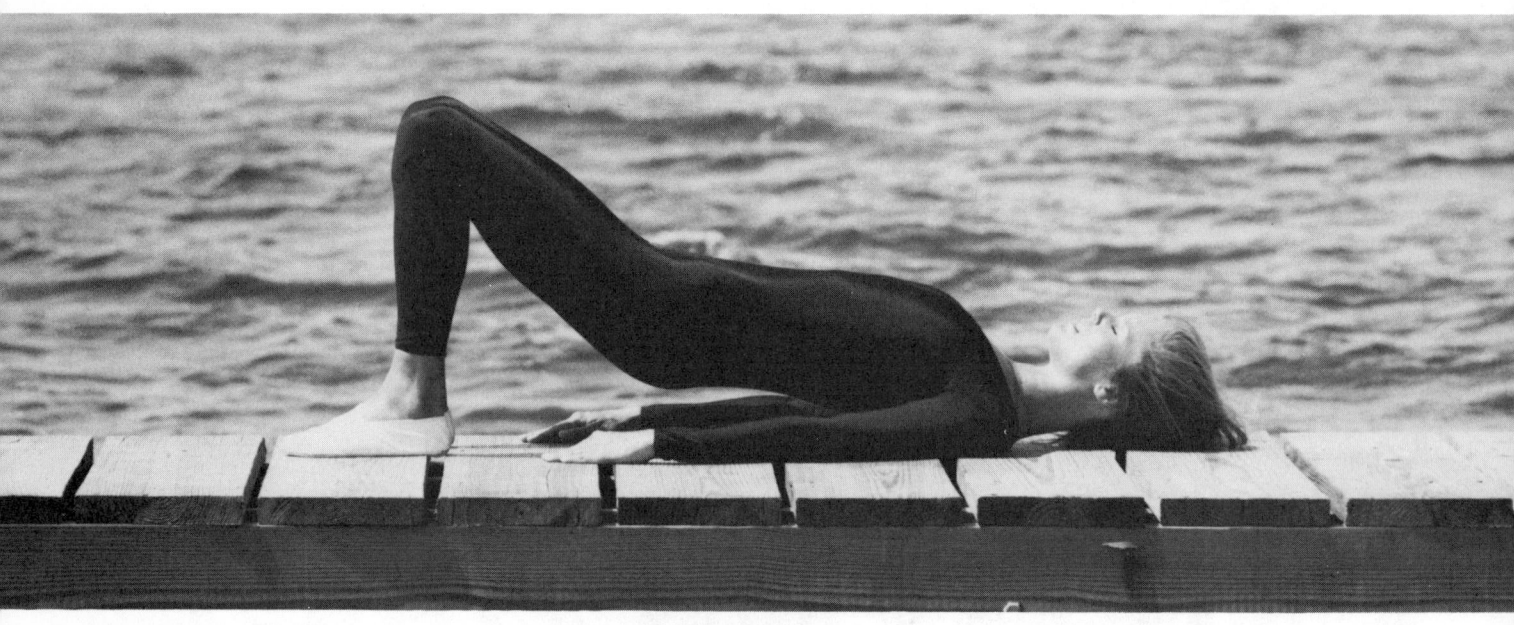

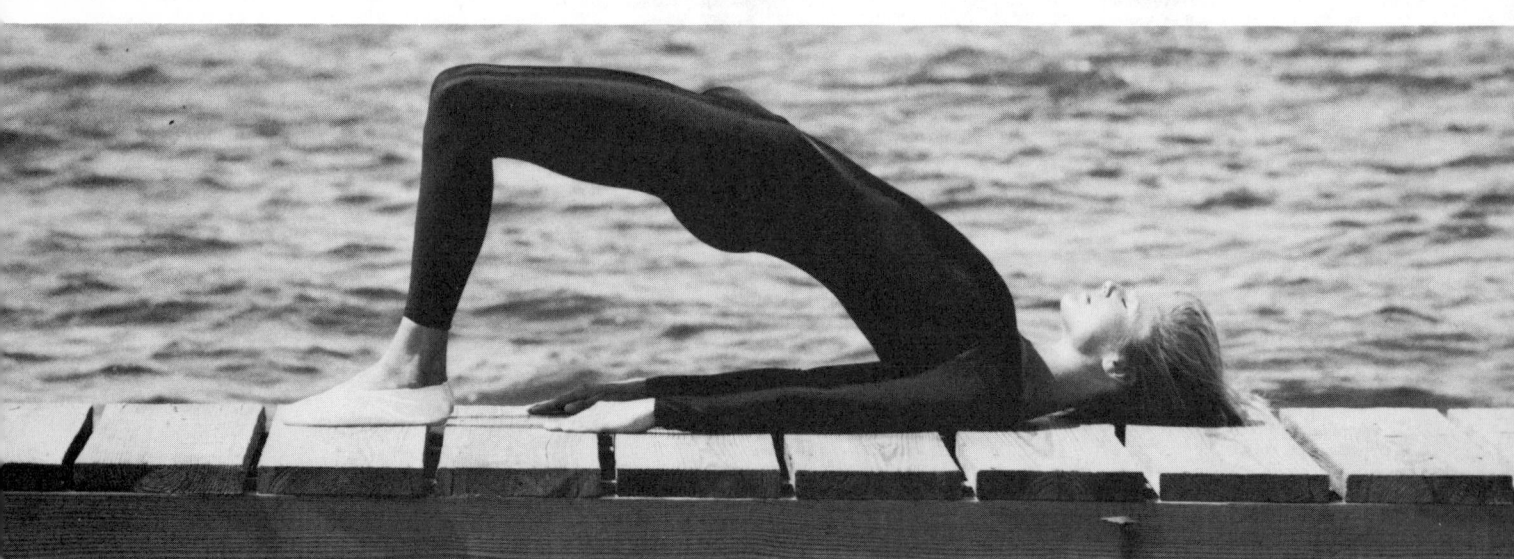

After working out it is important to cool down gradually. You can do this by repeating certain warm-up exercises—very slowly —to restretch your body.

COOL DOWN!

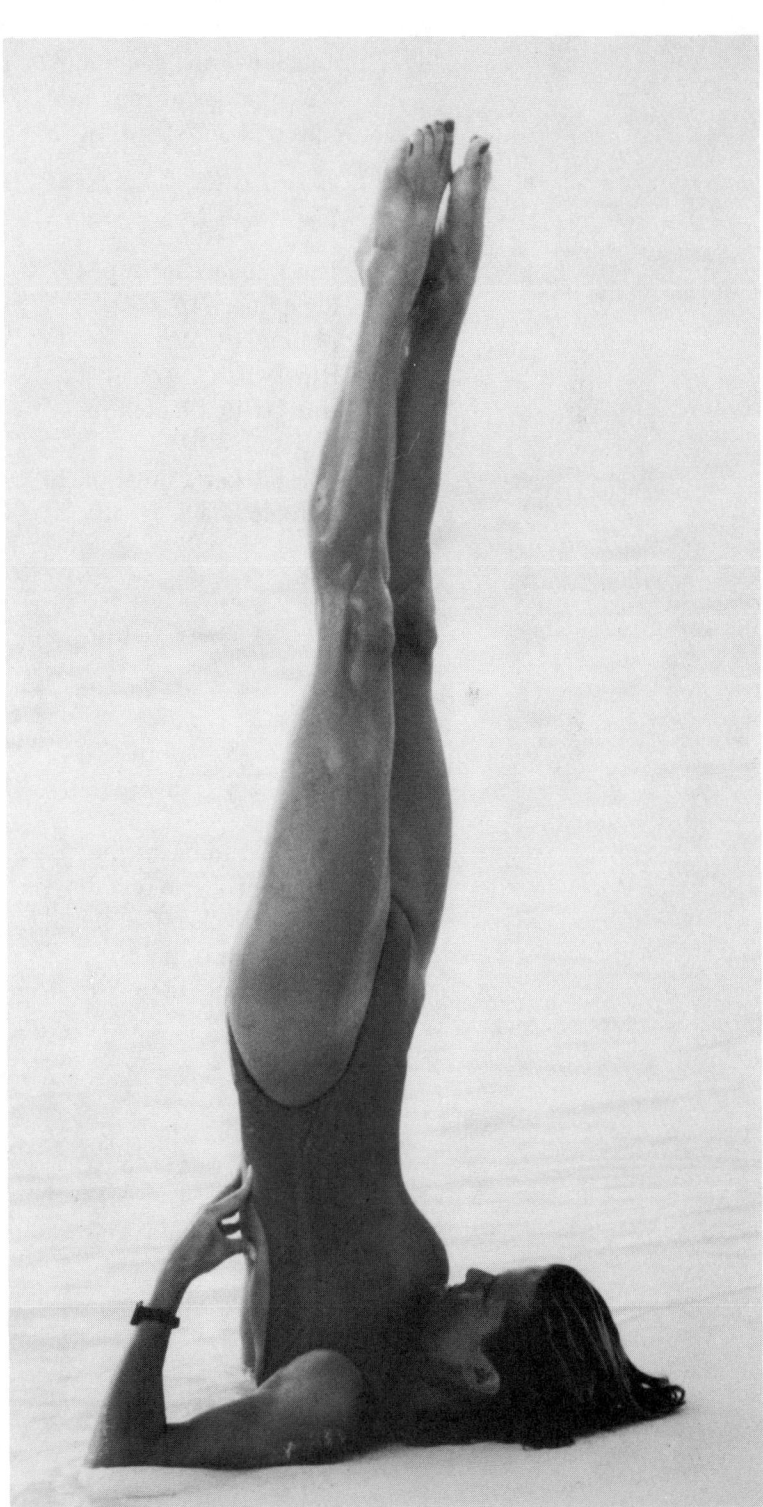

Yoga Shoulder Stand
A terrific cool-down is . . . the Yoga Shoulder Stand. This is great for circulation—therefore your complexion —as it relaxes and energizes.
1. Lie on your back.
2. Roll your feet up into vertical position, supporting your back with your hands—hold for 2 minutes.
3. Slowly lower yourself to starting position.

MY 45-MINUTE DAILY WORKOUT

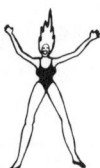

I try to do lots of different exercises every single day. I'm always consulting my exercise notebook for ideas. And I make a point of including a "fun" exercise like biking or riding or swimming in my daily routine. But if you're just starting out, you might find the following basic routine helpful. It should take about 45 minutes. It's much more fun if you put on some spirited music—just be sure not to get carried away and do the exercises too fast; form is important! These are the number of reps I do. If you are just starting out, do as many reps as you can without straining and slowly build up to the full number.

The Warm-Up

The Rubber Neck (p. 44)	30 reps
Rope Reach (p. 45)	15 reps
Oblique Stretch (p. 46)	10 reps
Hip Twist (p. 47)	15 reps
Hamstring Stretch (p. 49)	10 reps
Splits (p. 50)	10 reps
Aerobic Leg Lunge (p. 56)	20 reps
Aerobic Reach (p. 55)	15 reps

The Tone-Up

Jump Rope	5 minutes (build to 10)
Propellers (p. 57)	30 reps
Arm Tightener (p. 58)	30 reps
The Dizzy Dame (p. 60)	15 reps (each variation)
Lindy's Stomachache (p. 62)	20 reps
Lindy's Bicycle (p. 63)	10 reps
Ballet Circles (p. 68)	15 reps
Fran's Slant (p. 69)	10 reps
Pelvic Squeeze (p. 70)	15 reps

The Cool-Down (do these very slowly)

The Rubber Neck (p. 44)	15 reps
Oblique Stretch (p. 46)	5 reps
Hamstring Stretch (p. 49)	5 reps
Yoga Shoulder Stand (p. 71)	

Now don't you feel great!

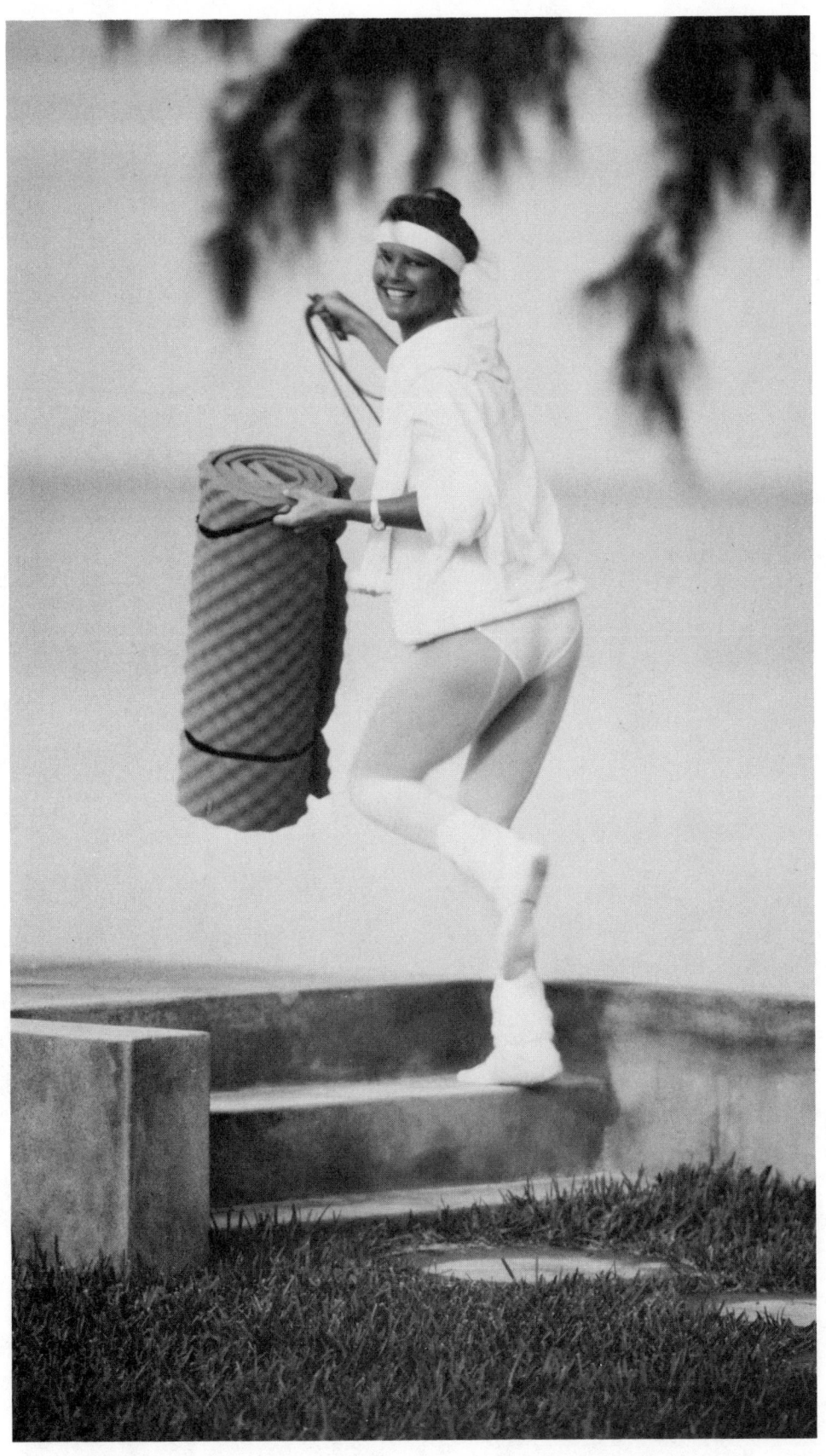

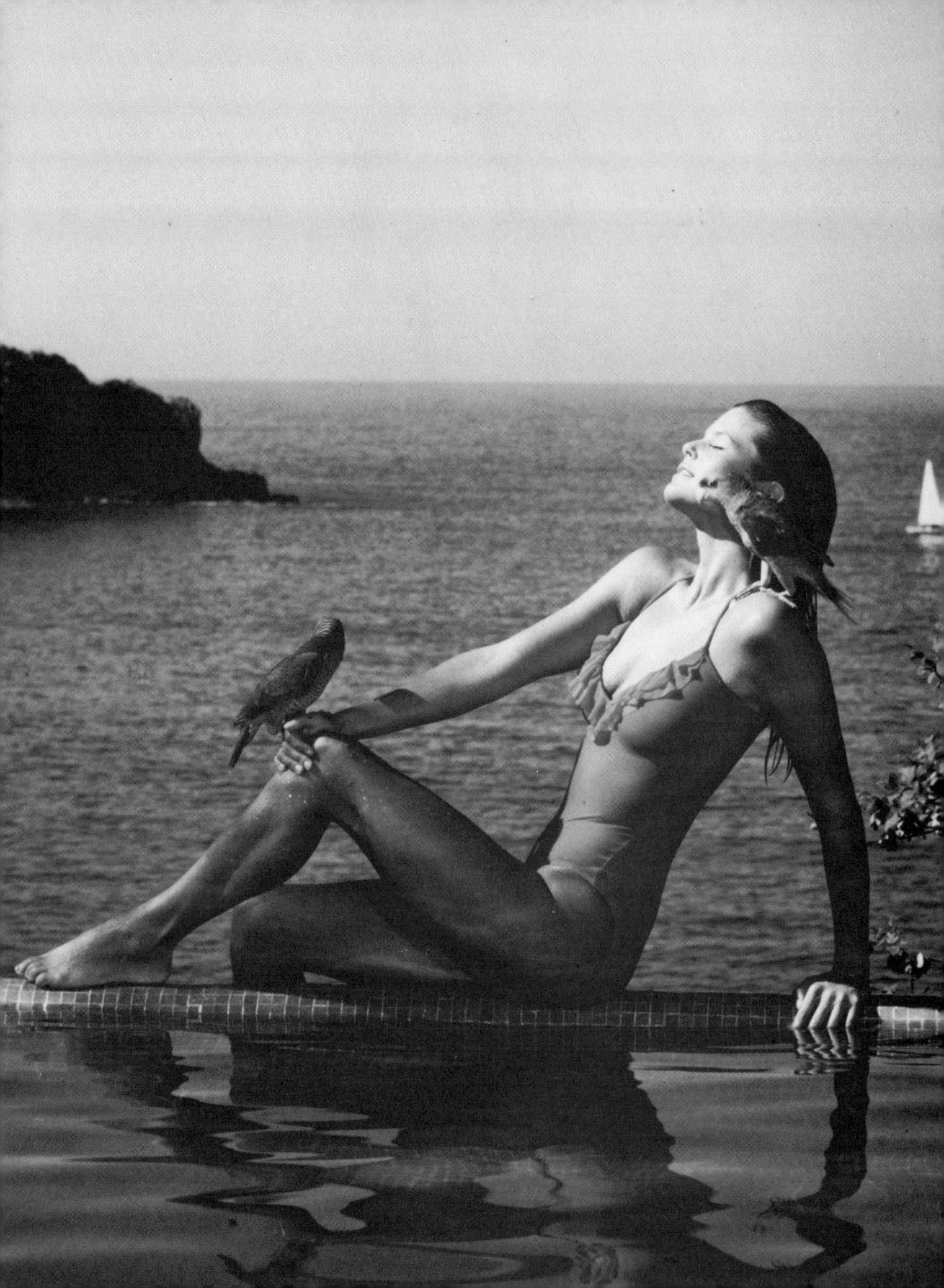

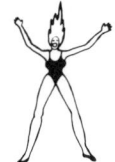

Buying a bikini can probably turn anyone into a criminal! You know the feeling, standing in the dressing room with a bikini top that fits and a bottom that won't get past your ankles, wondering if you'll be sent to prison if you're discovered switching the size 8 bottom for a size 14 to make both ends meet—so to speak!

Yes, the bathing-suit shopping expedition can be a traumatic event. Don't you wish they had locks on the dressing-room doors? Don't you wish they had flattering lighting?

Well, that's all behind you now. This time it's going to be fun because you've followed the diet and exercise section and you're in terrific shape! (If not, turn back a few pages and get started.)

And to keep you smiling once out of the dressing room, make sure you've chosen a style that's right for you. The goal is to accentuate the positive and minimize the negative. You can do this with the right combination of cut and fabric.

Short legs: If your legs are less than lengthy, try for a bathing suit that's cut high in the leg. This will make the line of your leg appear longer and give you a few precious added inches. Either a bikini or a one-piece suit will work but I think a bikini, by breaking up the body, draws attention away from short legs.

Heavy thighs: This is a common figure problem and there are two ways to handle it. If your thighs are firm and your legs are in good proportion to the rest of your body, you can try a one-piece with high-cut legs. This will elongate the leg and make it look slimmer. But if your thighs still need some firming up, you'd best stick with a suit with a brief skirt or short-type legs. Or you can always knot a scarf around your waist for some artful camouflage. It's a very pretty look.

Big bottom: If your derrière needs diminishing, try a suit—either a one-piece or a bikini—with detail at the side seams such as gathering that will draw the eye to your waist. A simple maillot can be very flattering. Just be sure to check the view from the back. The cut of the leg can make all the difference, but the right leg cut to minimize a generous bottom depends entirely on your unique shape, so try on a variety of suits.

Waistless: You'd do well to avoid a bikini, which would call too much attention to your waist. (Though if you're very trim a bikini can sometimes work fine, so try a few.) A one-piece suit with cutouts on the side can give the illusion of a wasp waist.

Too busty: If you've got a large bosom you'll be able to wear either a one-piece or a bikini. But be sure the top is structured. An underwire bra will usually be attractive and more comfortable than an unstructured top. If you choose a bikini, a low-waisted bottom will elongate your figure and de-emphasize your bust.

Small-busted: A bikini is often very flattering to a small bust. Look for a built-in bra that will keep its shape even when wet. Often a cotton or natural fiber is better than a stretchy one. One-piece suits can be fine if they have built-in bras and flatter the rest of your figure.

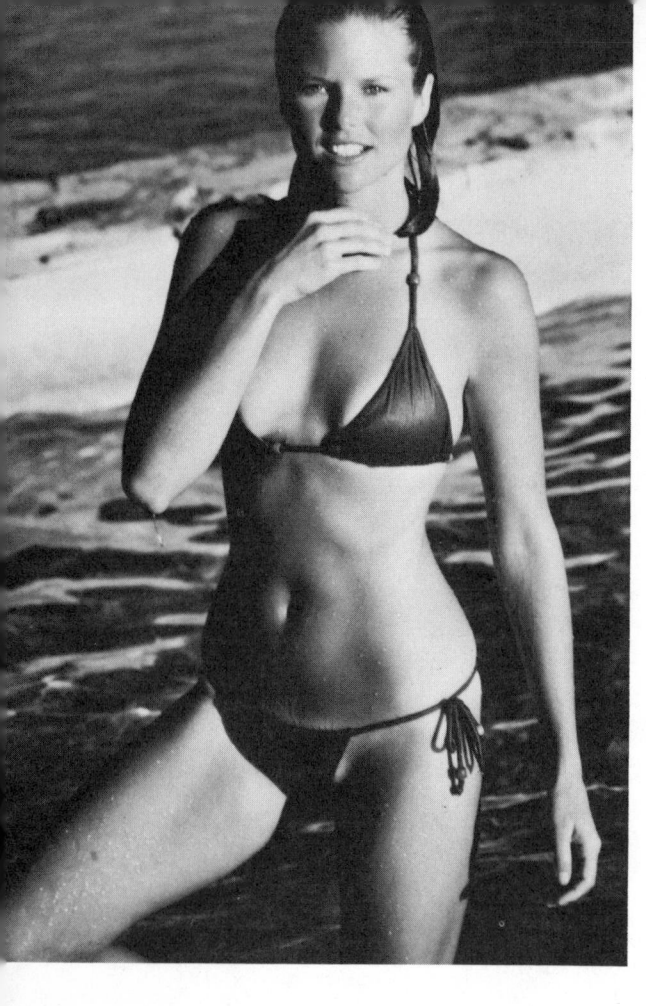

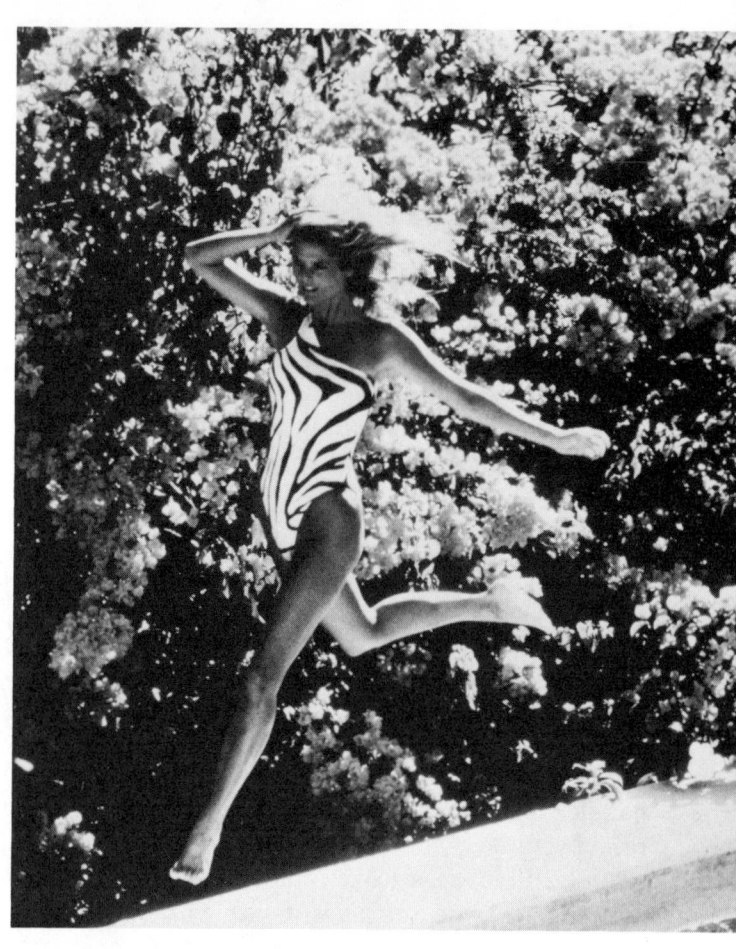

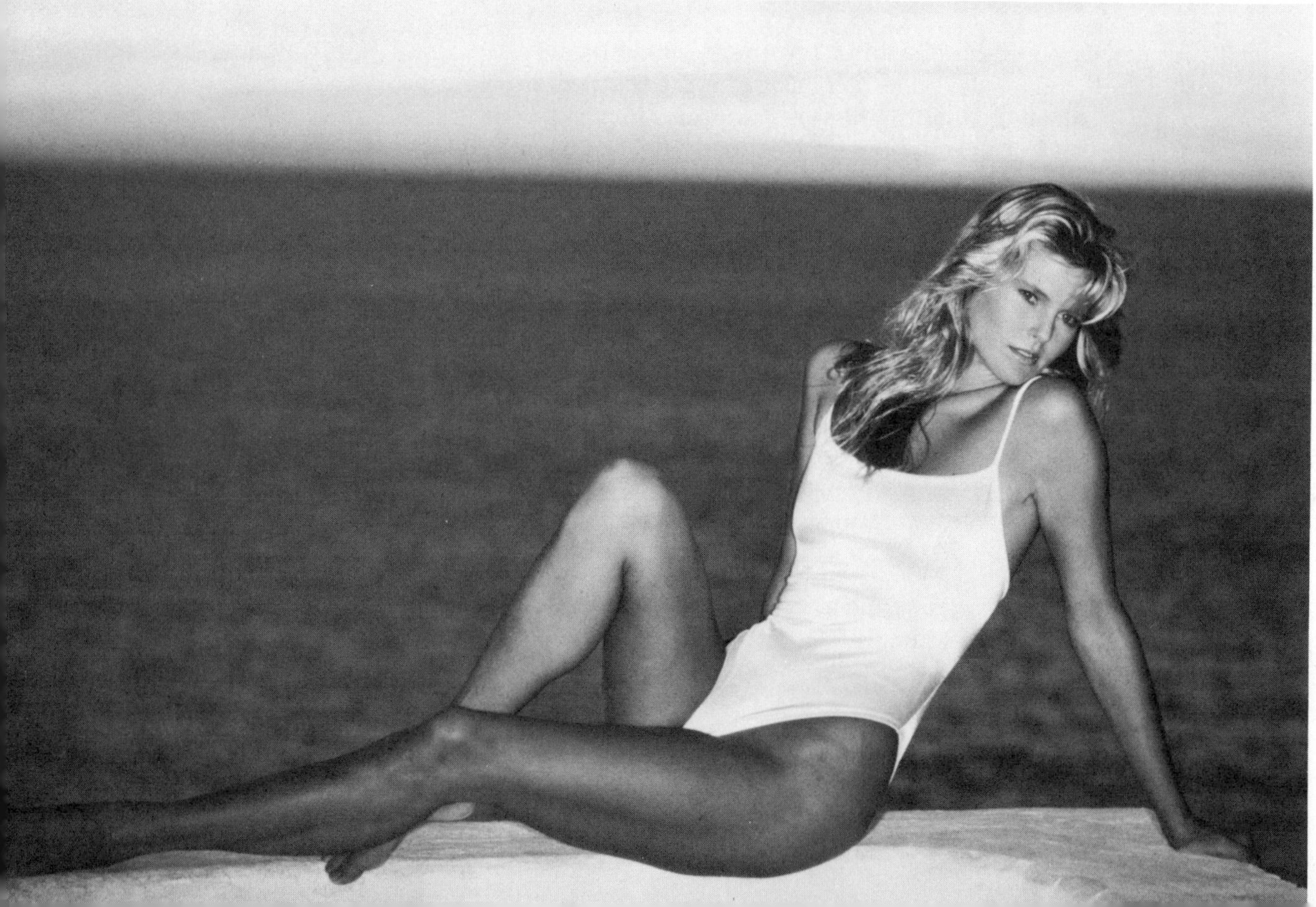

Too thin: A soft, detailed suit in a fabric that drapes or wraps will look super on you. It's best to avoid bikinis and tight maillots which will only emphasize angles. Though if your body has good proportions you might look smashing in a simple maillot in bright horizontal stripes.

When you're searching for a suit, think fabric as well as style. Stretchy, synthetic fabrics look great if you find a style that suits your figure. But they're not very forgiving. Every bulge will announce itself. Cotton and natural fibers will do a better job of hiding many flaws.

Once you've chosen your suit, take good care of it. Rinse it as soon as possible after swimming—a quick shower at poolside is best. And if you swim in chlorinated waters, take special care—the chlorine can take its toll on the color and life of your swimsuit. When you get home from the beach wash it in cold water and mild detergent and let it line-dry. And be sure to guard against snags and runs in synthetic fabrics.

Want to prolong the life of your swimsuit? Use my method: Have a swimsuit wardrobe! I like to have a few different suits. I change them frequently—sometimes a few times a day while sunning. Not only do they last longer, but I never get a dark tan line that makes it hard to change suits. An alternative to my system is to find one style that you love and that looks great on you, and buy two or three of the same suit in different colors.

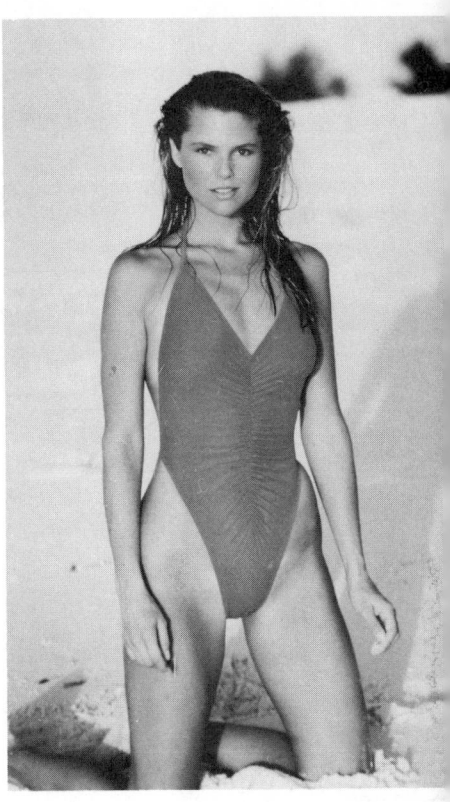

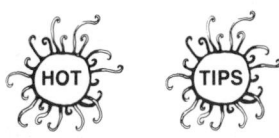

When choosing a suit remember that too many straps will leave funny tan lines on your body.

A striped bathing suit can leave you looking like a zebra when you take it off! A strong sun can actually tan you through the white stripes while the dark ones block the sun.

Beachwear

You've chosen your suit and it looks fabulous! But don't leave the store just yet. You need some cover-ups to keep you looking pretty, and to protect you from the sun.

So if you're planning a trip to a faraway island, add these items to your shopping list.

Giant T-shirts make great cover-ups. Get them in a really large size. That way you can belt them or tie them in knots or do anything your imagination inspires! I like them in black and white but bright colors are great fun, too. My favorites are my boxing T-shirts—they're terrific conversation starters.

Visit the men's department for a white, button-down shirt. Make sure it's in a comfortable fabric. Cotton is the best, and the bigger the better. You can then give it a hundred different looks with belts, scarves, etc. (You can also find great shirts in secondhand shops.)

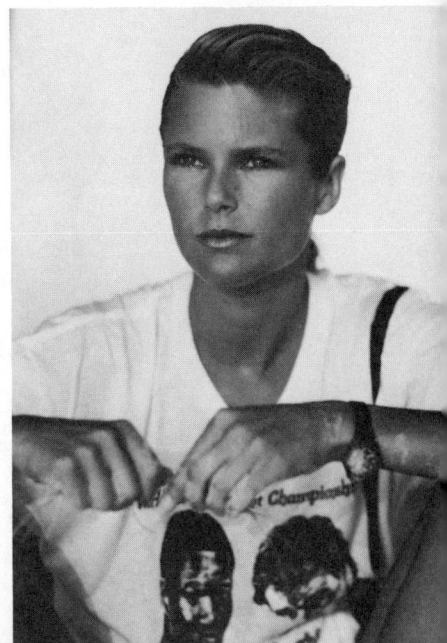

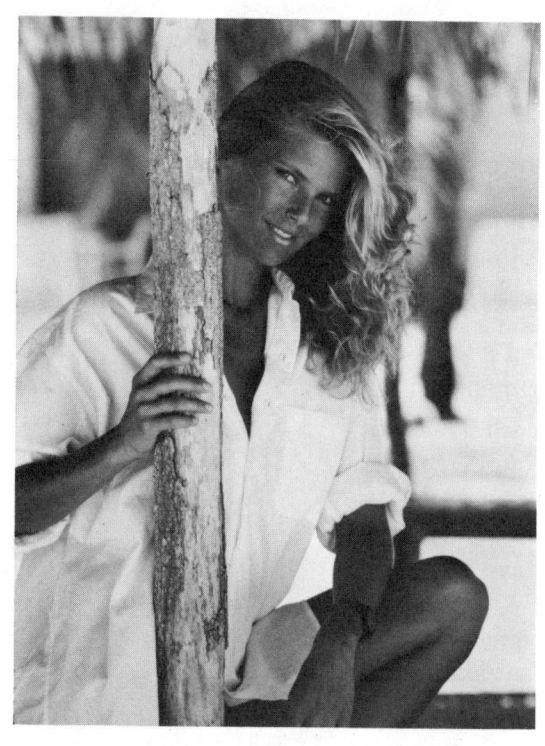
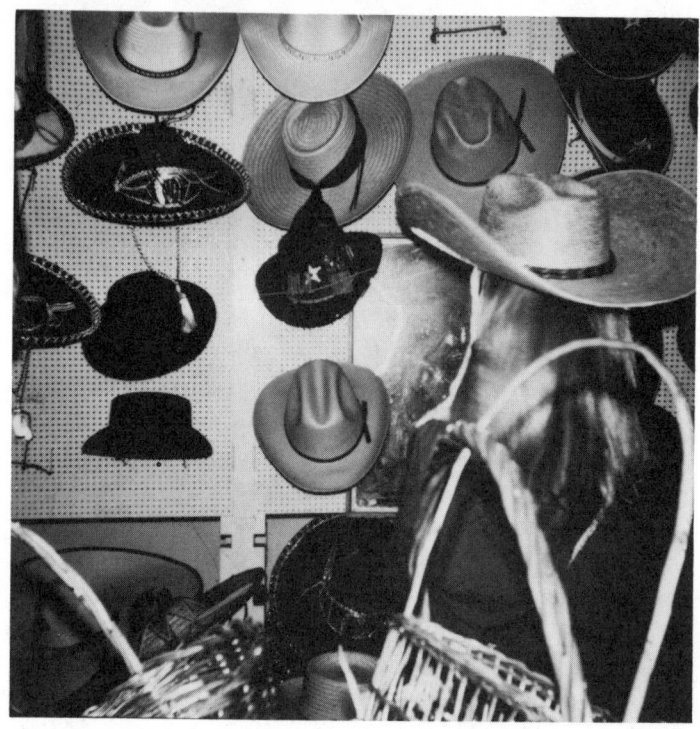

Hats! Before you leave the men's department, check out the hat section. Look for panamas and other styles that will be good on the beach. Visors, baseball caps, and of course the good old straw hat not only make you look good, but give you the necessary protection from the summer sun.

Gym shorts—great for running around!

"Local fashion"—while traveling always be on the lookout for local finds. Here I am in Morocco dressed like a native in comfortable "pooh pants."

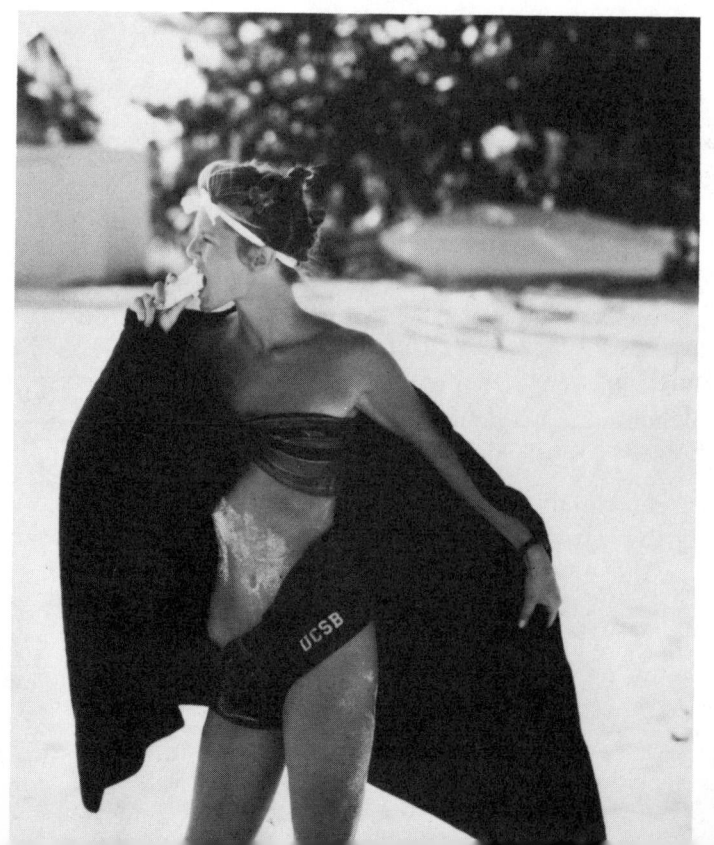
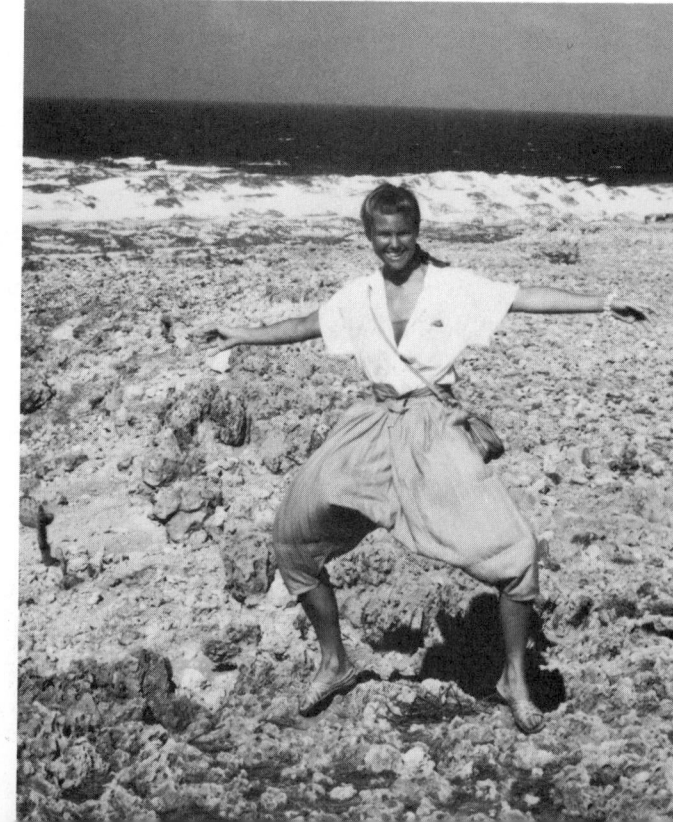

Scarves are a must. I have a collection from around the world in bright, beautiful patterns. They're in all different sizes and shapes and I can fashion a whole beach wardrobe from them. Just be careful about the fabrics and dyes on scarves you want to use at the beach because some colors will come off with the salt water. I've wound up with navy-blue thighs!

Scarf Wardrobe— How to Tie

DIAPER STYLE

For an instant bathing suit or sunsuit, just take a piece of fabric or a large scarf approximately 44 x 72 inches and, holding it lengthwise, wrap the fabric around your body and tie the corners together over your chest (1). Then bring the loose corners around to your back and pull the cloth through your legs back to front like a diaper and bring it up to your waist (2). Roll the scarf to fit, then bring the corners to the back and tie (3).

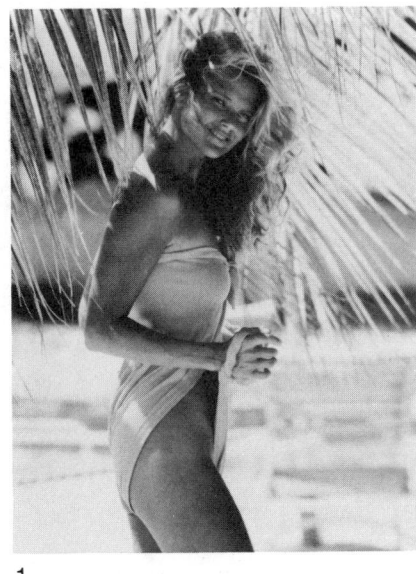

1

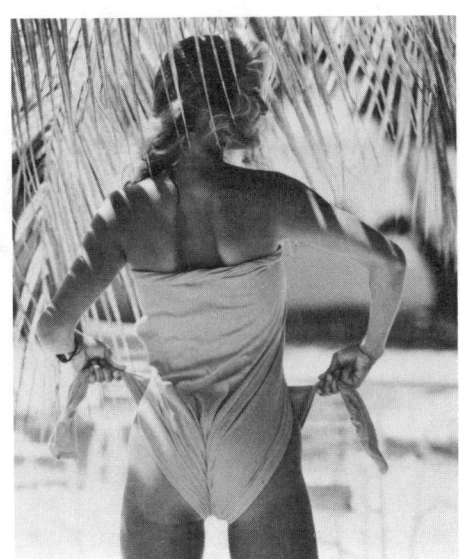

2

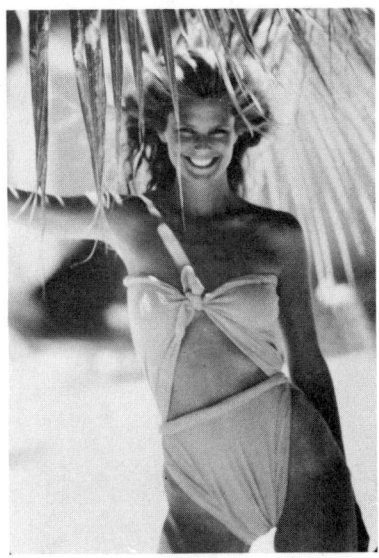

3

BANDEAU

This couldn't be simpler and it's a great way to top a bikini bottom, shorts, or skirt. Take a scarf or piece of fabric about 12 x 44 inches. Hold it lengthwise in front of you. Twist once, then arrange the twist between your breasts and tie in back.

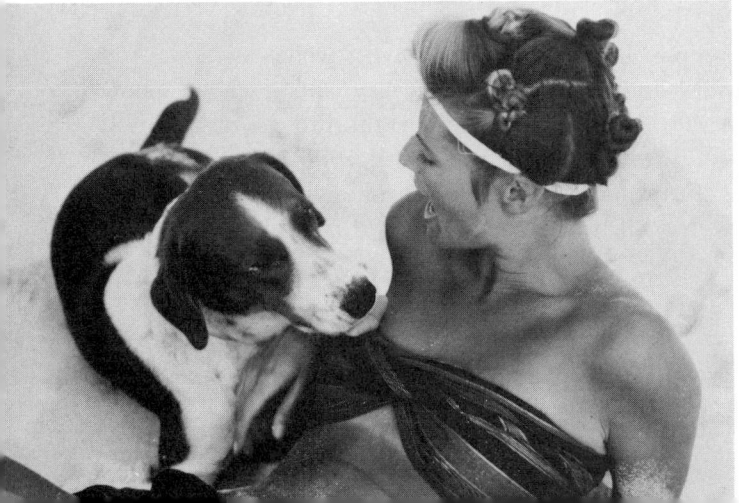

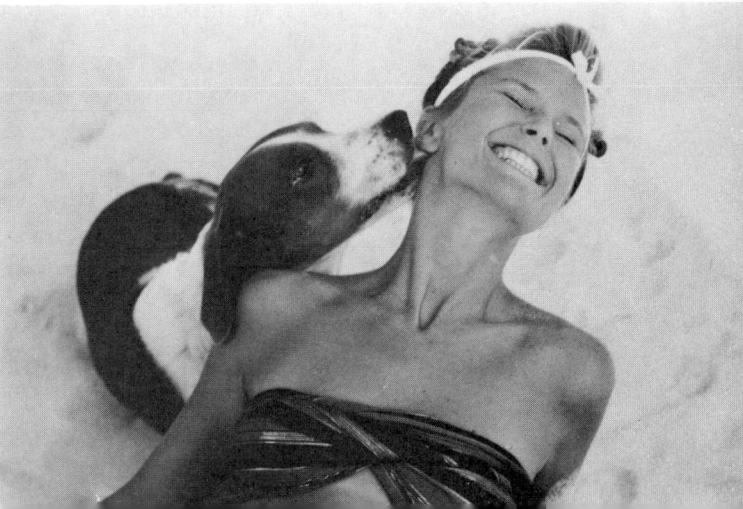

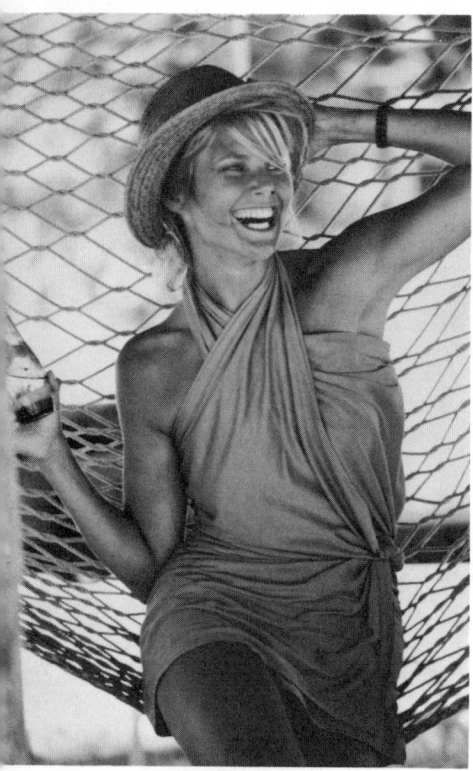

SARONG

This is good for topping a suit or just a bikini bottom. Take a piece of fabric about 36 x 45 inches. Hold the fabric behind you, bring the corners around to the front, cross over your chest and tie in back of your neck. You can then belt it or just let it hang loose.

Foul-weather gear. If you're planning a trip to an island, a light raincoat is a good idea. I always bring one—because if I don't, sure enough it always rains; when I do, it never rains. It's my way of ensuring great weather!

Now look for some shoes. Flat exercise sandals make great beach shoes. You'll want some rubbery shoes for seashell hunting—those French gumdrop shoes or tennis shoes are good. Just plain thongs are great all-around beach shoes. I've even worn windsurfing shoes at the beach—they look fine if you wear them with socks. And bring your topsiders, you never know when you'll be asked onto someone's yacht!

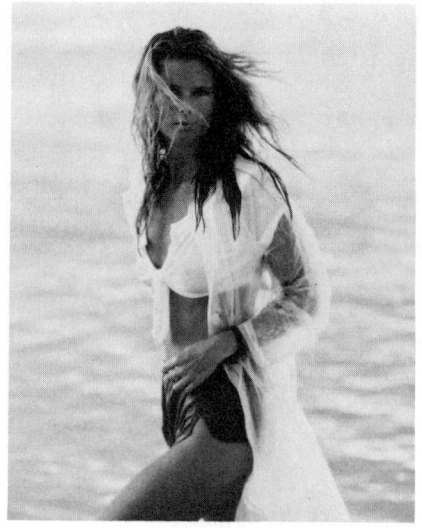
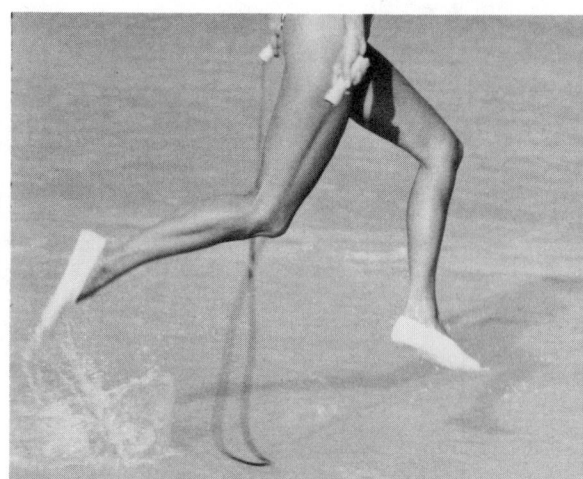

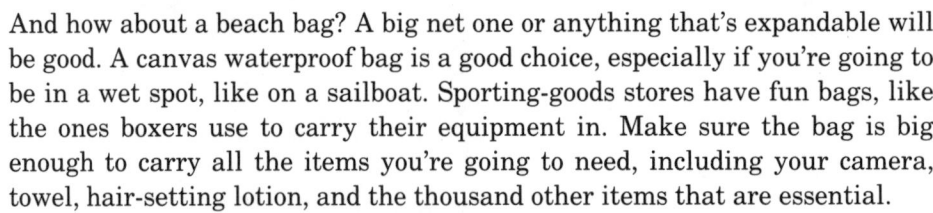

And how about a beach bag? A big net one or anything that's expandable will be good. A canvas waterproof bag is a good choice, especially if you're going to be in a wet spot, like on a sailboat. Sporting-goods stores have fun bags, like the ones boxers use to carry their equipment in. Make sure the bag is big enough to carry all the items you're going to need, including your camera, towel, hair-setting lotion, and the thousand other items that are essential.

Don't forget belts. You'll need them for your T-shirts and white button-down cover-ups. Try using a rope from the sail shop or hardware store, or twist a fishnet into a belt—both great nautical looks.

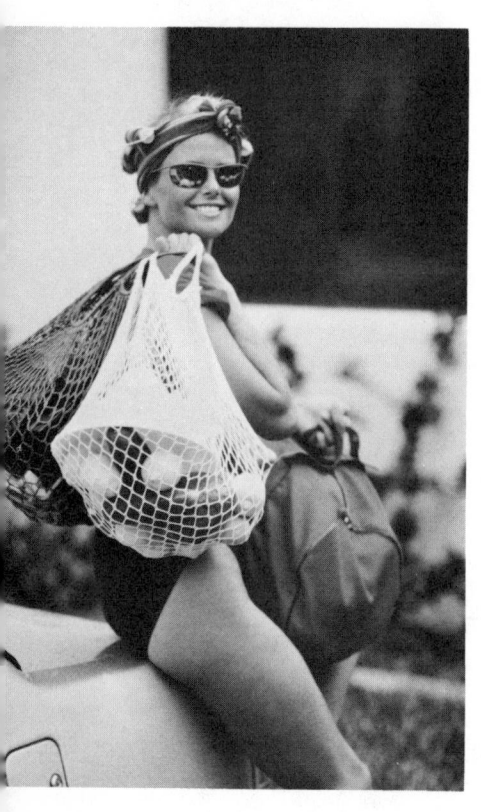

Beach jewelry? Keep it simple. Leave your expensive jewelry at home and have fun with beachy looks—inexpensive shell jewelry can be given a new look by spraying it with waterproof spray paint in bright, fun colors; gold and silver look great, too. Colorful rubbery or bright aluminum fish lures are eye-catching. (Be sure you carefully cut off the hooks so you don't catch anything else!) Beware of metal jewelry—if it doesn't sink you, it could become hot in the sun and burn you.

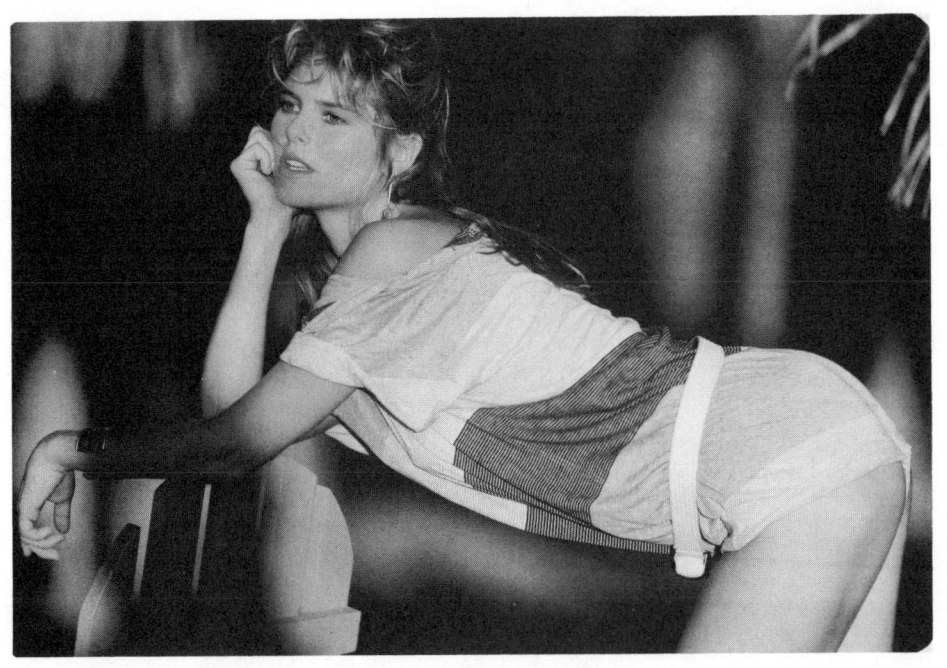

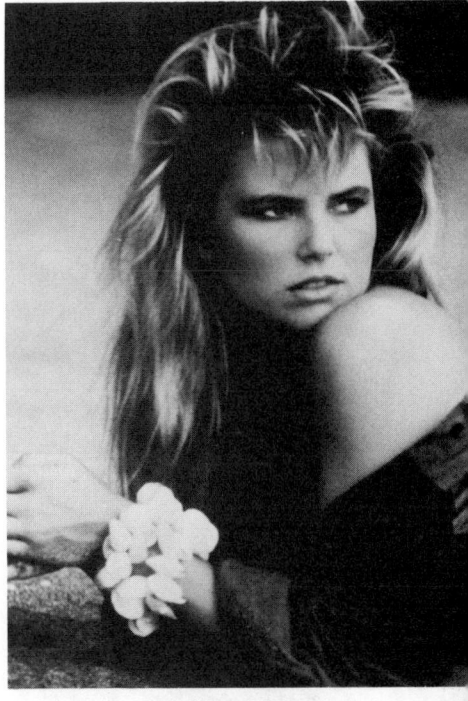

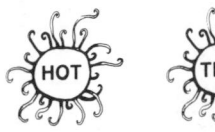

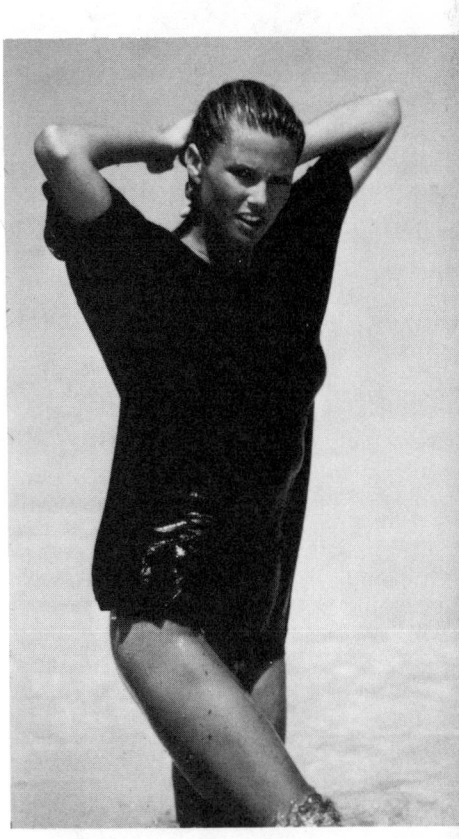

Skin very sensitive to the sun? The sun's rays penetrate lighter colors much more than dark colors. So if you need extra protection, a dark-colored cover-up is your best bet. Also, a fabric with a close weave will give more protection than a loose one.

Buying beach clothes? Natural fibers such as cotton and linen will keep you much more comfortable, because they allow your skin to breathe.

Your favorite suit stained by sunscreen? Buy some enzyme pre-soak from the detergent section at your grocery store. Make a paste with it and warm water. Wet the spot, rub the paste into it, and let it soak for a half hour. Pour clean water slowly to flood the stain and rinse out the pre-soak, then hand or machine wash in cold water.

SUMMER MAKEUP

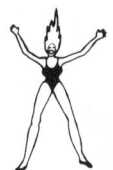

It's summer! Warm weather at last! Not only the temperature's changing, but your attitude, too. You feel fresh, carefree, casual, and ready for fun. You're thinking about beaches, boats, picnics, warm breezes, concerts in the park, and swimming pools. You're ready to break the bonds of winter and adopt a whole new lifestyle.

Flexibility is the key to a pretty summer look. You need to adjust your makeup to your summer lifestyle. How can you waterproof your makeup? How can you make a pale face look tanned? How can you continue to look fresh in 100% humidity? How can you cope with peeling or sunburned (ouch!) skin?

You want to be able to handle all these things easily and prettily, so here goes. . . .

Tools of the Trade

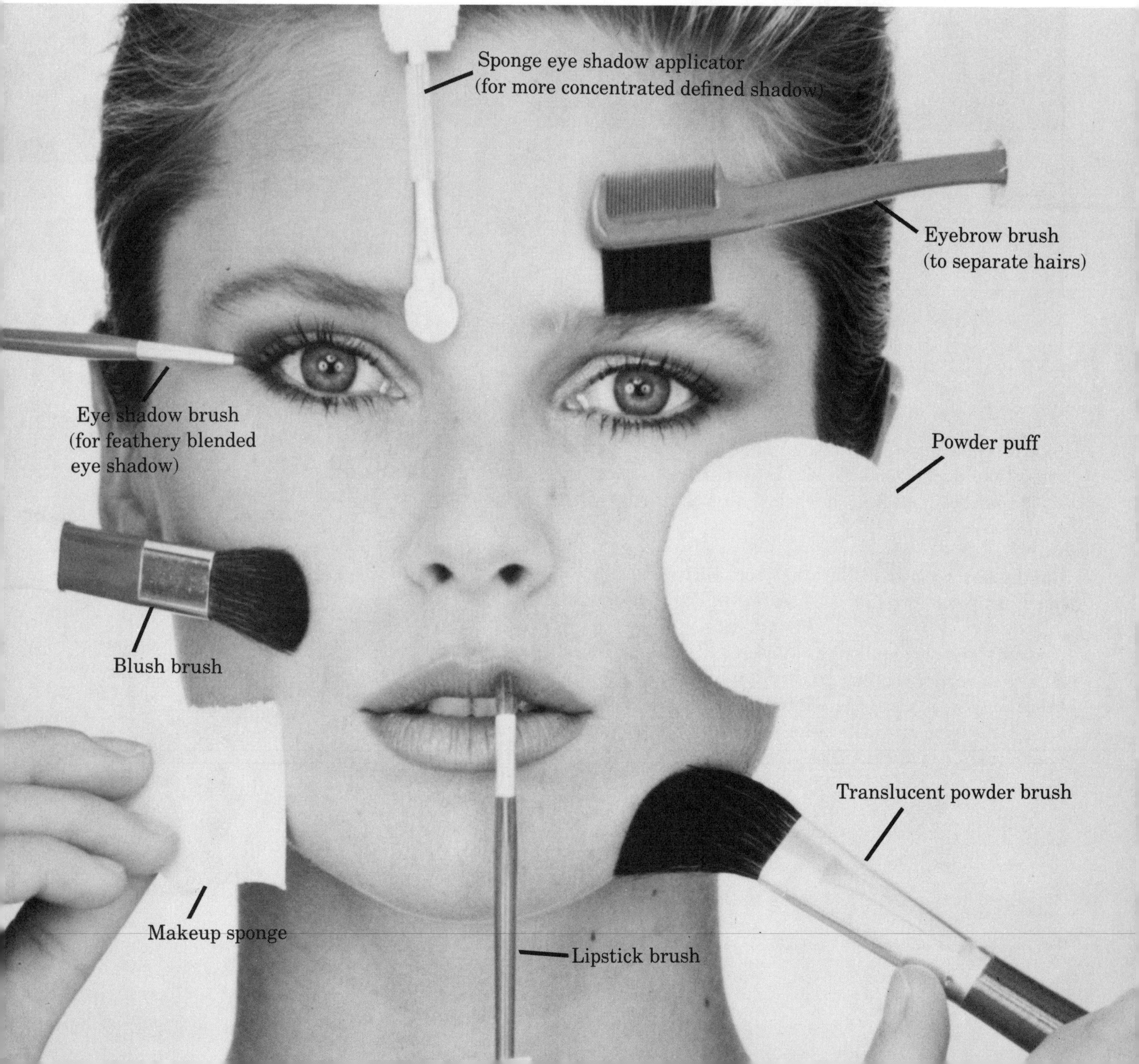

Sponge eye shadow applicator
(for more concentrated defined shadow)

Eyebrow brush
(to separate hairs)

Eye shadow brush
(for feathery blended
eye shadow)

Powder puff

Blush brush

Translucent powder brush

Makeup sponge

Lipstick brush

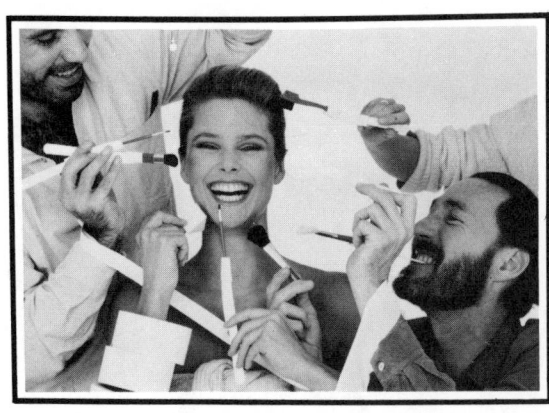
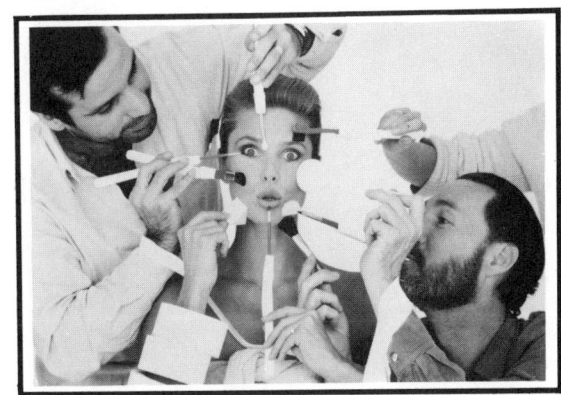
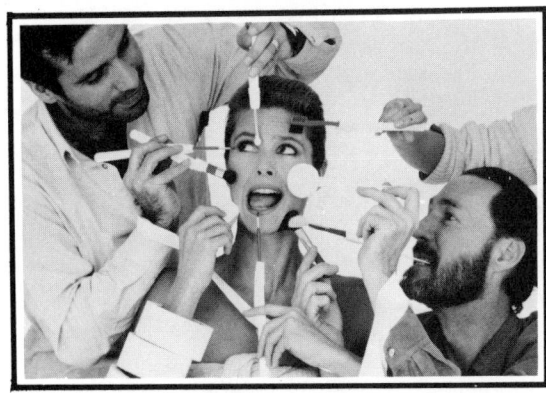
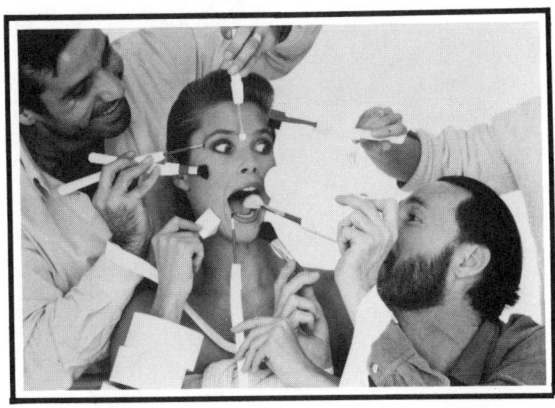
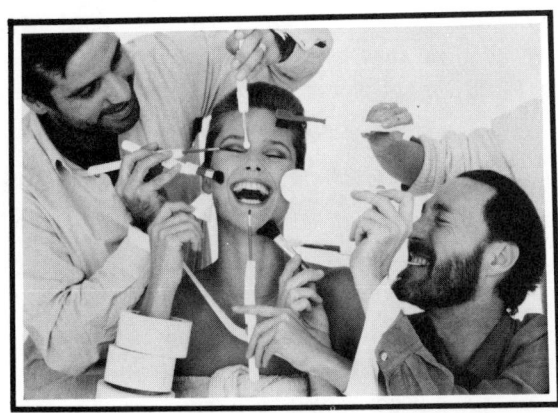
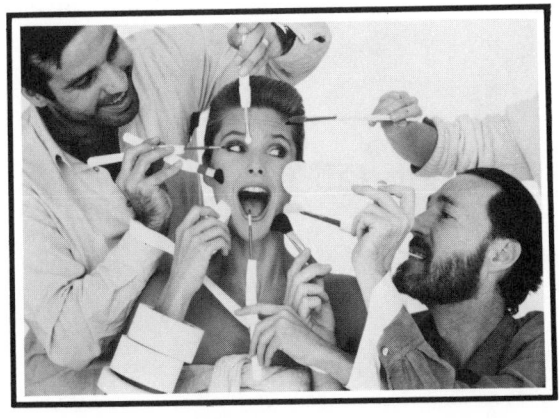

Here I am being made up by Vincent Nasso and Maury "Hops" Hopson.

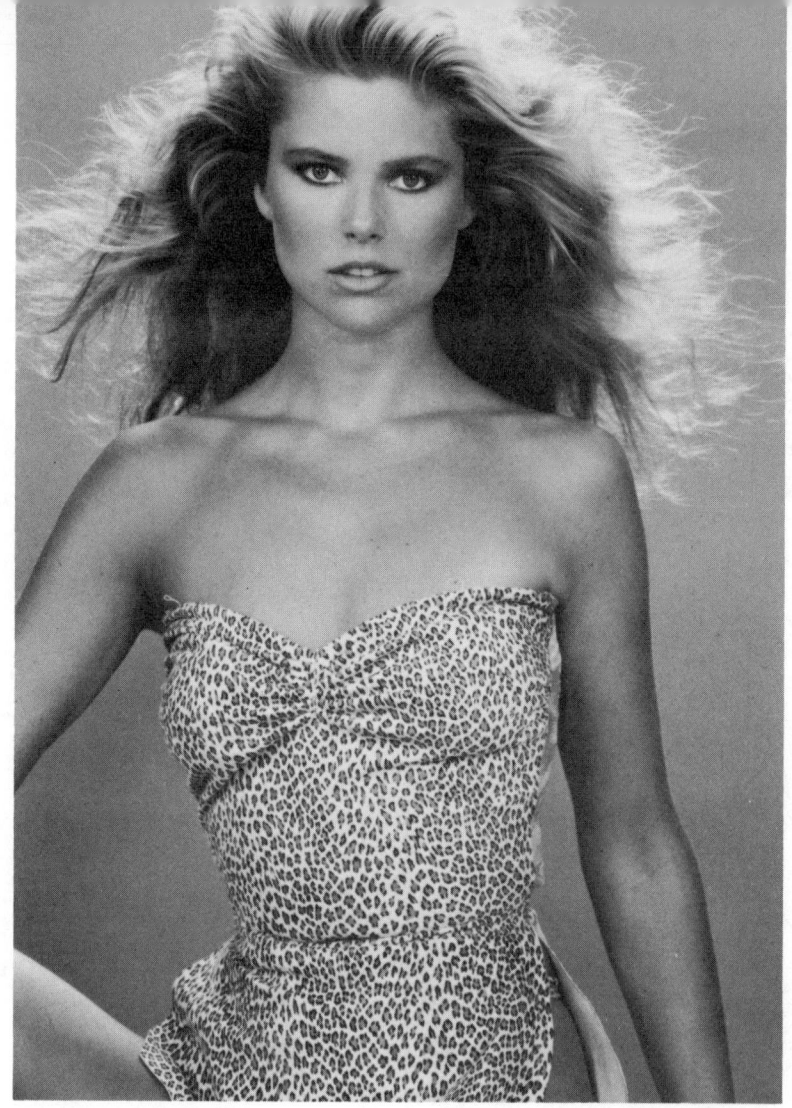

Lighting

For some reason, perhaps the abundance of natural light in a sunny climate, the correct lighting for your makeup is essential. I've often seen women emerge from hotels with broad stripes of color on their cheeks and eyes. I suppose they looked fine in the smoky light of the hotel bathroom but once out of doors they look like the old-fashioned "painted hussy."

I always put makeup on in the best light available. It's amazing how the quality of light can change the look of the makeup on your face. When I'm traveling, I bring a hand mirror along and prop it up near a window to put on daytime makeup. It's the only way I can be sure the sunlight will flatter my face. By the way, I never make up with a magnifying mirror as it can distort your features.

If I'm making up for the evening and even though I'm going to be in a place with muted light, I still try to apply my makeup in a good light.

Foundation

You should always start with a clean face before applying makeup. In "Cleansing Summer Skin" (p. 98) I go into detail on what I think is the best cleansing routine. Never skip a thorough cleansing. Because a tan face usually means warm weather, your face is perspiring more than usual. If you put makeup on top of a less than pristine face you'll clog your pores and encourage breakouts.

It's difficult to find a foundation that works well on a tan face. They often give a masklike look to your skin. I find if you *cover* your tan face with base it looks artificial. Everybody has tiny hairs on their face and once you're tan, unless your base matches your skin color perfectly, it will make those little hairs stand out and look strange. The important rule concerning foundation on a tan face is less is more.

Instead of covering my whole face with base, I mix the foundation with moisturizer in the palm of my hand. Then I dot it in certain spots around my face. I dab it under the eyes for highlight and along the length of my nose. I find that no matter how many hats I wear, my chin always gets a little more exposure than the rest of my face. Instead of trying to cover it with a light foundation, I dab on a darker one and it blends in fine with the rest of my face.

All the dots of base/moisturizer—on your nose, under your eyes, and on your chin—need to be carefully blended into the surrounding skin so the finish will look natural. I think that once your face is tan you'll want to avoid a very matte look with your makeup. A bit of shine looks more glowing and natural so don't worry that your forehead, for example, isn't covered with base.

Blush

You would think getting a rosy blush would be an easy matter when you have a tan, but it's where many women make mistakes.

The first thing you have to know is exactly what color your skin has become. In general, you'll want to go with sunny colors that will complement your hair and eyes, but everyone tans a different shade. Some people are gold, others cocoa-colored, and some get pink. You must be sure not to fight the color of your tan with the color of your blush. After the first few days in the sun you usually get a rosy glow which should be accented with a rose or pink blush. But as your tan settles in to stay, you will probably have to adjust your color. I find that my tan becomes somewhat orangy so that's the color tone I use for my blush. If I stuck with a rose blush I'd look like a clown.

You can apply a little more blush than you usually would because your face is darker and can probably stand the additional color. But be sure not to go overboard.

Eyes

I think that when your face is tan you should be using very little eye shadow. By using blush behind the brow toward the temple you liven up the eye and diminish the need for a bright shadow. I also think it's best to stick with a natural color. If you're using blue, for example, try a soft muted blue rather than a metallic one. You might try just a thin line of shadow above the lashes and a soft blurred line in the crease of the eye. Never smear your eye shadow all over the lid as it will look quite unnatural.

After your shadow you'll want to add some mascara. A light touch here is important. Lots of very thick, very heavy black lashes seem somehow unnatural with a tan face. If you're a blonde, use a dark-brown mascara; brunettes and dark-haired women can use black mascara, but only if it doesn't look too harsh with their complexions.

Lips

I think just a hint of gloss, perhaps in a transparent color, is all that's needed on the lips. A strong, bright color looks somehow wrong with a tan face. So stick to the light shiny glosses in a coral or pink shade.

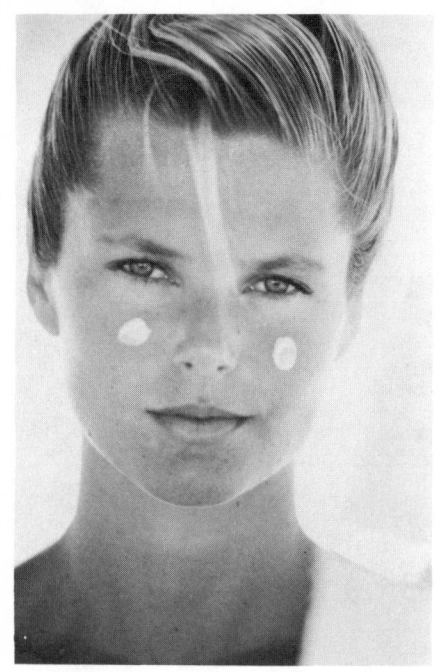

Step 1

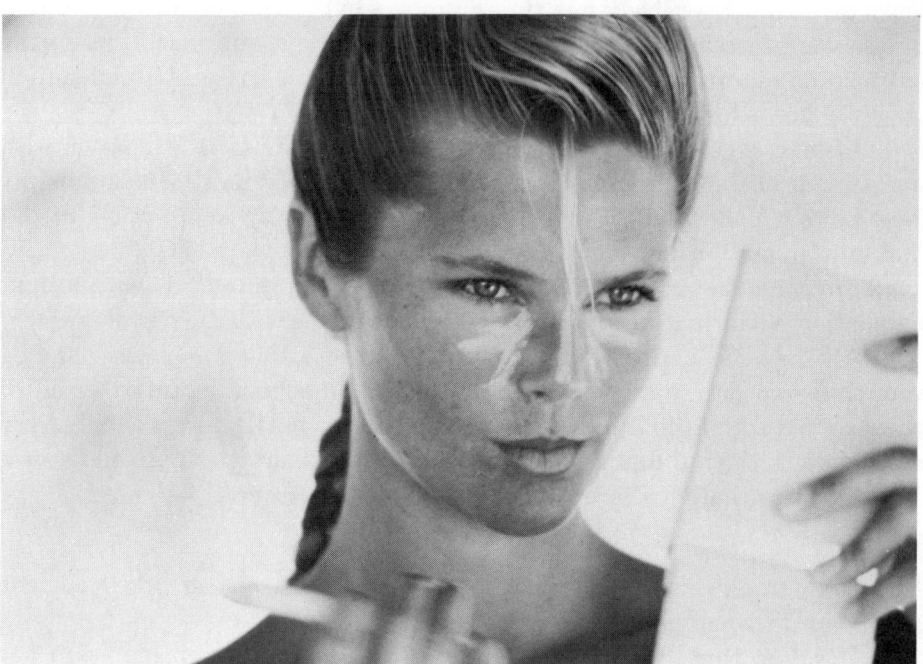

Step 2

How to Apply

Step 1. Moisturize.

Always start with moisturizer on a damp face; less in humid climates, more in dry climates.

TIP: If you're spending the day in the sun, use sunscreen as moisturizer! Or mix sunscreen in with your moisturizer.

Step 2. Makeup base.

Rather than cover your whole face with makeup base, which often ends up looking unnatural (especially in the sun), try covering only the areas where you really need it:

—under eyes, to make you look refreshed;
—to cover any blemishes or discoloration;
—across the bridge of nose, especially if it's sunburned, or a bit small like mine. Choose a shade just slightly lighter than your skin (except for chin, jaw, forehead—that should match your skin).
—in humid climates or for a waterproof effect I find stick and cream bases work very well;
—in dry climates I blend liquid base with moisturizer so I don't dry out my skin.

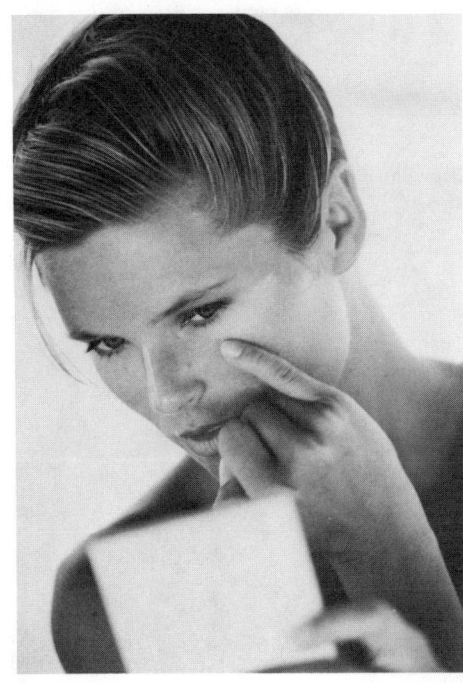 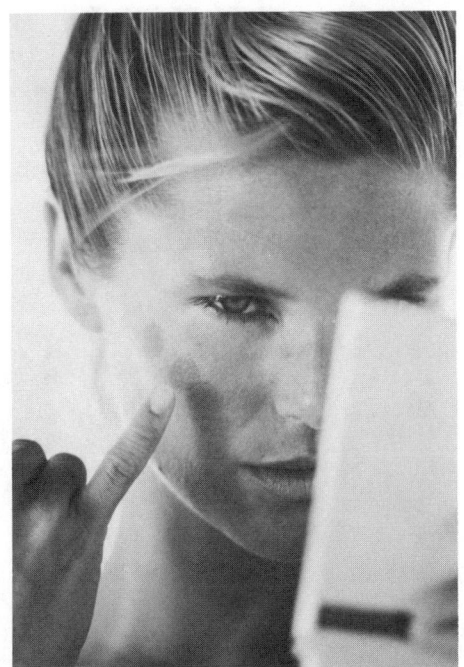

Step 3   Step 4

Step 3. Blend carefully.

The secret to a natural-looking makeup is blending. You want to look healthy and glowing, *not* made up.

Some professionals use cosmetic sponges to blend, but I prefer using my little finger in light strokes, blending the edges until they become invisible.

Step 4. Blush.

I don't care what shape face you have, in the summer in the daytime, I think the only place that blush looks natural is where the sun would have put it on your face—across your cheeks, behind your eye just below your brow, a touch on your nose, chin (earlobes for short-haired girls) and dusted lightly along your hairline—that's guaranteed glow! Once again, whether you're using cream blush for dry skin and dry climates, or powdered blush for oily skin and humid climates, blending is the way to ensure a natural look.

Choosing a color that is already present in your natural skin tone will also make it look like the blush belongs there.

TIP: When I'm being photographed by the sea, I use a cream blush. Then, in a matching color, I dust powdered blush on top. It seems to set the blush for good, as long as I don't rub it!

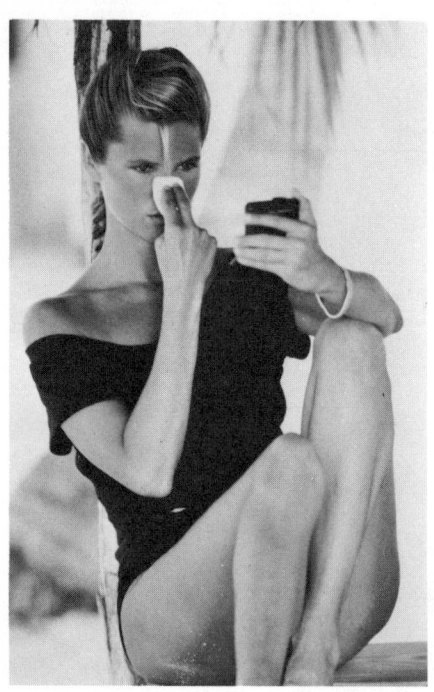

Step 5

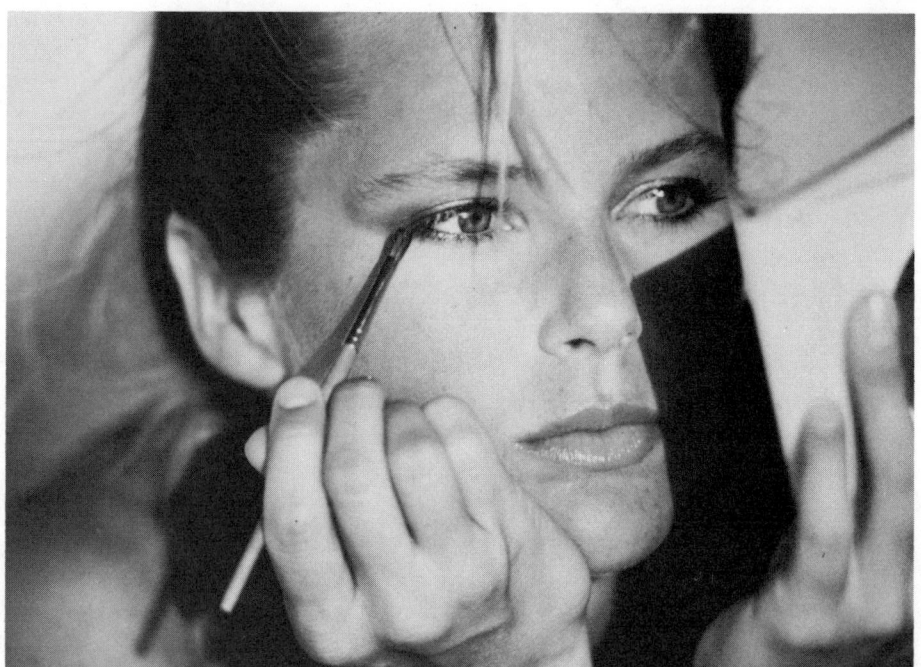

Step 6

Step 5. Powder *lightly.*

Now I apply *very* lightly a touch of translucent powder just around the *edges* of the blush I have applied, just to keep the makeup in place as I finish up the rest.

Most professional makeup artists use loose powder, but I prefer the control of a compact with a powder puff. If you're in a dry climate skip this step. You'll powder later.

Step 6. Eye shadow.

Eye shadow makes your eyes look larger by increasing the intensity of the shadow already formed by your eyes' shape. If you blend carefully you can exaggerate the shape and give your eyes more depth.

The most natural look is achieved by using "earthy" colors that blend easily with the skin.

Often I simply take my cheek blusher and brush it across my upper eyelid.

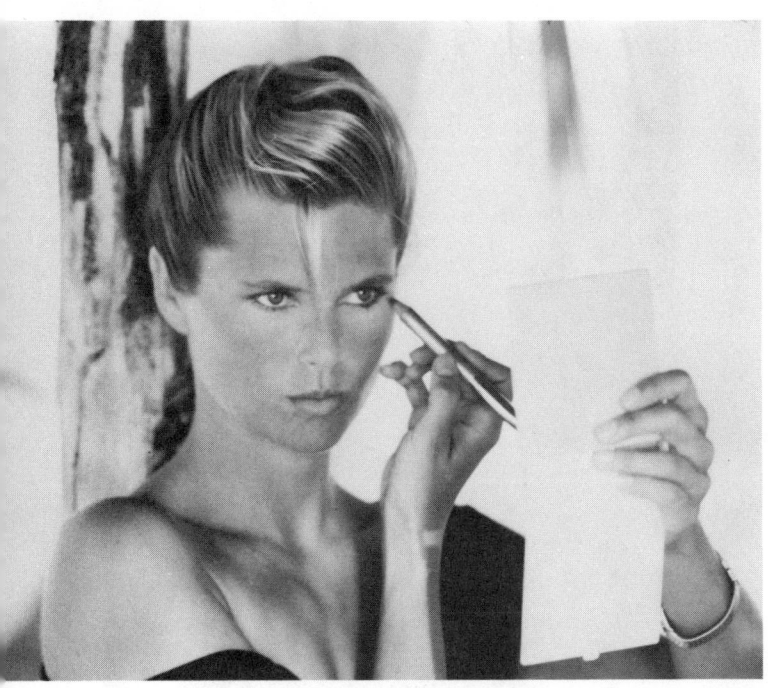

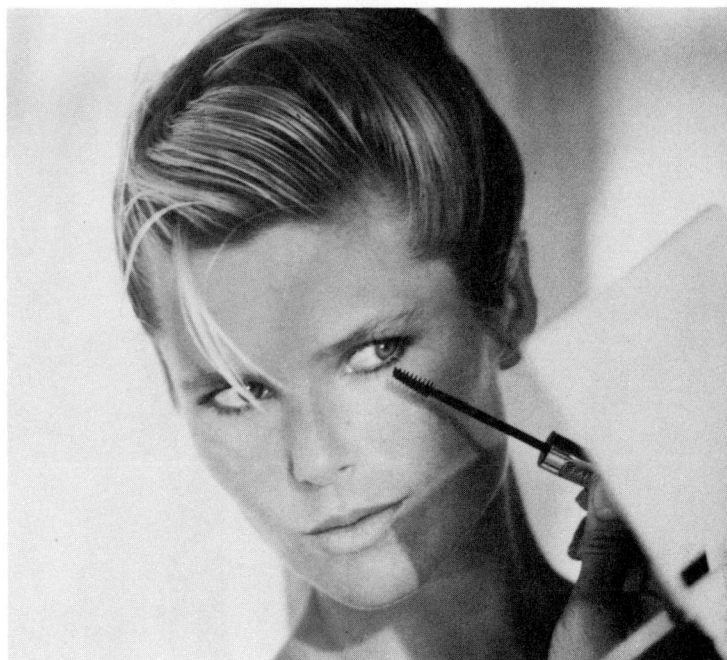

Step 7

Step 8

Step 7. Eye liner.

When used correctly, eye liner makes a nice frame for the eye. Incorrectly it can make you look hard and unnatural. I think pencils are the easiest to use. Choose a color that's flattering to your eye color and general skin tone. I usually use browns or grey-blue. I use the pencil to "fill in" where my eyelashes aren't thick enough. Then, using a spongy brush or my finger, I blend.

I use powder over my eye liner to give it the finishing touch which "sets" the liner in place.

Step 8. Mascara.

If you're going to be swimming make it waterproof mascara. Apply it a little at a time so you don't get big blobs of mascara sticking your lashes together. Use an old toothbrush on them after they've dried to brush off little chunks and separate lashes.

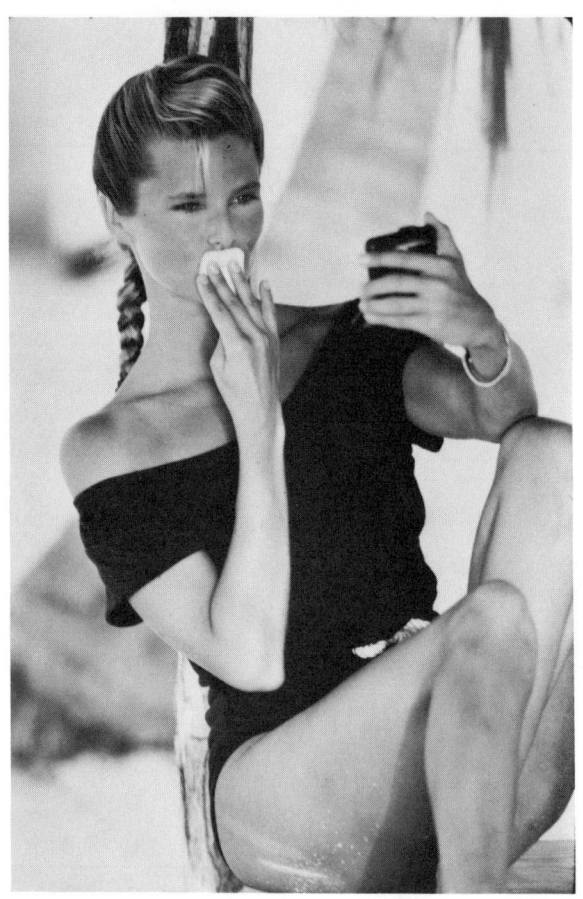

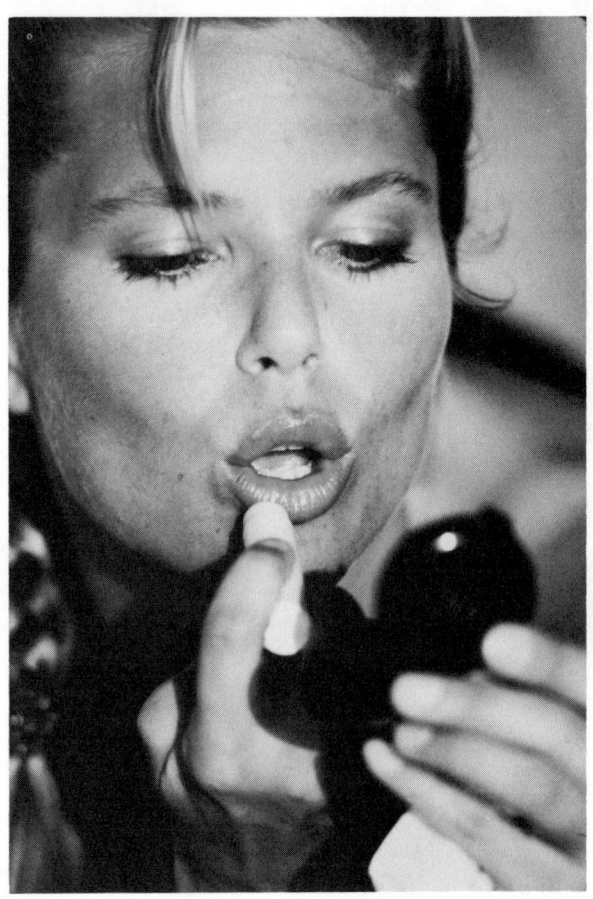

Step 9

Step 10

Step 9. Powder.

For daytime I never powder my whole face. I think a little shine looks most natural—especially in summer. I simply powder my nose, chin, the sides of my nose, and before applying lipstick I powder my lips to keep my lipstick from running!

Step 10. Lipstick.

If starting with lip liner, be sure to blend carefully so you aren't left with the "coloring book" look.

I find lip liners too drying for me and I feel I get enough definition just using a lipstick brush to apply the color.

I like my lipstick to look transparent so I can see the lip texture underneath.

And rather than use gooey gloss that just makes everything runny, I top it off with a lip balm with sunscreens—which protects and softens my lips, so they look just as good when the lipstick comes off.

Et voilà! It almost looks as if I have nothing on! (And that's what you should always try for.)

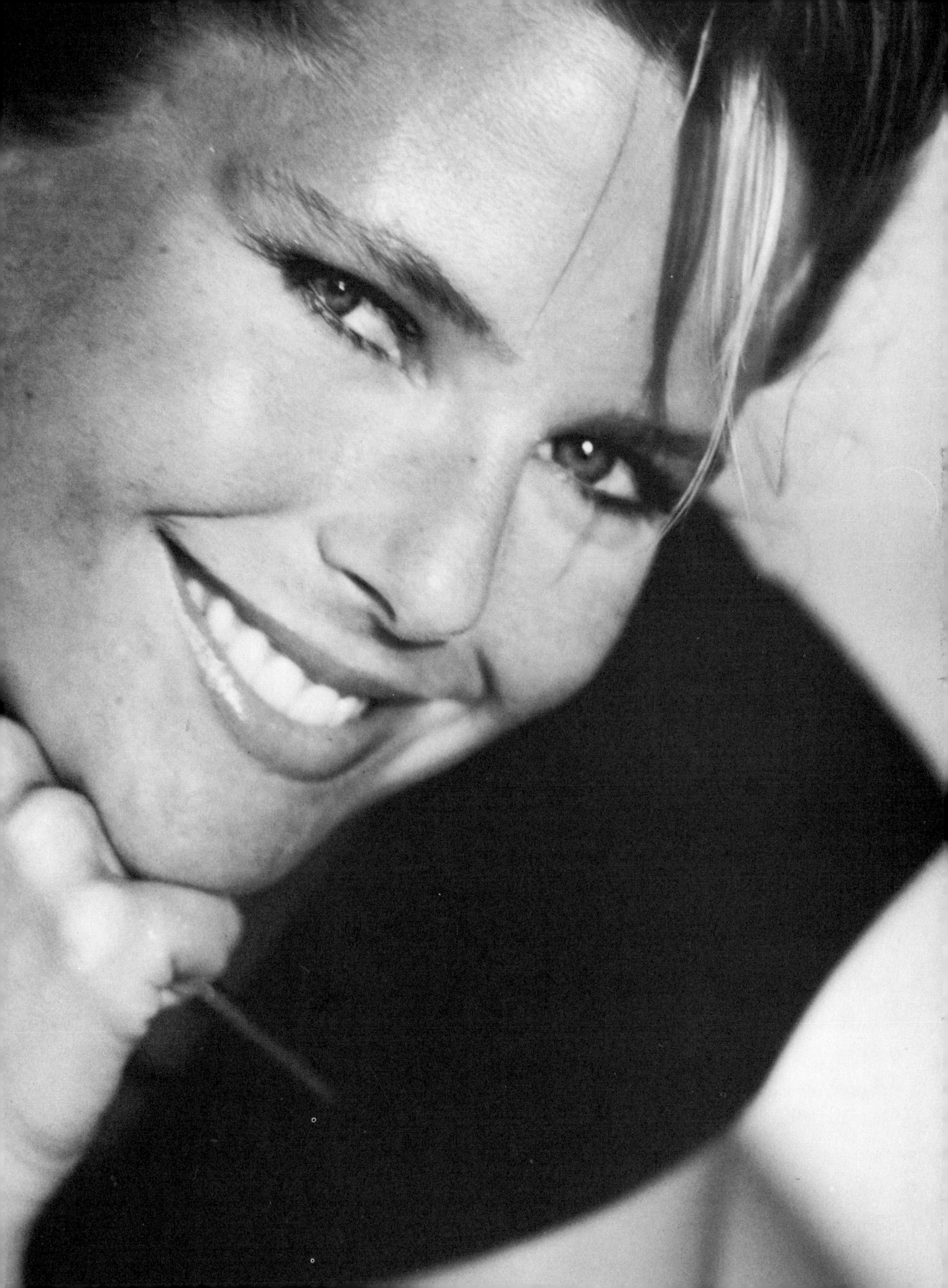

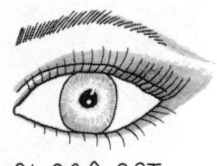

CLOSE SET

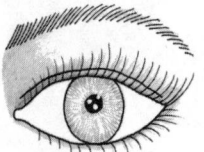

WIDE SET

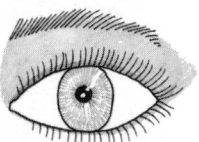

DEEP SET

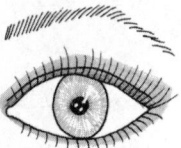

Shallow Set

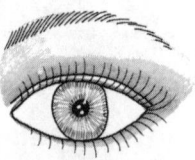

Small eyes

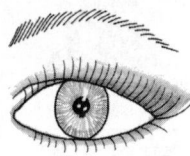

DROOPING eyes

Where to apply eye shadow
for different-shaped eyes

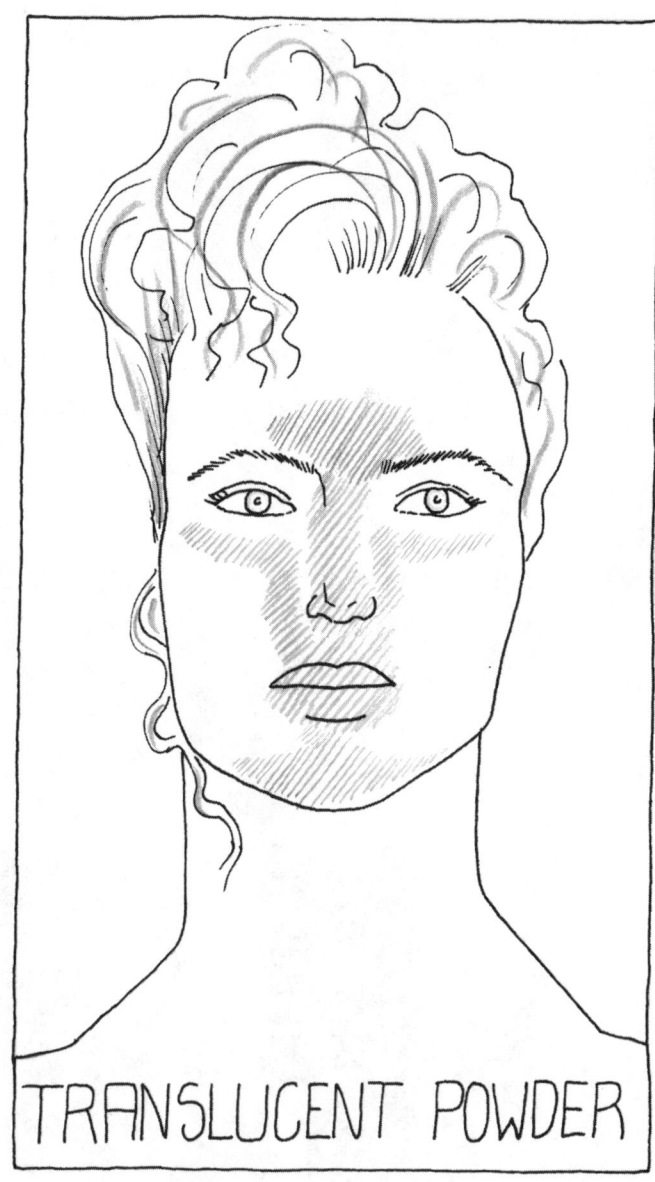

TRANSLUCENT POWDER

Where to apply powder

Artificial Tanners

These are the lotions or creams that you put on for a tan that will last about a week. These products contain a chemical that combines with a substance in the top layer of your skin to give you a darker color. Eventually it will wash off.

I've never used this kind of tanner but the biggest complaint I hear about it is that it can turn the skin an orange color. On the other hand, some women use it with success on their legs, for example, to take the place of stockings in the summer.

If you do want to use an artificial tanner, try it first in a place that won't show so you can see how the color looks on your skin and how many applications it takes to build up to the desired color.

Bronzers

Bronzers, which come in gel form, are a great way to even out your tan or give you a glow when you're feeling pale. Many cosmetic manufacturers make them, so you may have to try a few to get just the right shade for your skin: some of them tend to be brown, others red.

When you apply a gel bronzer, you'll want to put a light coating all over your face. Then highlight the places where the sun would naturally strike you: the forehead, the tops of your cheeks, your chin, and along the line of your nose. This will make the color look more natural.

Be careful about using bronzers in the winter. I don't think they really do a good job of faking a tan when you're truly pale, as they tend to streak. They're much more effective in the evening and for highlighting when you already have a bit of color. If you do choose to use a bronzer, remember a tan doesn't stop at your face: bronze your neck, ears, under your chin, and your chest and shoulders if they show.

Earth Dusts

Earth dusts are mixtures of clay and minerals (though some are made of artificial powders) that you can dust on your face to enhance a tan. I think, unless your skin is very dry, they work better than cream bronzers. However, they work best when your skin is already warmed by the sun. And they're just great for giving an extra touch of color, especially if your tan is fading.

Earth dusts are very potent so you need to use very little to get the right effect. Many of them are sold in small urns that you just shake and then use the tiny bit of dust that's accumulated on the cork stopper. A powder puff is the best applicator. Again, you'll want to highlight those places where the sun would naturally hit your face.

Earth dusts seem to be especially good for people with oily skin, as the clay in the dust absorbs the oil and keeps a nice finish on the face.

Makeup for a Pale Skin

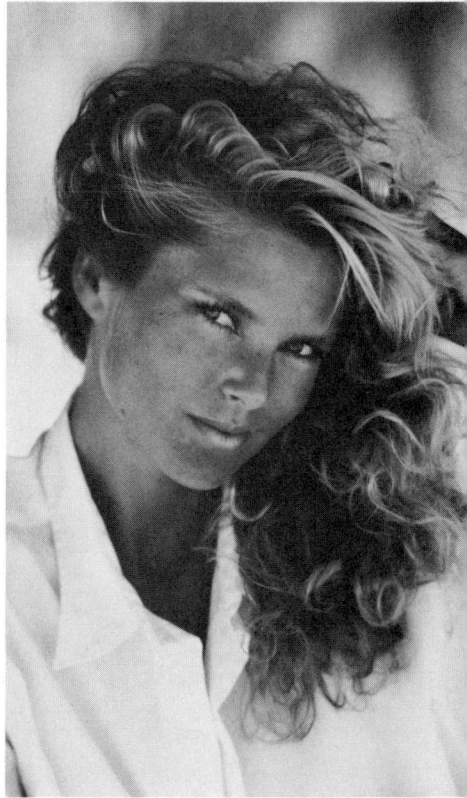

Makeup for a Very Tan Face

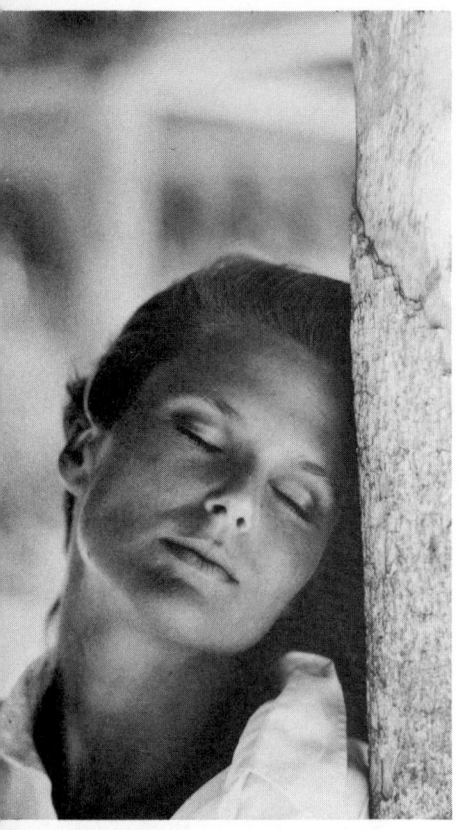

One of the best things about a tan face is that it needs very little makeup. The healthy glow of a tan usually doesn't need much help to make a pretty impression. Often, when my face is tan, I wear no makeup at all except for a bit of blush, some mascara, and lip gloss. But there are always those occasions when you really want to shine. Usually they are in the evening when even a tan face needs the amplification of some carefully applied makeup. Iridescent eye shadow in a light tone used on the brow of the eye adds lightness to a too-dark face. A great trick for the lips is to dab a dot of shimmery gold or silver eyeshadow in the middle of your lower lip—it adds fullness to the lip and makes it look wet like gloss but without the goo.

Remember that you can't just use your regular makeup routine on a tan face. The color and the texture of your skin are different and you have to adapt to them to get the prettiest and most natural effect.

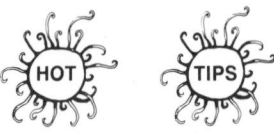

Makeup brushes and sponges can be washed in any cold-water detergent. Just soak briefly, squeeze gently, rinse and allow to dry away from heat or direct sunlight. Clean applicators will keep the colors clear and prevent bacteria build-up.

Whenever I travel and I know I'm going to be in the sun, I pour my makeup base out of its regular container and into a tiny plastic bottle. I bring three different shades of foundation along and as my tan gets darker I mix and blend the colors to keep up with my tan.

Waterproof Makeup

Going sailing? Windsurfing? Water skiing? There *are* times when it's nice to know you can count on your makeup even underwater. (And, of course, there are always those sad movies. . . .)

Here are some hints on using waterproof makeup:

Don't use a moisturizer under any waterproof makeup. It needs to lock onto your skin and the moisturizer keeps it from doing that.

When you put on waterproof makeup base, you should cover just a small area, only where you need coverage, and blend it very quickly. It dries fast and if you try to cover your whole face you'll never get a natural look.

Remove waterproof makeup carefully at the end of the day with soap or cleansing cream—whatever works best with your brand of makeup.

I don't think that even "waterproof" mascara will stay on through a typhoon, but it will get you through a day at the beach if you don't rub your eyes. But remember—it can be hard to take off. Make sure you have whatever you need

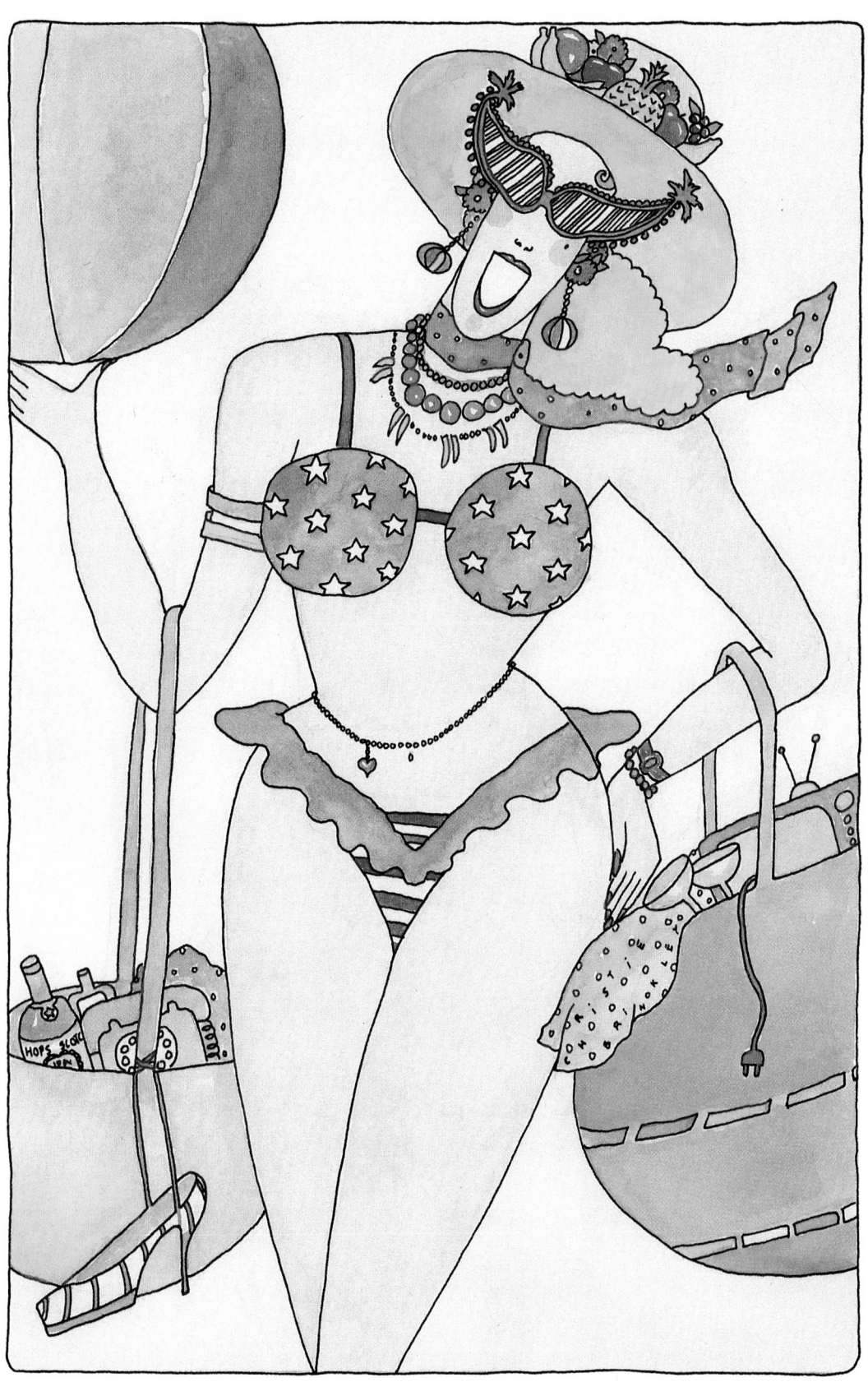

Don't overdo it! Keep your beach style simple and natural. Forget the heavy necklaces, dangling earrings, and major appliances. You don't want to scare the fish!

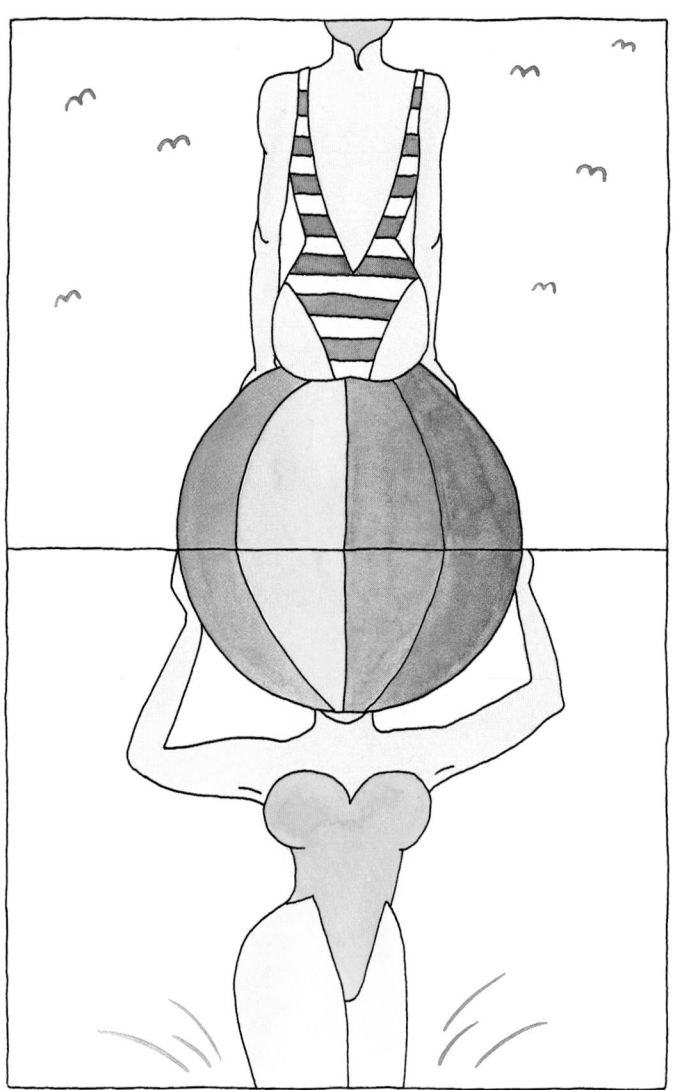

If you want to create the illusion of long legs, pick a suit that's cut high on the thigh. It will do for you what nature didn't.

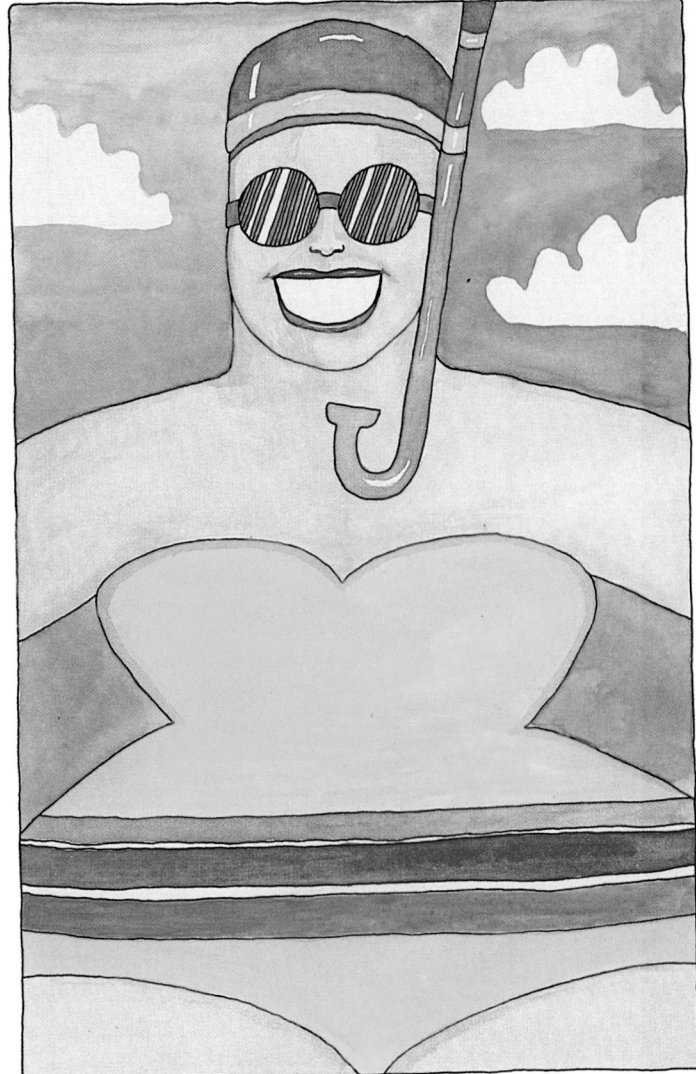

Are you hippy? Horizontal stripes are your worst enemy. Especially over the hips. They can accentuate any figure flaw. So best avoid them unless you're too thin and want to look rounder.

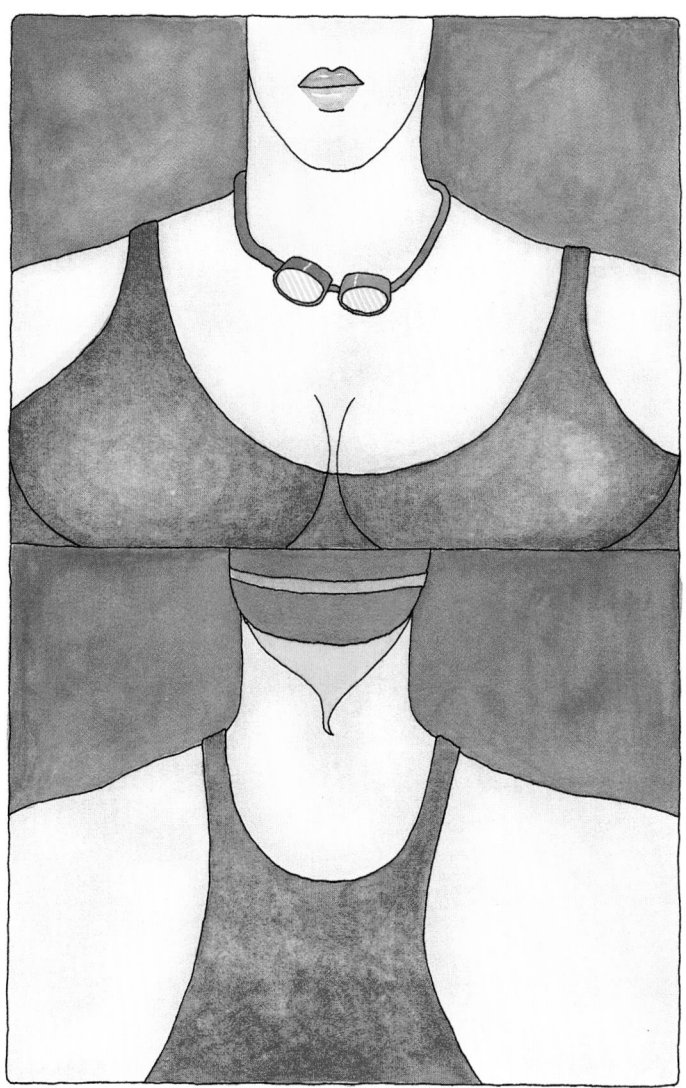

If your bosom is ample, you need suit support. Don't choose a swimsuit with an unconstructed top. Control's the goal!

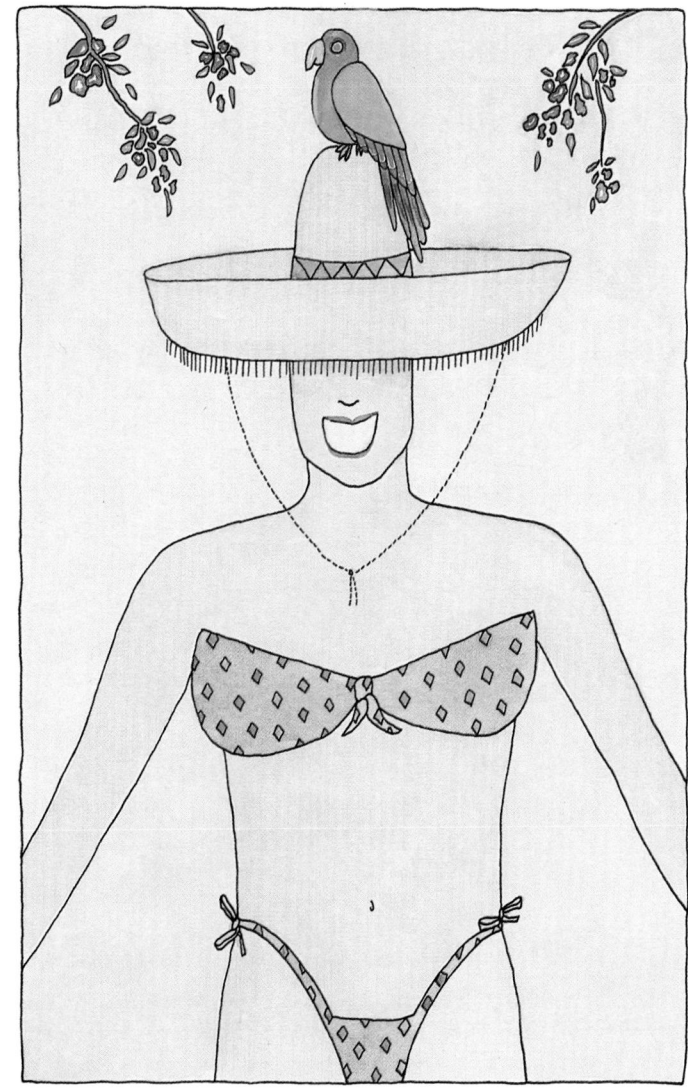

Still working on whittling your waist? If your waistline isn't your favorite feature, avoid bikinis. They'll call attention to your midsection. Opt for a one-piece suit.

GUIDE TO
THE PERFECT BEACH BAG

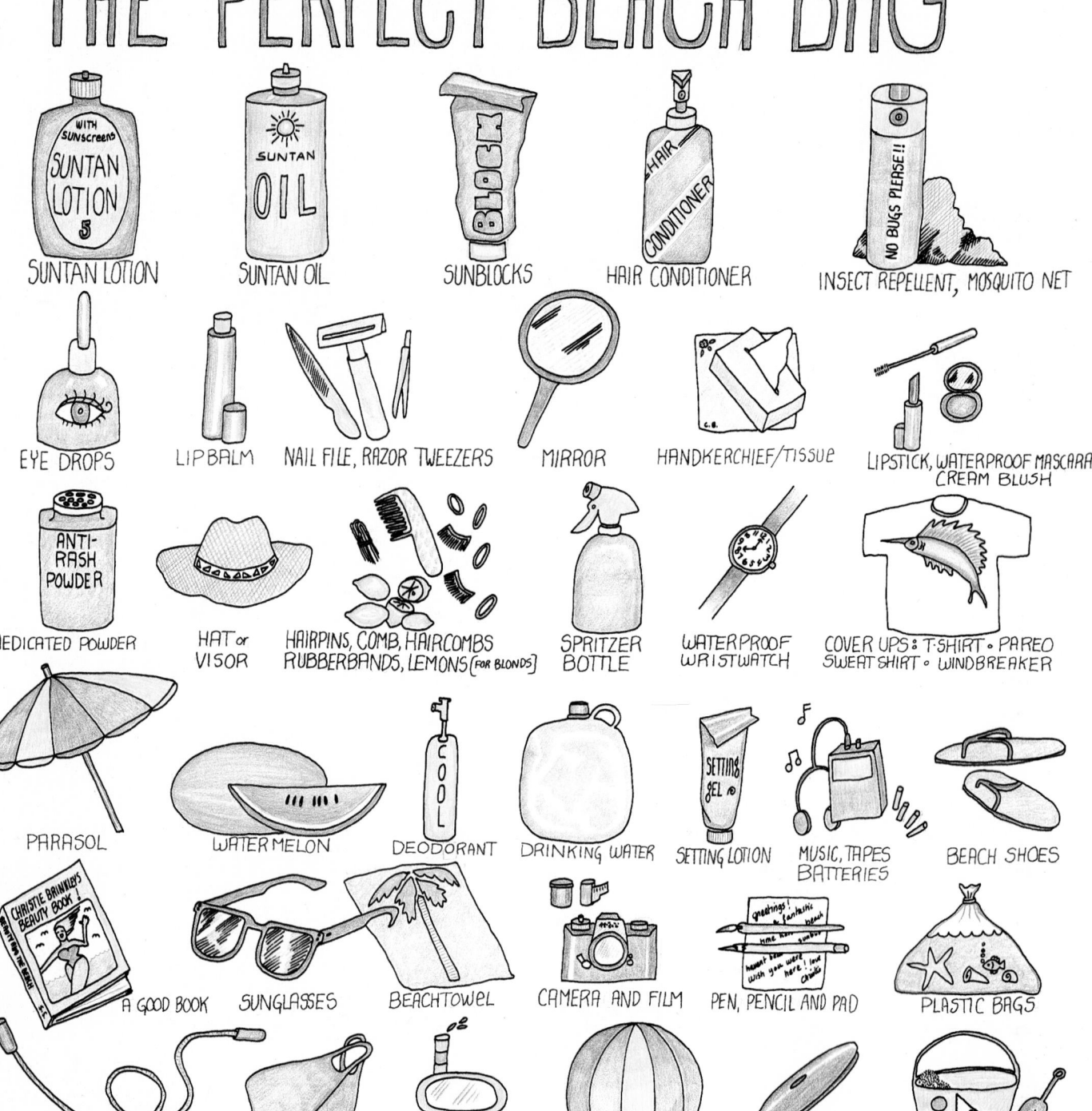

SUNTAN LOTION — SUNTAN OIL — SUNBLOCKS — HAIR CONDITIONER — INSECT REPELLENT, MOSQUITO NET

EYE DROPS — LIP BALM — NAIL FILE, RAZOR TWEEZERS — MIRROR — HANDKERCHIEF/TISSUE — LIPSTICK, WATERPROOF MASCARA CREAM BLUSH

MEDICATED POWDER — HAT or VISOR — HAIRPINS, COMB, HAIRCOMBS RUBBERBANDS, LEMONS (FOR BLONDS) — SPRITZER BOTTLE — WATERPROOF WRISTWATCH — COVER UPS: T-SHIRT • PAREO SWEAT SHIRT • WINDBREAKER

PARASOL — WATERMELON — DEODORANT — DRINKING WATER — SETTING LOTION — MUSIC, TAPES BATTERIES — BEACH SHOES

A GOOD BOOK — SUNGLASSES — BEACHTOWEL — CAMERA AND FILM — PEN, PENCIL AND PAD — PLASTIC BAGS

JUMP ROPE — FINS — MASK, SNORKEL — RAFTS, KICKBOARDS, BALLS — FRISBEE — FOR THE KIDS — HAVE FUN!

Christie

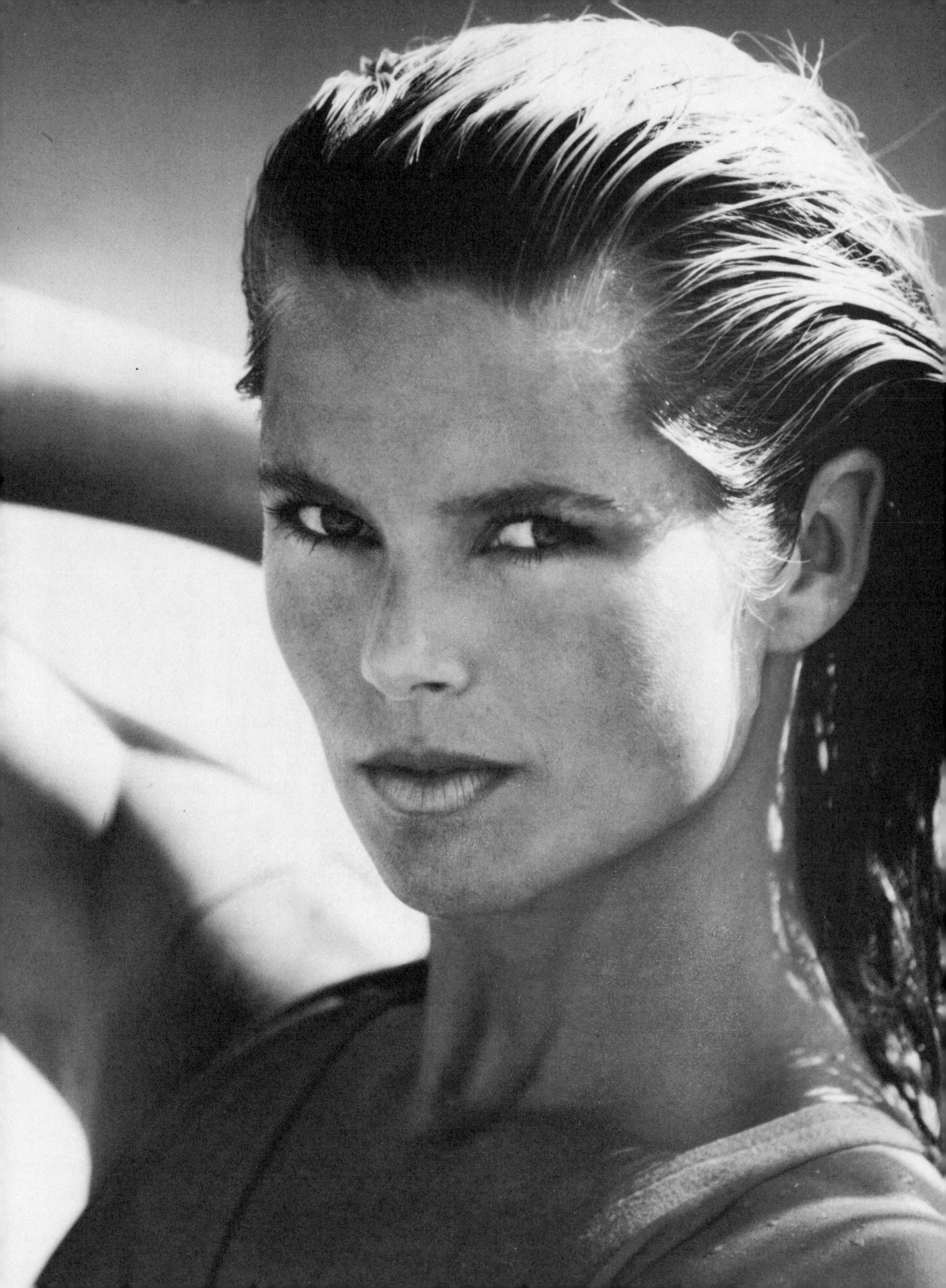

to do the job—oftentimes it requires a special remover, so look for one when you buy the makeup. And don't forget to bring the remover when you travel! (In a pinch, you can try using vegetable oil as a remover.)

I find waterproof makeup base too drying for my skin, so I've developed a "waterproofing" routine using my regular makeup which keeps it looking fresh and in place in or out of the water. The only product I use labeled "waterproof" is mascara.

Here's how you do it:

—use *cream* makeup base only where necessary (cream bases have more staying power than liquids);
—use a cream blusher on your cheeks and eyelids just under the brow;
—now "set" your cream blusher with a powdered blush of matching tone;
—powder your face with translucent powder—this will *also* help "set" your blush in place and will smooth out any unblended edges;
—use a pencil to line your eyes. Blend and "set" with matching color of powdered eye shadow;
—waterproof mascara and a nongreasy lipstick with lip balm as gloss polish off the look;
—now spray your entire face with a light mist of mineral water (I use Evian atomizer, available in beauty supply stores). This will keep it all in place.

Remember after swimming, don't rub your makeup off on your beach towel—let your face dry naturally.

Dyed Lashes

Having your lashes dyed at a salon is one way of having permanent color, though frankly I'm not really an enthusiast of this procedure.

I once had my lashes dyed navy blue (they said black would be too harsh) and I didn't really like the effect. Since a lot of the dye accidentally got on the skin below my eyes, it made me look as though I'd just gone 15 rounds with Sugar Ray Leonard! Moreover, it made me look as if I always needed to have the rest of my face made up.

The other drawback to lash dying is the products themselves. Some of the dyes contain coal tar ingredients which are dangerous to your eyes. Even though these dyes have been outlawed in the U.S., some salons still use them. If you are going to have your lashes dyed, be sure that the dye being used is free of any coal tar ingredients.

Seasonal Skin Care

Your skin is very sensitive to its environment and it's constantly changing to adjust to temperature and humidity. Heat, cold, dryness, and humidity all make different demands on your skin.

To care for your skin properly you need to be aware of your environment and adjust your beauty routine accordingly. Here's a chart to help:

DRY SKIN	*OILY SKIN*

HOT AND DRY
(deserts/overheated apartments/warm, windy days/airplanes/western states)

• humidify sleeping area • use moisturizing masques • use moisturizer, even under makeup • drink lots of water! • use mineral-water spray after applying moisturizer • use a "spot masque" (see p. 100) only on breakouts • use cream cleansers • use eye creams and lip balms	• take advantage to rid skin of excess oil • moisturize eye area and use lip balm • clean frequently but gently • eliminate astringent if it's too drying and switch to skin freshener

HOT AND HUMID
(tropical places/Manhattan in summer—yuck!/the South)

• use a dry-skin soap or special cleanser • a scrub is important, as pores are open and perspiring • use astringents around nose and chin • steam face to clean pores • fight breakouts with a masque in spots or a "T-zone" masque • moisturize eye area and lips	• use astringents throughout day • use drying masques regularly • if prone to breakout, ask doctor for special cleanser • use slightly abrasive scrub on face to keep skin fresh • steam face regularly to cleanse thoroughly

COLD AND DRY
(skiing/Himalayas/eastern cities in windy winter/airplanes)

• moisturize, moisturize! • always use mineral-water spray after moisturizing • use moisturizing masques • use cream cleansers	• use light moisturizer • don't forget lip and eye areas: moisturize! • use gentle cleanser • use skin freshener instead of astringent

Covering Scars

If you have a scar that you want to cover for the beach, there is one product that seems to be especially effective: Lydia O'Leary's Covermark. It comes in different shades and can be blended to match your skin tone. Just be sure to apply it in a good light so it will look natural once you get to the beach. Covermark is available at many pharmacies.

If you have a severe scar, there is a special line of cosmetics called Corrective Concepts that is sold through the burn units of many hospitals. If you can't find the product, have your doctor contact: Ms. Pat Patrek Henderson, Patee Products, European Crossroads, Bordeaux Building/Suite 218, 2829 West Northwest Highway, Dallas, Texas 75220.

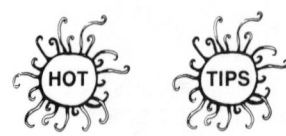

Avoid bringing creamy makeups to the beach. The very high temperatures can "curdle" them and change the texture so they're unusable.

If, like me, you are allergic to many things, here's great news. Some cosmetic manufacturers will work with your doctor in trying to track down specific ingredients in their product that you are or may be allergic to. These companies will send lists of ingredients and even special testing kits to your doctor. When they do isolate the offending ingredient, they'll mix up a batch that's safe for you.

　　If you have a cosmetic you would especially like to use, first try a patch test (see p. 123) and if you get a reaction, write directly to the manufacturer to see if they offer this kind of help.

CLEANSING SUMMER SKIN

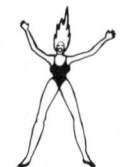

Careful cleansing is the best thing you can do for your skin all year round, but it's especially important when you're tan and the weather is hot. As your skin darkens it hardens slightly and dead cells accumulate on the surface. If these cells are not washed away your complexion can develop a dull, lifeless look.

Six Steps to a Clean Face

Here's the weekly routine I like to follow for deep-cleansing my tan face:

　　1. Once a week I give myself a facial steaming. The moist heat helps dissolve the oil and dirt that have accumulated during the week. The steam opens the pores and gets them ready for a serious cleaning.

　　2. Next, I like to use a facial masque. A clay masque is especially good for a deep cleansing. A gel masque is usually better for cold-weather gentle cleaning but if you have very dry skin it might be a good choice in any weather. Follow the directions on the masque of your choice. Since a clay masque can be drying, I use it only on the forehead, chin, and nose, and while it's working I use the time to moisturize the eye and lip areas.

　　3. After I rinse the masque off, I use a Buf-Puf or an almond scrub. I think that, unless your skin is terribly sensitive, a certain amount of light abrasion is good for it. In a pinch you can simply use a washcloth. They say, by the way, that a man's face ages more slowly than a woman's because every day while shaving he removes some dead cells and renews his skin.

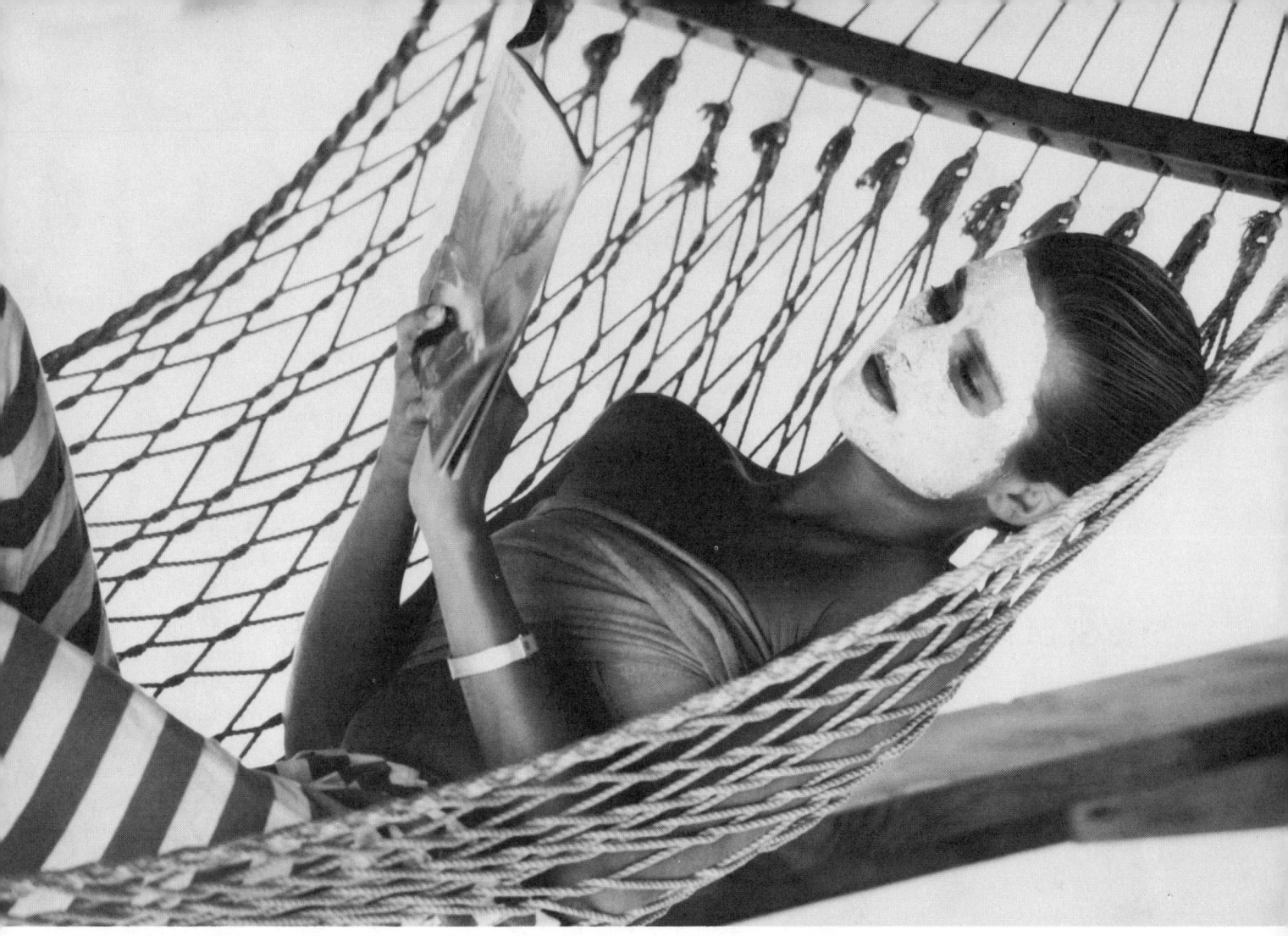

Relaxing in an almond scrub

4. After rinsing off the scrub I apply astringent to any area that is especially oily—usually around the nose and chin, but always avoiding the delicate skin under the eyes. Then I apply freshener to the rest of my face to remove any residue.

5. Before I use any moisturizer I spray my face with mineral water, pat it dry (leaving the skin slightly damp), and then apply the moisturizer. By wetting my face first the moisturizer will help to seal in the additional water and keep my skin moist and dewy.

There are two kinds of moisturizer: *humectants*, which help to seal in moisture already in the skin, and *emollients*, which attract moisture from the atmosphere to your skin. I don't recommend this type for humid climates where it can make your skin literally drip with moisture. I inadvertently used one on a tropical island and couldn't keep my face dry until I washed it off!

6. Finally, I use a slick or colorless lip balm on my lips and I'm ready to either put on fresh makeup or go to bed. Before going to bed I may dab on some eye cream or a light oil (sesame or vitamin E) around my eyes.

My Daily Cleansing Routine

In the A.M.

A. Splash water—that's it!
B. Then apply moisturizer

In the P.M.

A. Remove all eye makeup with special eye-makeup removal cream.
B. Use cream makeup remover all over my face.
C. Splash off with water. If skin feels oily use skin freshener.
D. Spray entire face with mineral water.
E. Then apply moisturizer on entire face except lips.
F. Use petroleum jelly on lips.
G. And finally, if certain areas of my face seem very dry, I apply petroleum jelly to those areas.

The Spot Masque

I'm always running around the house with a polka-dotted face. I may look pretty funny (especially to my doorman and messengers)—until I take it off! It's a great beauty secret. The dots are actually a masque for extremely oily skin. They soak up excess oil and work on those breakouts. Many women when they see a blemish make the mistake of grabbing their masque and smearing it all over their face. But why dry up the areas that don't need it? Simply dip your fingertip into the masque and put a dab on the blemishes only. Put a little eye cream near your eyes and some lip balm on your lips and you'll be doing three jobs at once!

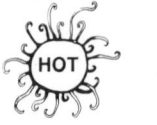 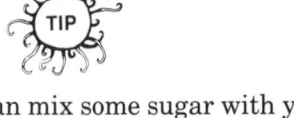

If you left your face scrub at home you can mix some sugar with your soap and use that. Just be sure the water is cool or the sugar will dissolve and you'll have a glazed face!

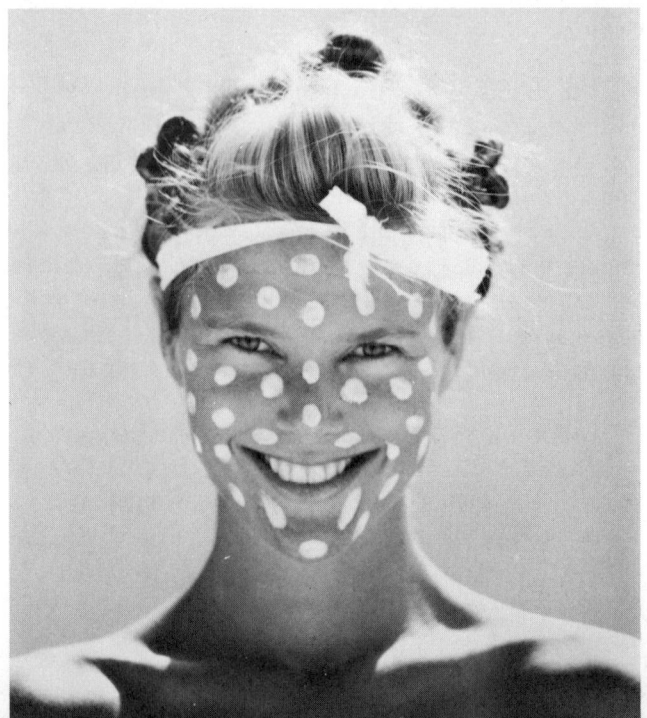

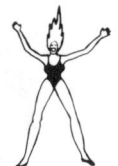 My eyes have a tendency to get puffy, especially in humid climates. I try to sleep with a large pillow to elevate my head a bit in order to keep the fluids from settling there. And I try not to drink too much before I go to bed. But I still usually have to wake up two hours before I'm having a photo taken so I can get the fluids redistributed. It helps to cut down on your salt intake, but you have to be careful if you're in a hot or humid climate where you might be sweating a great deal.

Here are some solutions:

A cool used tea bag on the eyes will help. The cheaper tea bags seem to work better—they have more tannic acid. The only "good" tea that seems to work is camomile.

A slice of cucumber on the eye will help with puffiness and feels so refreshing!

Cotton pads saturated with milk left on the eyes for about 10 minutes will depuff and are also good for allergies.

I always sleep with a humidifier in the room when I'm in a dry place. I make a special point of it in winter when rooms are dry and overheated.

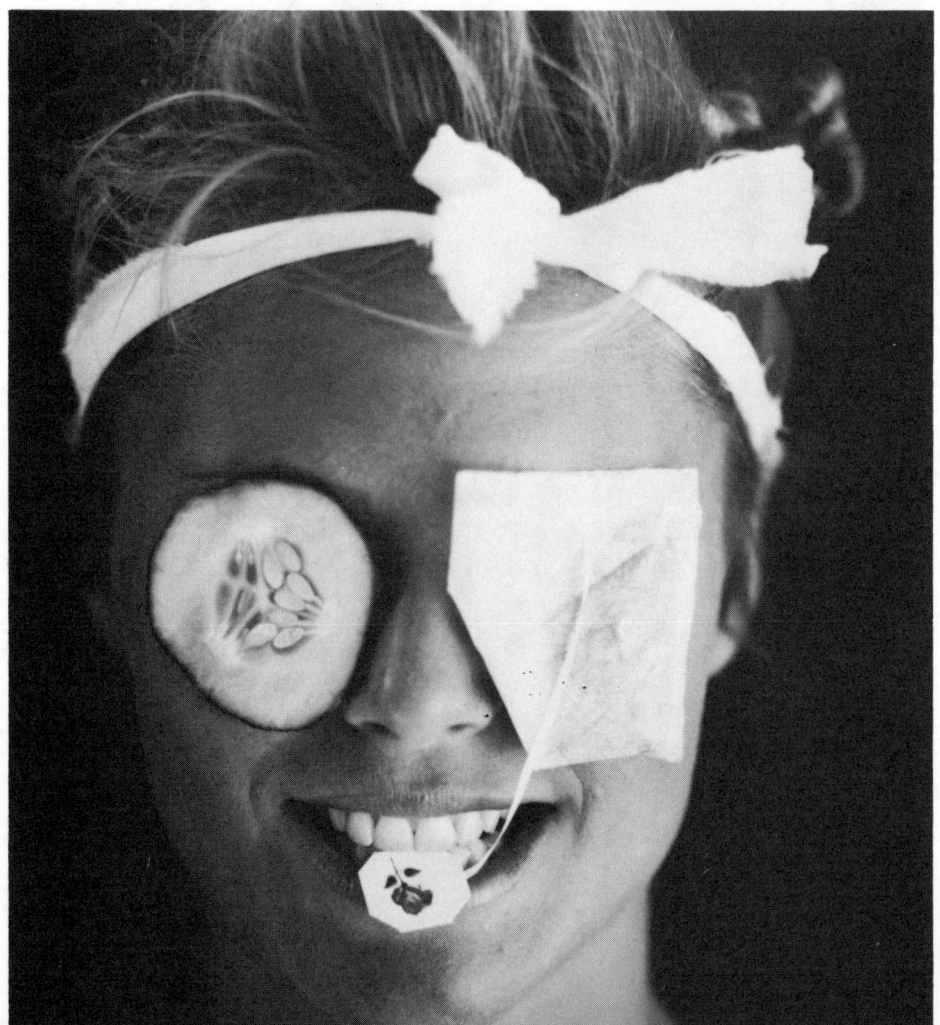

WATER—MY BIGGEST BEAUTY SECRET

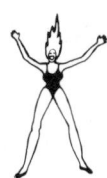

When I was filming the movie *National Lampoon's Vacation* in Arizona, the role called for me to be tan and happy—on vacation —all the time. I was being careful about my skin because the climate was so dry, but one morning I woke up and my skin was as tight as could be and totally parched. When I went to be made up, the makeup just sat on my skin and wouldn't sink in. I tried everything I could think of to get my skin back to normal. I bought a humidifier and slept with it in the room. I sprayed water on my face and sealed it in with petroleum jelly. I rubbed aloe vera cream on my face. I found that eventually my face became more elastic—after all, by then I had more oil on it than they have in Texas!

But it wasn't until I remembered to do the most obvious thing that my face felt like my own again: I started *drinking* the water! I had gone from hot, humid Manhattan to hot, dry Arizona and hadn't increased my intake of water!

Even though we later traveled (humidifier by my side) to a still drier location where I got tanner and tanner, my face never became totally dried out again. The humidifier and the water drinking paid off. And ever since, water has become a really big part of my beauty routine.

Now I drink at least eight glasses of water a day. I mix water with my fruit juice to make it less concentrated or I might add a slice of citrus fruit to fizzy water. It's low in calories and tastes great!

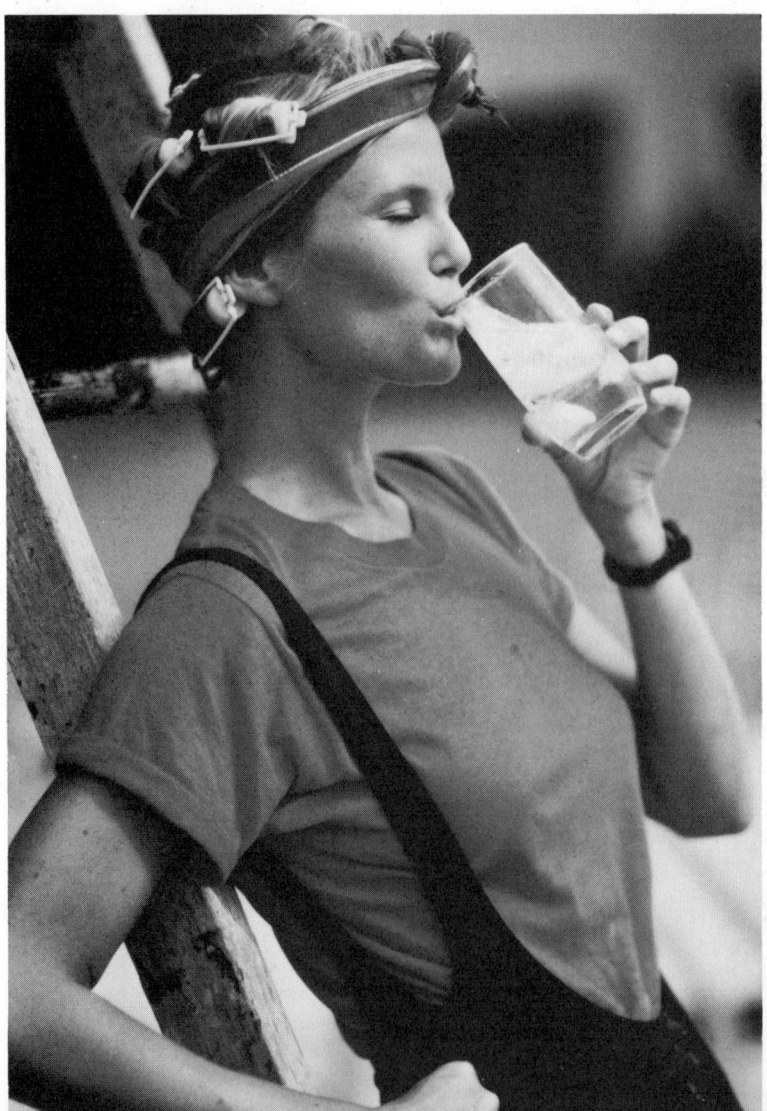

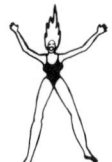

Here are some of the most popular hair-removal techniques. If you're already using one you might like to switch to another for the beach. For example, some women shave in the winter but wax in the summer. But before you try any new method, make sure there's time to recover if it doesn't work as planned. Once I was going to do a bathing-suit modeling job for *Vogue* and they sent me for my first and last leg waxing. Unfortunately, because my skin is so sensitive, I wound up looking like a plucked chicken!

Shaving

This is the most common way to remove unwanted hair and it's my favorite and usual method because it's the fastest. I find that the best time to shave is in the shower when my hair's been softened by the heat and moisture. It's best not to shave first thing in the morning because after all those hours in bed your skin is puffy from fluids beneath the surface. If you *must* shave in the morning, do your exercises first. Also, you won't get a really effective shave after a long tub bath—your skin will be too wrinkled!

Always use a fresh single-blade razor when shaving—the twin-bladed men's type is much too abrasive—and use lots of soap lather on the area to be shaved. If your skin is sensitive or you're shaving a delicate area like the bikini line, it's best to shave first in the direction of the hair growth and then against it. This seems to prevent those little bumps caused by ingrown hairs.

I think you should always moisturize after shaving but be very careful what kind of moisturizer you use. Some contain ingredients that can irritate the skin—especially after shaving when the skin is slightly irritated anyway. Test any new moisturizer on a small area after shaving and give it an hour or so on the skin. If no reaction develops, it's probably safe.

One last thing: If you do tend to get ingrown hairs, try washing the shaved area with a washcloth while bathing or showering; the slight abrasion of the cloth can help prevent the hairs from getting trapped beneath the skin.

Waxing

Waxing seems to be more popular these days and there are some new methods that make it more effective and less risky. The time-honored method is to heat a special kind of wax until soft, then apply it to the skin in the direction of hair growth. Once the wax cools and hardens, you pull off the wax and the embedded hairs are removed as well. Because waxing removes the hair root, regrowth is slow—it takes from three to six weeks to come back. But of course the hair follicle remains so it *does* grow back.

The advantages of waxing are that it leaves you hair-free for quite a long time and, because the hair that's growing in is a new one rather than a cut-off one, it won't be stubbly like after shaving.

The disadvantages are that it can be irritating to sensitive skin, as you'll recall from my own waxing story. It can also be a little painful and a bit tricky to use—the wax has to be just the right temperature. There have been some waxing breakthroughs lately which make the job easier. There is a cold wax that eliminates the danger of burns, and there are strips that already have the cold wax on them—you simply press in place and zip them off.

If you want to try waxing, I suggest you have it done at a salon the first time around. That way you'll know how your skin reacts and what's involved. You can always go solo if everything works out. Most beauty salons do waxing and it's not terribly expensive.

Depilatories

Depilatories work by dissolving the hair so it can be wiped away. I've used them with some success, though you do have to be careful when applying them to cover just the areas you have in mind—no more, no less. And be sure to do it *before* showering—the dry hairs absorb the product better, and since the products never smell very good, at least *you* will!

Bleach

I was born with fair hair so I've never had to cope with a moustache, but I've roomed on jobs with other models who devote a certain amount of time each week to bleaching the hair on the upper lip. Bleaching of course doesn't remove hair, but it lightens it and makes it less apparent. There are a number of hair-bleaching products on the market geared for different parts of the body —legs, arms, face, etc. Again, before you try them be sure to do a patch test (see p. 123).

Electrolysis

This is the only known permanent method of hair removal. The hair is pulled, theoretically never to reappear. I say "theoretically" because the regrowth rate is about 50%. This means that most hairs need to be treated at least twice.

The advantage of electrolysis is that it's permanent: no more shaving, bleaching, or waxing. Unfortunately, the disadvantages rule it out for many people. It's expensive, somewhat painful, time-consuming and, if not properly done, it can scar the skin. Most people who have electrolysis limit it to their face.

If you're interested in electrolysis ask your doctor to recommend a reputable operator and try to find a customer to interview so you can learn what to expect and how successful the treatment's been.

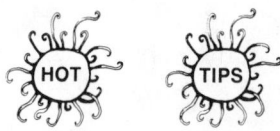

A loofah, a natural abrasive sponge, used daily in the shower will help get rid of ingrown hair and rough bumps. The Swedish models I work with often have a "dry brush" in their suitcases. They use it to brush their bodies before showering to remove dead cells that cause the skin to harden and bump. I took their advice and use one along with a loofah. It keeps my skin very soft and is great when my skin is tan and tends to roughen up.

Never, never tweeze hair out of a mole. And don't use depilatories on it either; the chemicals are too strong. Instead, just clip it off if it bothers you.

Ouch! Styptic pencils—those little white pencils the man in your life uses to stop the bleeding when he nicks his chin—work equally well on your legs.

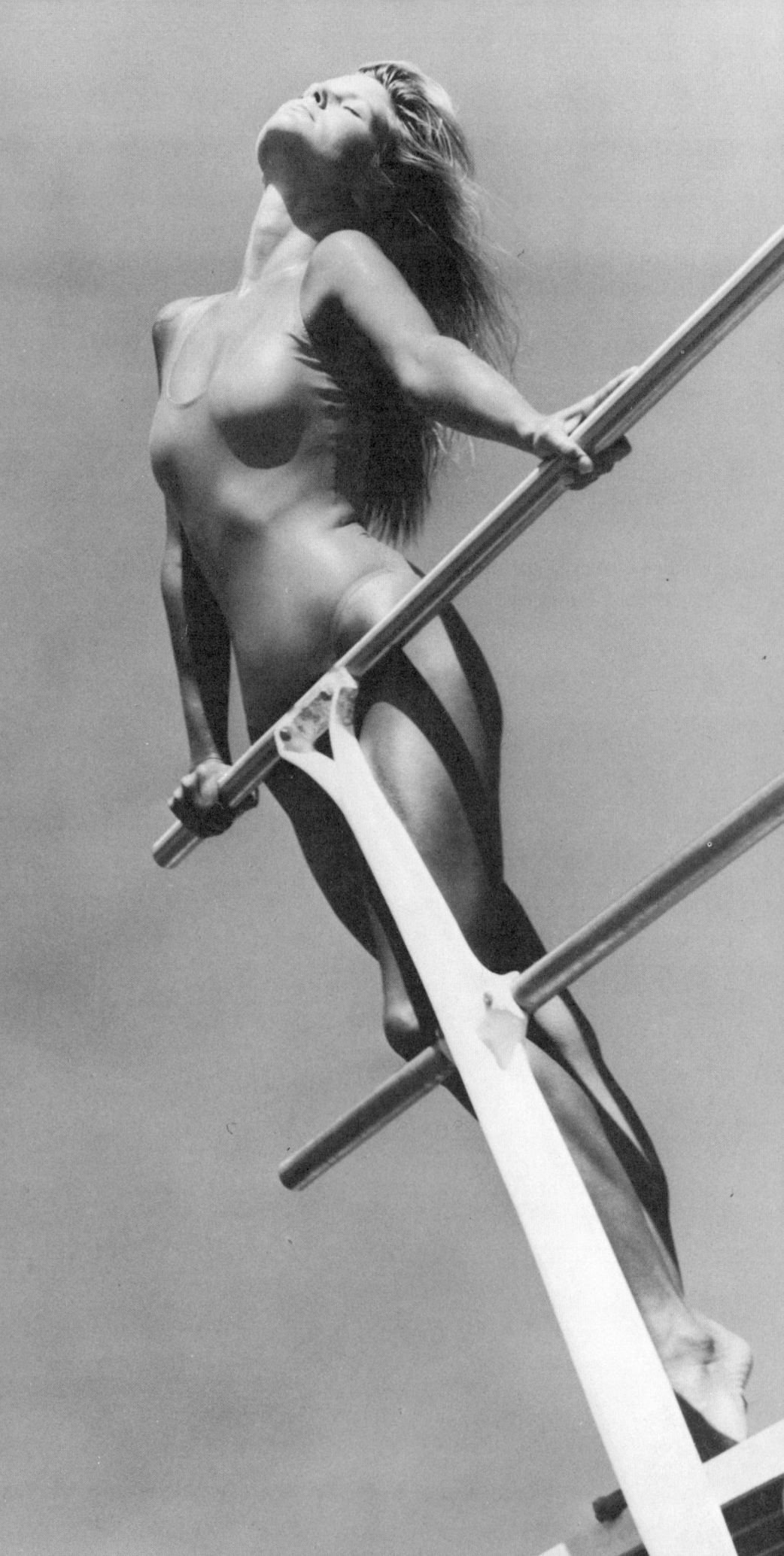

THE SUN

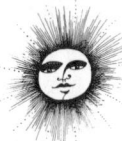

WORKING ON A TAN

I'm so lucky! You've heard the expression "work on a tan"? Well, I've actually been paid to do it! Many bathing-suit assignments on exotic islands start with that request. So off I go to "work" at the beach. It's my favorite assignment, but I've seen it become a hazardous occupation for other models who took the job too lightly. Many, hoping to look golden brown for the photos the following day, have overdone it to the point of not being able to be photographed at all. Their red, swollen faces clash with the clothes! Some days the client, seem-ingly oblivious to the weather, will say "get a tan." But even with an overcast sky I can still manage to get at least a little color. (The trick is to keep drops of water on your skin after it's been oiled. The droplets magnify the sun.) So because of my occupation I do take tanning very seriously. Knowing how the body tans helps me to do it the right way.

You need extra protection while "working" on rafts. . . . All that water reflection can easily give you a nasty burn.

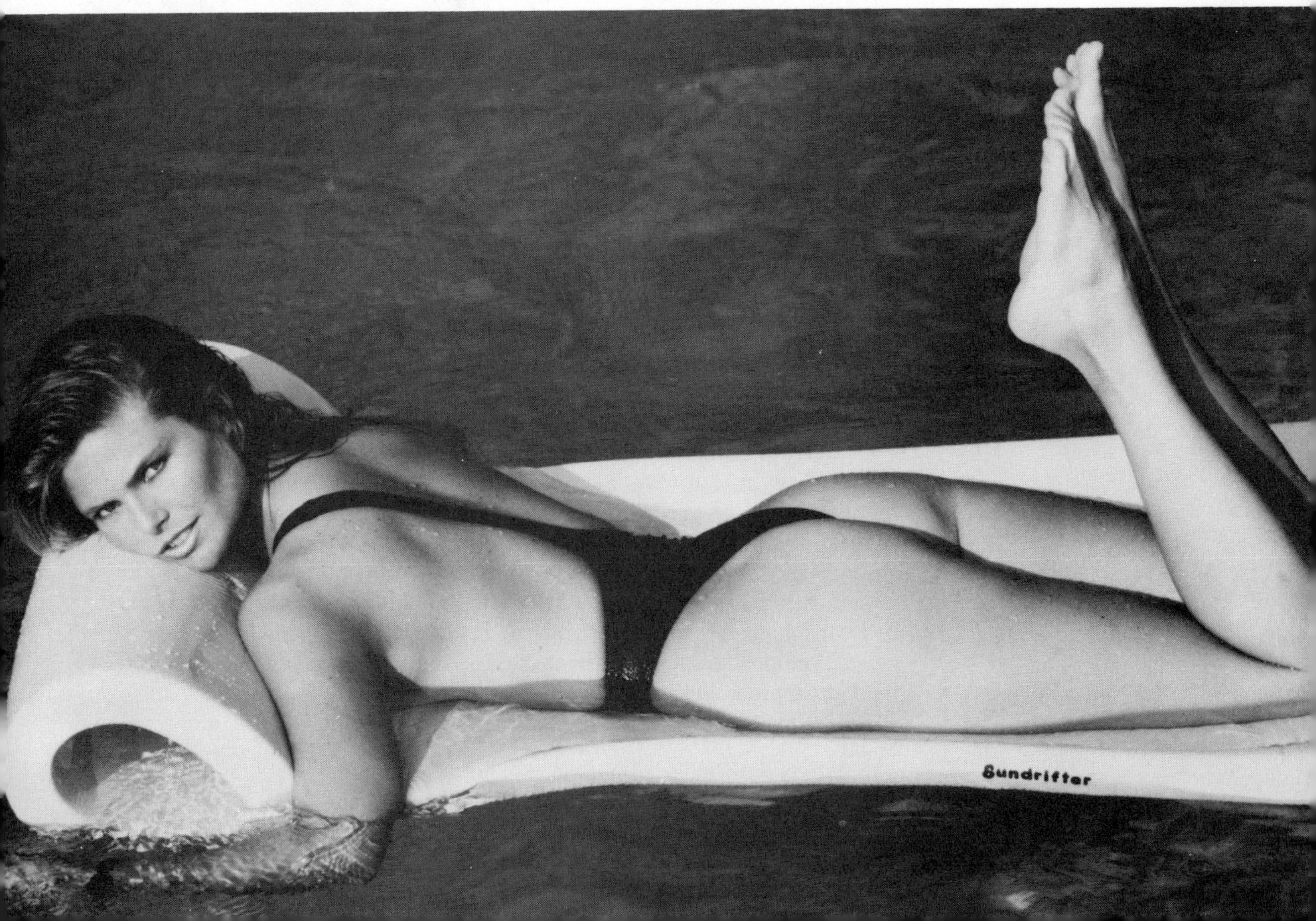

HOW YOUR BODY TANS AND BURNS

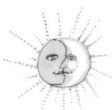

The first thing to remember about sunning is that a tan and a burn are two totally separate, unrelated reactions to sunlight. A tan is caused by one kind of ultraviolet ray while a burn is caused by another. I was amazed to learn this. Some people think that a burn is inevitable at the beginning of the season and that it eventually turns into a tan. Not so! A sunburn and a suntan are not the same thing. It may seem as though they're connected because if you get a slight burn it will disappear in a few days and by then the tanning process which began as soon as you were exposed to the sun will show up as a light tan.

So remember, you do not have to burn in order to tan. You *never* have to burn if you take the right precautions.

Your skin is really a protective organ. Tanning is the skin's way of protecting itself from the sun. As you probably know from experience, a good tan can help protect you from a burn: Once you have a tan you can stay out in the sun for longer periods with no ill effects. Tanning occurs when the ultraviolet rays of the sun stimulate the production and spread of the body's tanning pigment, melanin. Everybody, with the exception of albinos, has a certain amount of melanin constantly present in the cells of the skin. But the sun's stimulation produces more melanin and spreads it throughout the skin, giving it that familiar sunny look. It takes three or four days for the tan color of one sunbathing session to fully emerge.

While a tan is the skin's natural protection from overexposure, a sunburn means that the skin has lost its battle. Sunburned skin is injured skin. A sunburn forces the tiny blood vessels near the surface to swell. As they grow larger and more porous they begin to leak blood into the surrounding tissue. And we are left with the awful symptoms: pain, redness, blisters, and swelling.

THE GOOD NEWS

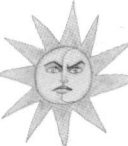

But don't worry, there is some good news about the sun. You're probably already familiar with one of the major benefits of sunbathing—it makes you feel good. I know that nothing relaxes me more than a day in the sun on a beautiful beach listening to the waves. For all the relaxation the sun gives me, I'm sure it's actually saved me from some wrinkles!

Now scientists confirm what we always suspected: The sun is necessary for a sense of well-being. In fact, though they don't understand exactly how, researchers tell us that increased exposure to the sun can help people who are suffering from severe depression.

Want some more sunny news? The sun increases your sex drive. I've always thought that was true because you're spending all day at the beach relaxing so you have time to think of other things besides work! It turns out that the truth is a bit more technical, but the sun does have a measurable effect on our hormones. They've even done experiments which revealed that certain Eskimos who live where there is a long winter with short days and little or no sun are virtually celibate until spring brings more sunlight. So when a young man's fancy turns to romance in the spring, it's not just because the flowers are in bloom.

If it's not enough that the sun makes you cheerful, relaxed, and sexy, it also helps the body produce vitamin D—the "sunshine" vitamin. And it may be helpful in the treatment of acne. I say "may" because this is a controversial issue. Some people with acne find that exposure to the sun helps clear their skin. It helps by drying, peeling, and healing it. On some people it seems to slow down the oil production while drying up the oil that's already there. This temporarily helps to clear the skin. But others react to sunshine with skin flare-ups. If you have acne, pay careful attention to how the sun affects your skin and modify your exposure accordingly.

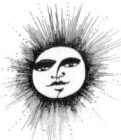 It's so hard to believe that your skin could be damaged by something as fun and relaxing as sunbathing. And besides, you look so good with a tan, right? Well, here's how you can look into the future and convince yourself. Just compare the skin on the back of your hand, which is frequently exposed to the sun, to that on your breast or bottom. Compare the color, the texture, and the number of lines. Unless you're very young or constantly sunbathe in the nude, you'll probably see a dramatic difference. Well, now imagine the skin on your hand ten or twenty times worse. If you continue to have lots of unprotected exposure to the sun, that's what your skin will look like in ten or twenty years. And not just on your hand. Your face will have a wrinkle for every carefree or, rather, careless summer sunbath! Believe me, it's not worth it and I'm going to give you lots of tips on how to enjoy that glorious sunshine without sacrificing your skin.

A GLIMPSE INTO THE FUTURE

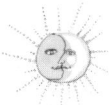 Now that you know that a tan and a burn are two different things, you should make a resolve *never* to burn! There's no reason to. A burn damages your skin and then peels right off, leaving you pale and disappointed.

Here's how to get a tan that lasts and lasts:

FOR A LASTING TAN

GO SLOW!

The watchwords for a great, long-lasting tan. Pay attention to such factors as location, time of day, altitude, etc.—and slowly, slowly build up your tan. The best way to do this is with what I call "sun rationing." If I know I have three weeks to spend on a beach and I'm starting out pale, I strictly ration my sun time. The first three or four days I'll spend no more than fifteen or twenty minutes in the sun, and *never* in the midday danger hours. I split that time between morning and afternoon. By the fifth day I'll have a nice light tan so I'll spend almost as much time in the sun as I want, still avoiding the midday sun. By the third week I find I can be in the sun most any time but never, never in the whole three weeks am I in the sun with no protection whatsoever.

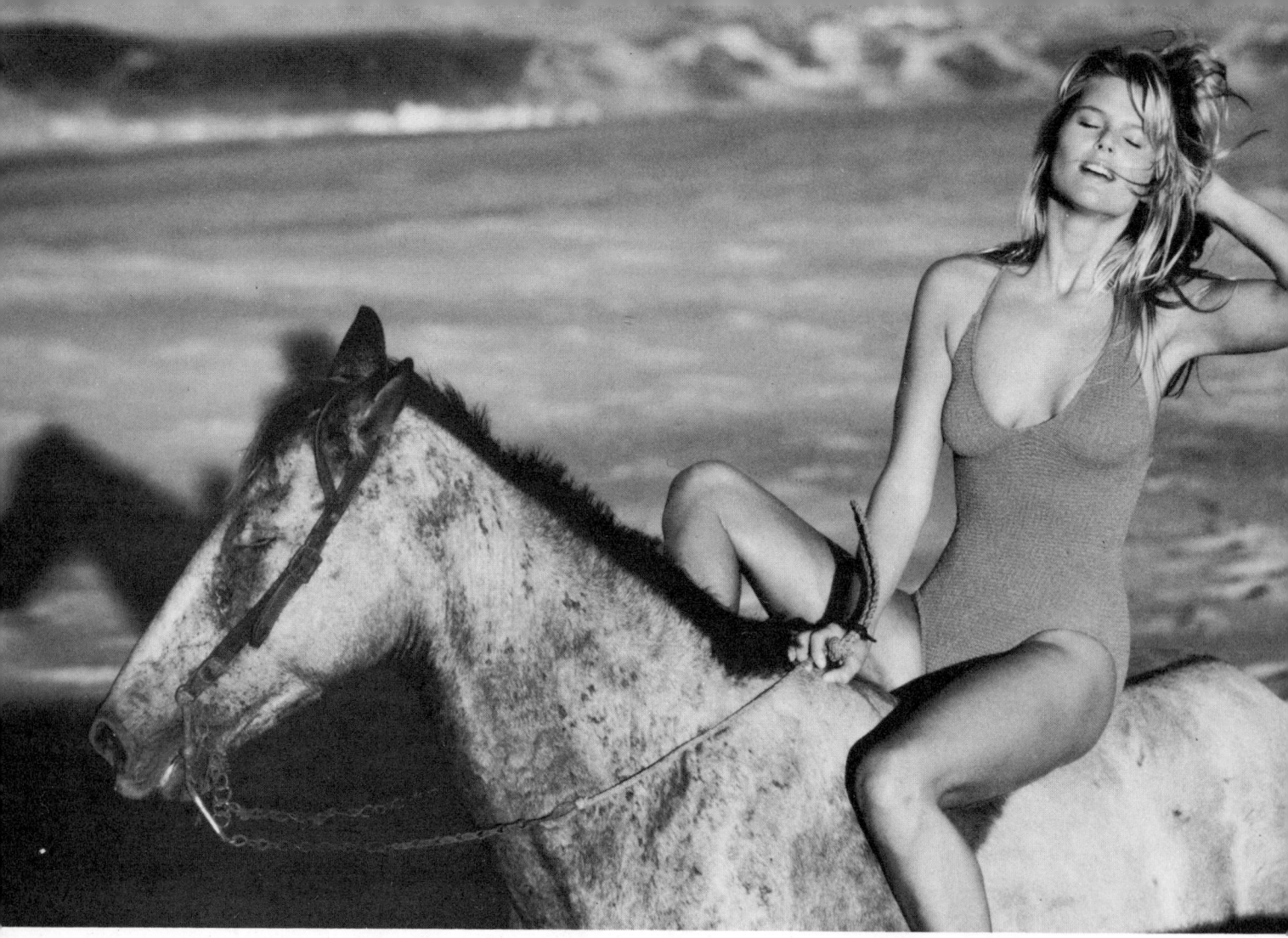

On an early-morning ride I get all the color I need on my face—then it's hats and sunblocks the rest of the day.

TIME OUT!

That means avoiding those burning midday rays! If I'm going to be in the sun for just a few days I modify my sun rationing with slightly longer morning and afternoon sessions but *never* any midday sun.

Sometimes when I'm on a job I have only a day or two to get a "healthy glow" for the photos and I have to do this without any burning. Makeup just won't go on a burned face; it sits on top of the skin and looks like a mask. I find that if I take about an hour of sun in the early morning and another hour late in the afternoon, I get enough of a "glow" and avoid a burn.

The point of sun rationing is to be aware of what your total exposure is going to be right from the beginning. Then regulate that exposure by avoiding the most damaging sunning hours and always using protection of some kind. After all, your goal should be a long-lasting, healthy tan. Once you've got that tan there's no need to get any darker. You don't want to push your skin to the limit and pay for it tomorrow; you want to look great today!

PROTECT YOURSELF!

Use the proper sunblocks and sunscreens that you've chosen from my chart (see p. 121). Adjust the SPF (Skin Protection Factor) to the weather, time of day, location, and reflection factors, and apply them often. Put extra sunscreen on your face and shoulders before you go in swimming. Whenever you're in the sun—at the beach, playing tennis, skiing, or just walking—certain parts of your body get more punishment because they're so frequently exposed. These areas include your shoulders, the tops of your breasts, your lower lip, nose, knees, the tops of your feet and ears, and your neckline area. Be sure to protect these areas with hats, cover-ups and sunscreens. Even if you're already tan, these areas need some protection.

Also take special care if you sunbathe in the nude. Any part of your body that has not had much sun exposure can burn very quickly, so use a high-factored sunscreen on those places. The area around the nipples (the areola) has more pigment than the rest of the breast so it won't burn as quickly, but it still should be protected with sunscreen.

Don't forget to reapply sunscreen after you come out of the water. Being near the water is like sitting in a giant reflector—allowing the sunlight to bounce all over you.

RINSE!

Whenever possible, rinse yourself free of drying salt and chlorine.

MOISTURIZE! MOISTURIZE!

Immediately after showering, before you're completely dry, slather on that moisturizer. It's a skin saver! There are lots of products on the market that are geared for *après* sun. Try them. Your skin will thank you and your tan will hang around for more!

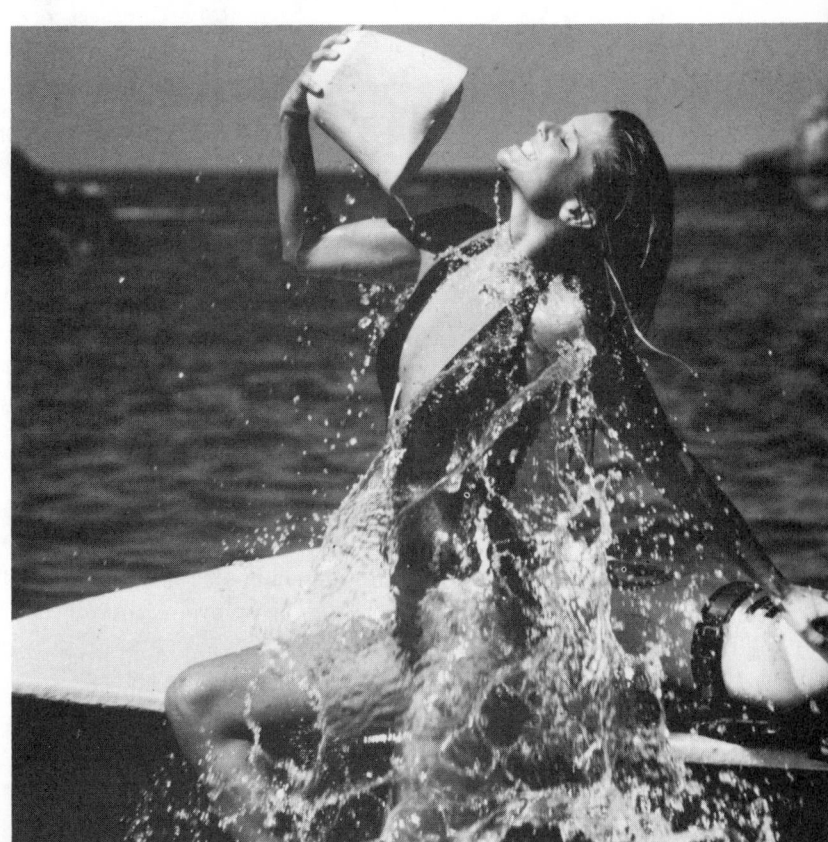

SIX CRUCIAL TANNING FACTORS

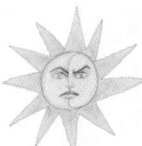

As children, no one could pry my brother and me out of the water! We were always the first ones in and the last ones out. When the surf's up, no time to stop at a sink—we'd even brush our teeth in the sea! "Fishy" was a good way to describe us. One summer we went to the island of Tobago swimming and snorkeling and, zowie—I became a lobster! Stupid! Tobago is very close to the equator and the nearer you are to the equator the stronger and more damaging are the rays of the sun.

The most important lesson I learned in Tobago was that sun, and your susceptibility to sunburn, depends on many things, including the time of day, the weather, the time of year, the location and, of course, your skin type. When I visited Tobago I knew my skin type but nothing else. Now I know the other factors that can affect my sunbathing and I take them into account. Moreover, I know that the sun affects my skin *all year long* and sunbathing isn't the only activity that requires caution. Here are some additional things you should know about the sun:

1. Water transmits the burning rays of the sun. You need protection even while swimming—and even more so if you're near the equator.

2. June 21 is the most dangerous day of the year for sunbathers. That's because in the northern hemisphere at least, June 21 marks the summer solstice—the day on which the sun's rays are the most intense. A bright sunny day in mid-May or mid-August is not as dangerous as one in mid-June.

3. Atmosphere counts. I'm not referring to the "ambiance" of your sunning spot but to the *air*. At higher elevations the air is thinner and you'll burn faster. This is something to remember all year long: You can get a burn on a skiing vacation if you're schussing at a high elevation. One last thought on atmosphere, and probably the only good news you ever had on air pollution: All those pollutants in the air screen out a lot of damaging rays. So city folk have a tiny bit of protection that disappears at the beach or in the mountains where the air is cleaner.

4. Reflection is important. Most people think if they crawl under a beach umbrella they're protected from the sun. Not so! A very white beach can reflect up to 50% of the sun's rays; a typical sandy-color beach reflects about 20%. On the other hand, dry grass will reflect only about 3%. If you're a ski enthusiast you should know that fresh snow reflects 85% of the sun's rays! That can mean a bad burn if you're unprepared.

5. Calculate the time of day. Here's the factor that can make the difference between a rosy blush and a bad burn. Most people are so eager to tan quickly that they'll soak up as many hours of sun as possible right from the start. I know people who I think would sunbathe 24 hours a day if the sun would cooperate. But if you want to tan *safely* and get a tan that *lasts,* you should avoid sunning between 10:00 and 2:00—the hours when the sun's rays are the strongest. This is especially important for your first few exposures; once you've built up some color, that melanin is doing its protective job and you can *cautiously* enjoy the midday sun.

6. Most important of all: your skin type. Your vulnerability to the sun depends on the amount of melanin present in your skin. Melanin, as I mentioned before, is the pigment in the skin that gives you color. If you have a lot

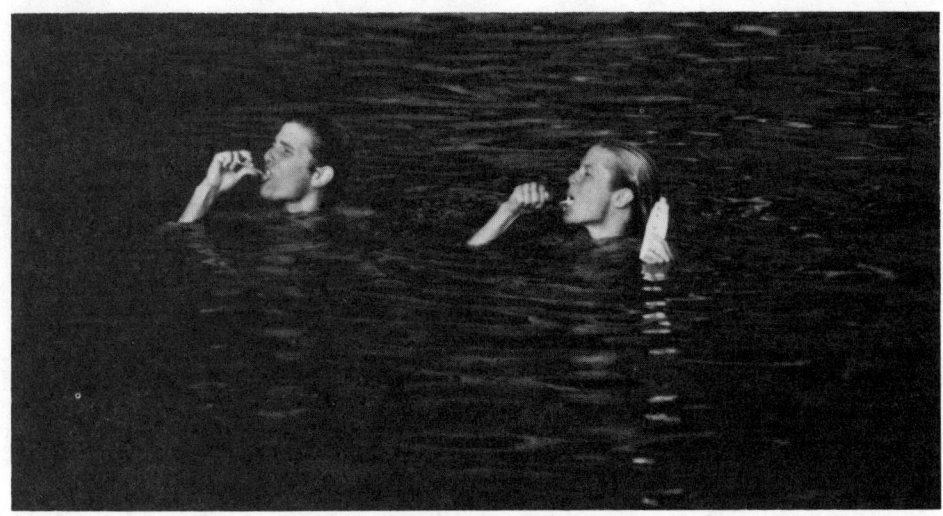

We haven't changed much—except nowadays we don't burn!

of melanin, you'll tan quickly and rarely burn, whether you're a blue-eyed blonde or a black-eyed Latin. Many people think that you can judge just by hair and eye color but this isn't the full picture. After all, I have blond hair and blue eyes and my skin is not especially sensitive to the sun. The hair/eye color guide is only part of the story. The best basis for judgment is your past tanning history. The chart on page 121 will tell you what skin type you are and what kind of sun protection you should be looking for.

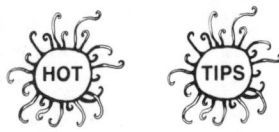

While the body is tanning it's using up more B vitamins than normal, so help bridge the gap by taking extra B vitamins when you're working on your tan.

Baby oil, alone or mixed with iodine, does nothing to help you tan. Though iodine can temporarily dye your skin, the oil will not protect you from the sun and, in fact, can clog your pores and even cause an itchy rash.

That cooling breeze feels great when you're in the sun but it can be an ill wind. It can make you feel so cool and comfortable that you don't realize you're getting a bad burn. Moreover, though scientists don't really understand *how*, the wind can increase the burning effect of the sun's rays! So grab that sunscreen!

Never use a sun reflector on your face. It will magnify the sun's rays and make them even more damaging. Worse yet, it directs those rays at areas that usually aren't exposed to the sun—under the nose, ears, and chin and around the neck—and can give you a very bad burn.

THE SUN AND YOUR SKIN

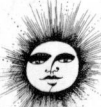

You've probably noticed that the sun has been getting a lot of bad press lately. It's certainly true that the sun is the villain in many serious skin problems. But I think it's important to remember that most of these problems occur when we overdo. If we're sensible about tanning and time spent in the sun, it can be a source of great pleasure and relaxation. And with what we know today about the effect of sun on the skin and how to regulate it, there's no reason to totally avoid the sun even if you prefer to remain peach-blossom pale.

Overexposure to the sun is, without question, the major cause of premature aging of the skin. Though it may take 10 or 20 years for the cumulative damage to show up, it will—in the form of leathery, toughened skin, with mottled coloring and lots of wrinkles.

The skin is made up of two parts: the epidermis, or outer layer, and beneath that, the dermis. The top layer, or epidermis—the skin you see—is really dead cells. These cells are constantly being washed or rubbed away. The dermis contains two things important to every sun worshiper—collagen and elastin. These substances give your skin elasticity, tone, and suppleness. They're like the water in a waterbed. The ultraviolet rays of the sun will eventually damage the collagen and elastin, and then your skin will be like a waterbed that's been drained—wrinkled, saggy, and droopy.

THE SUNBURN

A sunburn is a serious matter. A bad one can cause chills, fever, vomiting, and delirium. Blisters will often form and, while they're always ugly, sometimes they can get infected and even cause scars. So a sunburn is not a matter to take lightly.

If you're lying in the sun, keep checking your hand mirror and do a "fingerprint" test often. Just press a finger against your skin. If a white mark remains against pink skin and you feel a slight tingling sensation, it's too late: You're already burned. Your skin will react right away if it's burned. If you're very fair, it can happen after 20 minutes in the noonday sun. After the pinkness appears you should get out of the sun immediately. Even though you may not be uncomfortable at that moment, you will be later.

It takes 2 to 6 hours for the redness of a sunburn to blossom into its full painful glory. After 15 to 24 hours you will be feeling at your worst, but the symptoms can hang on for 3 days.

First Aid for Sunburns

1. After removing yourself from the sun the next thing to do is take a bath in tepid or lukewarm water. Hot or cold water will be too painful. I find that adding some apple-cider vinegar—a cup or two—to the bath water really helps in soothing a burn. Oatmeal added to the bath is also helpful. The oatmeal reduces the redness. I've also used baking soda in the bath water and found that it gives some relief from the swelling.

2. Moisturize! After your bath, while your body is still damp, apply a body lotion. Use a light nonoily type. The heavy oily kinds seem to just sit on top of the skin and make you feel worse by holding in the heat of the burn.

They can also cause water blisters. I like moisturizers that have aloe vera in them as I think it's really soothing.

3. Don't get chilled. A sunburn chills your body so you don't want to emphasize this problem. Keep comfortably warm. Avoid air conditioning or turn it down for the duration. In the first stages of a burn I usually feel warm and have often left for dinner in a cool blouse—only to get chills later and spend the evening shivering. So remember to take a light, soft sweater. Sweatshirts are great!

4. If you're really swollen, use cool compresses. Dip a towel in a mixture of cool water or milk to which you've added some cornstarch. Rest the compress on your burn for 15 or 20 minutes. Follow with a soothing moisturizer.

5. Take two aspirin (unless you're allergic). It helps relieve the pain.

6. I advise you to steer clear of the products that are made for "sunburn pain." Most of them have ingredients that end in "-caine" and these ingredients can irritate your skin, which is the very last thing you need when you're sunburned.

7. If you develop bad blisters, see your doctor. You've got yourself a serious sunburn and you need some professional help.

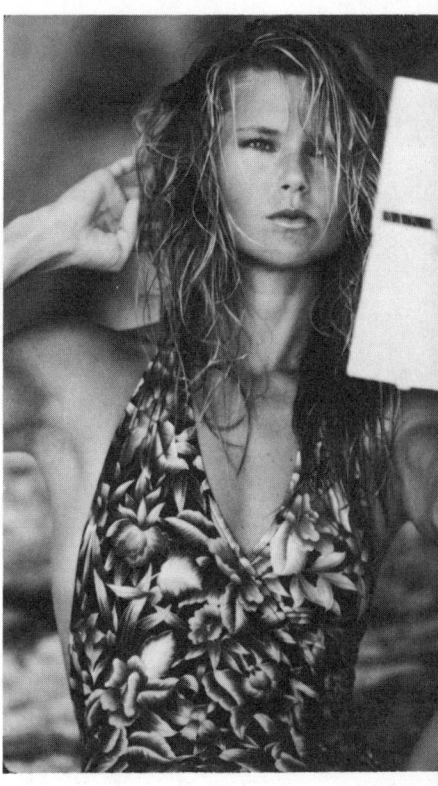

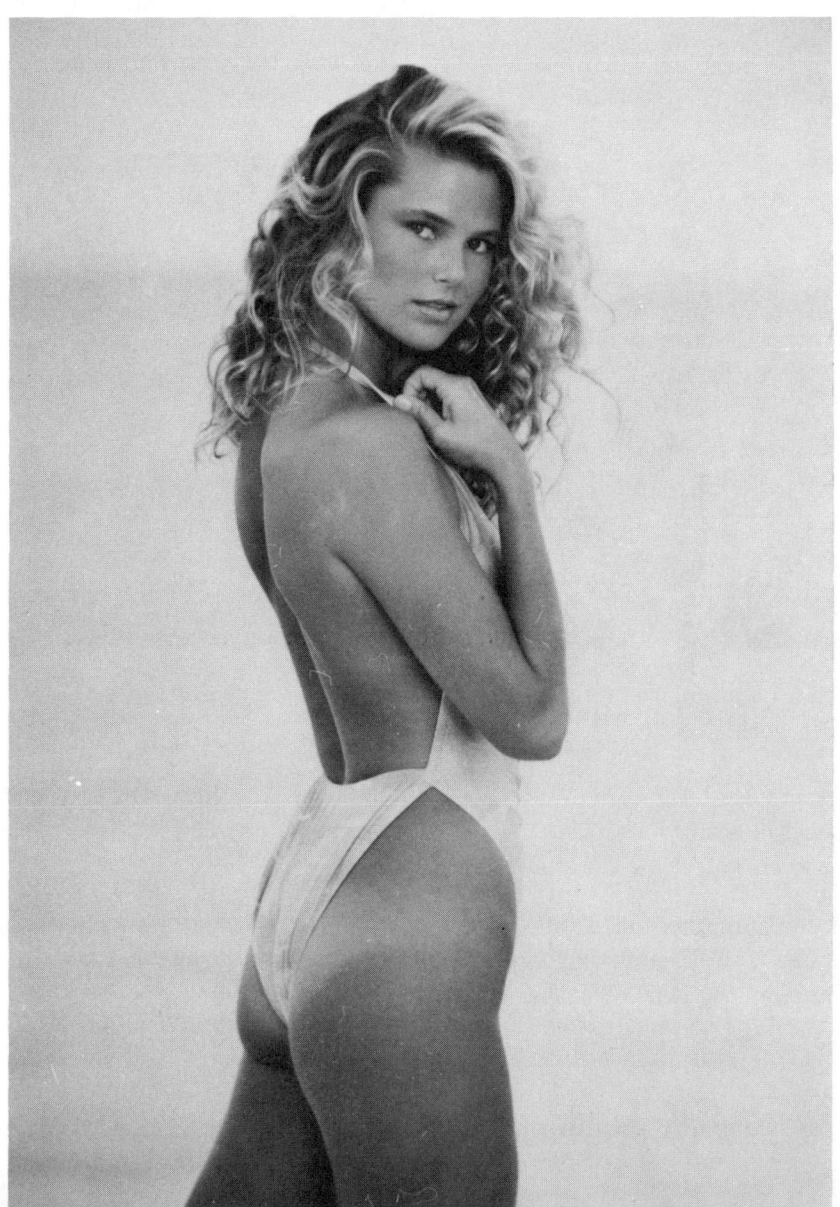

8. Stay out of the sun. Do you wince as you read this? I do. At least when I remember how the sun feels on sunburned skin. The last thing a sunburn victim longs for is a day at the beach. But there's always somebody who can't bear to stay home and for you this advice: Go shopping, see a movie, visit a museum, but stay out of the sun at least for four days following your burn. That will give your skin a chance to recover.

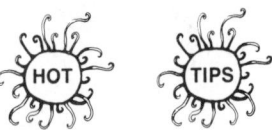

You probably already know that on a cloudy day you can get a burn. In fact, 50% of the ultraviolet rays are getting through. But the bigger danger is a *hazy* day, when virtually *all* the ultraviolet light is wreaking havoc on your skin!

If you do get a sunburn, sprinkle some talcum powder between your sheets at night. It will feel very soothing.

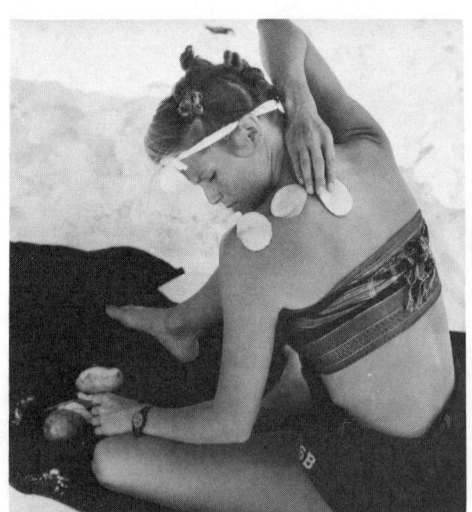 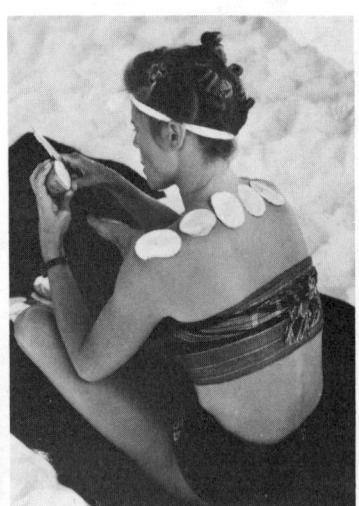 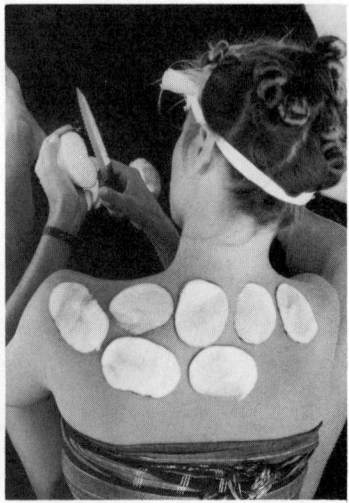

Slices of raw potato placed on a sunburn will take the heat right away. (Potato chips won't work!)

Did you know that those big, puffy, cumulous clouds up there can increase your chances of getting a sunburn? They're reflecting even *more* sunlight back to you. So keep squeezing the sunscreen!

Your pet can sunburn, too! That's right, dogs and cats can get an uncomfortable sunburn if they're left in the direct sun for too long. If your pet gets his coat trimmed in the warm weather, he's even more vulnerable.

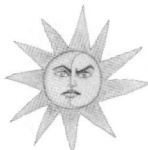 Back in the fifties and sixties, if you wanted to spend a day in the sun you could almost count on a sunburn. The only way to avoid one was to be under your beach towel, or throw in the towel and go home. Suntan lotions were really moisturizers that kept skin from drying out but did little to protect from a burn. Zinc oxide, that white gooey stuff, was the only effective sunblock but only lifeguards and little children endured it—and then only on the tips of their noses. All my childhood beach photos feature bikini bottoms and a white nose!

When better sunscreens, including PABA (para-aminobenzoic-acid), were developed, human skin began to have a fighting chance. Finally in the mid-seventies the government required that manufacturers label their sunning products with an SPF or Skin Protection Factor number. The numbers range from 2 to 15. They refer to how long you can safely stay in the sun while using that product. The glory of these sunscreens is that they *do allow you to tan* (unlike zinc oxide which gave you a white nose before, during, and after using it!). The lower range of SPFs block out only the harmful ultraviolet light while allowing the tanning rays to do their job. The very highest numbers, like zinc oxide, block out everything. Because you can be so selective about the amount of protection you're getting, there's no longer any good excuse for a sunburn.

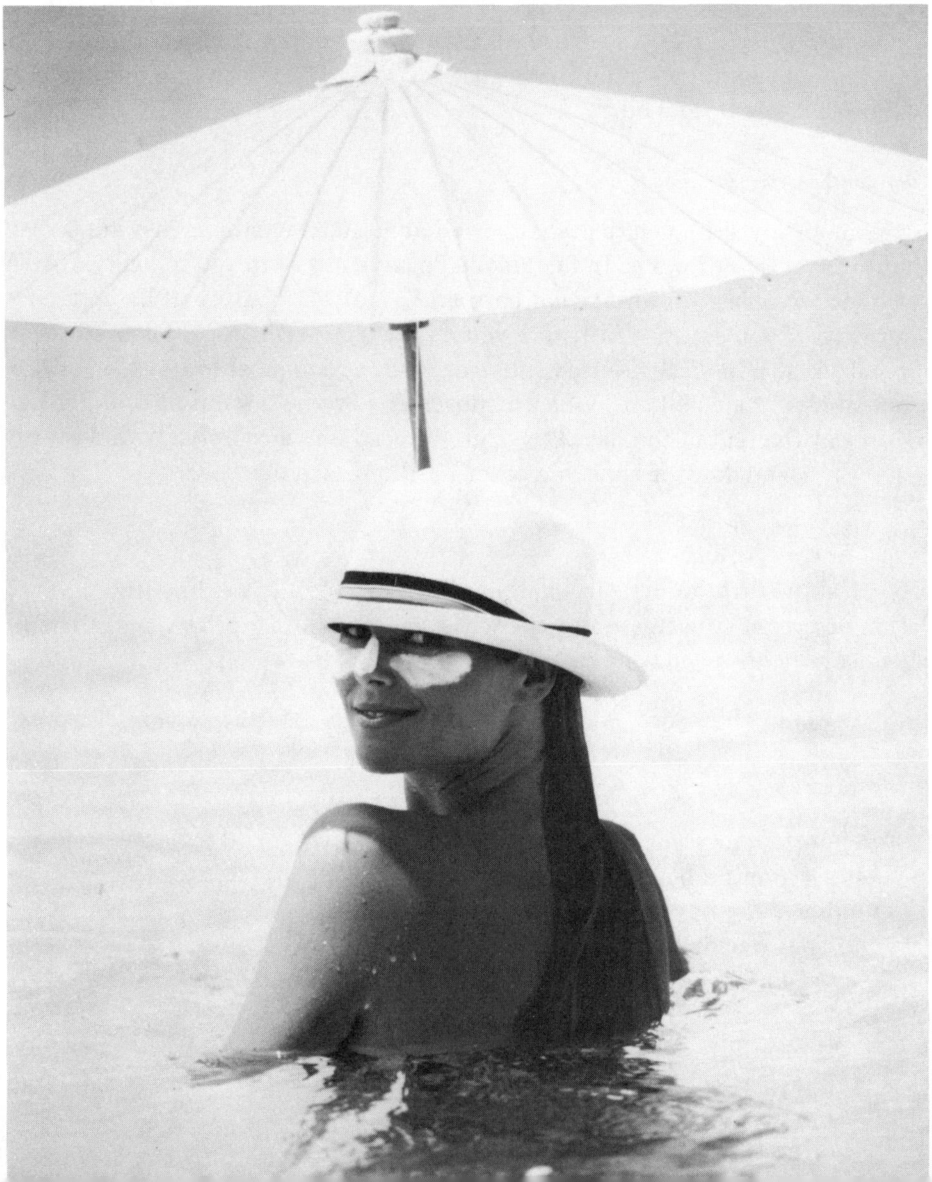

SUNBLOCKS AND SUNSCREENS
What They Are

Selecting a Sunscreen

Flexibility is the key with sunscreens, and I think if you are regularly in the sun you should have an arsenal of screens that you use interchangeably. For example, during your first exposures, before you have any color, you should be using a high-factored sunscreen. If you would ordinarily use a 5, then use an 8. And be especially careful of shoulders, nose, tops of breasts, and tops of ears. You might want to use an even higher-factored sunscreen in those spots. (Remember that even though you're using sunscreen, you're avoiding the mid-day sun.) After three or four days you should be able to drop down to your normal SPF number *but* you should still pay special attention to your nose, shoulders, etc.

Sooner or later, depending on your skin type, you'll achieve your ideal color. Do you throw away your sunscreens? *No!* Though a tan does give you some protection from burning, it's really only worth an SPF of 3 or 4, which isn't all that high. So continue to use the lowest number possible that will keep you from burning *and* keep you from getting too dark. And continue to pay special attention to your nose, shoulders, etc.—any area that gets maximum exposure. A sunscreen forms a chemical bond with the outer layer of your skin. If you apply it about an hour before you go into the sun, it has a better chance of bonding to your skin and keeping it protected.

Beyond SPF: The Right Sunscreen for Your Skin Type

There are other considerations than numbers when you choose a sunscreen. You have to look for a screen that's good for your skin type as well as one that will protect you from a burn.

Oily Skin

If you have oily skin, you're probably well advised to avoid a greasy sunscreen that could clog your pores. In fact, if you do have oily skin you're lucky: PABA seems to work best in an alcohol base and an alcohol base will be better for your skin. If you skin is really oily you might try PABA in gel form. It's even more drying than alcohol-based sunscreens. But remember to use special care when applying alcohol or gel-based sunscreens or you'll wind up looking like a zebra at the end of the day. Cover all exposed areas completely and evenly —have a friend do your back and other hard-to-reach places.

Dry Skin

If your skin starts to dry out or if you have dry skin to begin with, choose a lotion or cream sunscreen and check the label—the nongreasy moisturizing chemical *urea* is a good one to look for.

Your Own Personal SPF

Here's how to figure out which SPF you should be using:

1. Determine how long you can stay in the sun without burning—say, 15 minutes if you have fair skin.
2. Then decide how long you want to stay in the sun—say, 3 hours.

3. Divide your "safe time" (1) into your "intended time" (2) and you'll have your SPF number, in this case 12.

$$180 \text{ minutes} \div 15 \text{ minutes} = 12 \text{ minutes}$$

The following chart will help you determine the correct SPF for your skin type.

SUN TYPE 1	SUN TYPE 2	SUN TYPE 3	SUN TYPE 4	SUN TYPE 5	SUN TYPE 6
Characteristics:	*Characteristics:*	*Characteristics:*	*Characteristics:*	*Characteristics:*	*Characteristics:*
Very sensitive skin; creamy white; always burns; never tans	Sensitive skin; very fair; often burns; rarely tans	Normal skin; burns moderately; tans gradually	Skin not overly sensitive; tends to be darker in exposed areas than #1 and #2; burns minimally; tans well	Skin is light brown on exposed areas; it's not especially sensitive; rarely burns; tans very well	Skin not very sensitive at all; deeply pigmented; rarely burns
SPF:	*SPF:*	*SPF:*	*SPF:*	*SPF:*	*SPF:*
#15	#8	#6	#4	#2	#2
Product Code: Ultra	*Product Code:* Extra	*Product Code:* Moderate	*Product Code:* Minimal	*Product Code:* Minimal	*Product Code:* Minimal

180

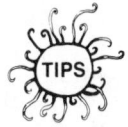

If you carry those little tins of cocoa butter to the beach, try to keep them upright in a cool or at least shaded place. Otherwise the cocoa butter melts and when you open the tin you can get a nasty burn if the hot stuff spills over.

Keep moving your bathing-suit straps around so you don't get white suit marks! Forgot? Then try an "instant tan" product to fill in the gap, but experiment before your big night out to be sure the color works on your skin. As an alternative you can also use a cosmetic bronzer that will wash off, but make sure it doesn't stain your clothes!

Don't forget to use a sunblock on the part in your hair. Otherwise you can get a burned stripe on your head and a few days later you'll have a peeling scalp that will resemble the worst dandruff you've ever seen.

Eight hours of sleep is the best thing for your skin. (I never skip!) But if you're on the beach and you want to nap, *move to the shade!!*

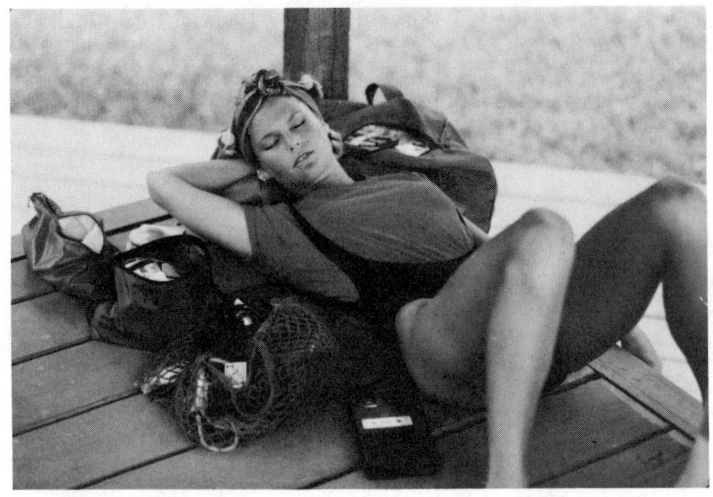

If you have short hair, don't forget to sunscreen your ears. Do remember your boyfriend's ears, too!

Avoid taking sunscreens or tanning products in aerosol cans to the beach because in the intense heat of the sun, those cans may explode!

SUNSCREENS AND ALLERGIES

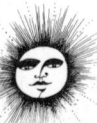 I've saved the worst sunscreen news for last: Some people are allergic to them . . . like me!

I was sent to St. Bart's on a modeling job for *Glamour* magazine. The editor decided that it would be a good idea to shoot a series of photos that showed exactly where to apply sunblock. So they put extra heavy stripes of white sunscreen in upside-down rainbows beneath my eyes, along my nose, and in big stripes on my cheeks and forehead. Instantly my face started stinging! I rushed to wash the stuff off. As I rubbed the white stripes off I found underneath they'd been replaced by *red* stripes of burning skin! (Very patriotic—but not the look we were after!) I wound up at the local hospital where they said I had the worst allergic reaction they'd ever seen. (Luckily, it did clear up in time to do the magazine cover!) Since then I've been very afraid of sunblocks and have relied on big hats and cover-ups to keep me protected. But this year, with so many new products to choose from, I bravely stuck my elbow out (for a patch test) and came up with a variety of products right for me.

If you have an allergy problem, don't give up. Here are the new ingredients to look for when buying sunscreens. It could be that even if you react to PABA, one of these will be safe for you:

1. padimate 0
2. ethyl 4-[bis(hydroxypropyl)] aminobenzoate
3. glyceryl aminobenzoate
4. menthyl anthranilate

How to Give Yourself a Patch Test

If you want to test a new sunscreen but you tend to have allergies, you should always give yourself a "patch test." Put a bit of the new sunscreen on the inside of your elbow where the skin tends to be sensitive. Cover the sunscreen with a small bandage and leave it on for about 24 hours. When you take the bandage off, check for any reaction such as bumps, swelling, redness, or rash. If your skin's clear, the sunscreen should be safe for you.

PEELING: THE TAN THAT GOT AWAY AND HOW TO LIVE THROUGH IT

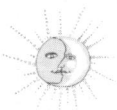 Once on holiday in Mexico I wanted to return to L.A. (where tans are status symbols) as dark as could be to impress a new boyfriend. On the first day out I burned, but it turned to a tan. I thought I'd been spared. I continued to work on my tan and by the time I had to leave, it was gorgeous! But on the airplane it began to peel—and by the time I was ready to pick up my luggage, I had a patchwork face!

Is there any way to avoid peeling? The sad answer is no. Once you've gotten a sunburn you've damaged your skin. After the swelling goes down, that top layer of skin is going to peel off. It looks ugly, it feels uncomfortable, but you're going to have to live through it.

The one thing that you can do for your skin while it's peeling is moisturize it. It won't change the rate of peel but it will keep your skin looking smoother and make it feel softer.

I also think it's a good idea to use a loofah *very gently* in the shower while you're peeling. You don't want to *scour* the skin. You just want to loosen any flakes that are about to fall off anyway. And, of course, be sure to moisturize after the shower.

Whatever you do, don't start peeling your skin yourself! Though sometimes you can do it safely, other times the skin that is exposed will be raw and sore and very vulnerable to sun damage or irritation.

While you are peeling, stay out of the sun entirely or else use a high-factored sunscreen or sunblock. Otherwise your skin will begin to tan unevenly and you could have real trouble getting it back to one color again!

And in the meantime, use earth dusts and bronzers to give yourself a smooth, even color.

CHEMICALS AND THE SUN

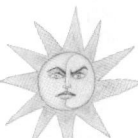

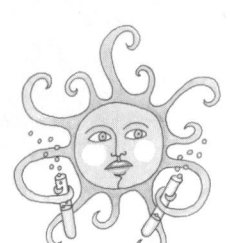

Phototoxicity? It sounds like a rare disease that models get from being around too many cameras! Well, it's not a disease. And it's not limited to just models either! Phototoxicity is actually an unwanted reaction due to the combination of certain substances and the sun. Fortunately not everybody has adverse reactions to these things but in any case, it pays to be aware of what *could* cause a problem. Here are some substances that can be phototoxic. If you use them, be especially careful about using them in the sun.

Plants. Limes, figs, parsley, carrots, fennel, celery, and dill can give you a reaction. But they have to be applied externally while in the sun for that to happen. That shouldn't be too much of a problem unless you wear your salads at the beach.

Limes & company. I mention limes again in its own category because it's one of the most phototoxic substances. And it's not only a problem in your gin and tonic. Lime juice is often an ingredient in perfumes, skin fresheners, and after-shave lotions. Using any of these products in the sun can cause a phototoxic reaction. Be sure to tell your brothers and boyfriends about the lime after-shave danger—they can be having a reaction on their sensitive, just-shaved faces and not know what's causing it.

Perfumes. You should never wear perfume at the beach! An ingredient in perfume—oil of bergamot—is phototoxic. Not only can it cause an allergic-like reaction on your throat, wrists, and between your breasts—the common places to apply perfume—but it can leave permanent discoloration of the skin even after the rash clears up. Watch out for any item which has perfume in it, like hand lotions and the like, and avoid using such things at the beach.

Deodorant soap. I was surprised to learn that deodorant soaps can cause a phototoxic reaction. It's because of the special chemicals like hexachlorophene that they contain. In fact, many hotels in sunny resorts no longer provide deodorant soaps in their rooms. The problem can be compounded because during the summer or in warm, sunny places people are more likely to worry about perspiration and so would be more likely to want to use a deodorant soap. But if you're spending time in the sun, be sure to avoid such soaps so you won't be the victim of an uncomfortable rash.

Cosmetics. Some cosmetics contain ingredients that are phototoxic. This includes some shampoos, some hair conditioners, some medicated cosmetics, and some medicated lotions and creams. Not *all* hair conditioners contain phototoxic ingredients, and everyone reacts differently to such substances anyhow. If you've spent time in the sun and you notice an odd reaction—an unusual sunburn, a rash, redness or swelling—your cosmetics could be the culprit. You have to experiment and by process of elimination see if you can pinpoint the problem. I always think it's a good idea to write to the manufacturer of any suspect cosmetic and see if they can help. Most cosmetic manufacturers are eager to keep their customers happy and if you explain your use of the cosmetic and your reaction to it they can sometimes tell you why you reacted and how to avoid such reactions in the future.

Diet drinks. Yes, that's right, those delicious low-calorie diet drinks that you sip all summer long can make your skin photosensitive. The artificial sweeteners they contain, including cyclamates and saccharin, can give you an especially bad burn and, like perfume, can leave permanent dark marks on your skin. But unlike perfume, you're not affected if you dab diet drinks behind your ears! You can only get a reaction after drinking, not wearing, your soda. Not everyone is vulnerable to this, but if you are and don't know it, the results can be most unpleasant.

Medications. This is a very important category because the consequences from the combination of too much sun and certain medications can be quite dangerous. The drugs in question can harm you by making your skin very photosensitive or by making your body especially vulnerable to heat. In the former situation you can get a rash or a very bad burn, in the latter you can actually suffer heatstroke because your body isn't properly retaining fluid. Either way you can have a serious problem.

Birth control pills are common offenders. Because of the increased estrogen in the body, some women taking the pill (or if they are pregnant) find that they develop brown splotches called cloasma (the mask of pregnancy) on their faces, especially the upper lip and cheeks. When these splotches are exposed to the sun they can become dark and unsightly. Some doctors recommend that sunbathing patients take the pill at night so their hormone level will be highest when they're *not* in the sun.

Other drugs that can cause problems include some tranquilizers, some antibiotics including certain tetracyclines, and some antihistamines. These drugs don't cause adverse reactions in everyone, but if you do take any regular medication, even something other than the ones I've mentioned, be sure to ask your doctor about any potential problems with the sun and/or warm weather. It's especially important to do this if you're going on vacation from a cold place to a warm place, which will already cause a shock to your system.

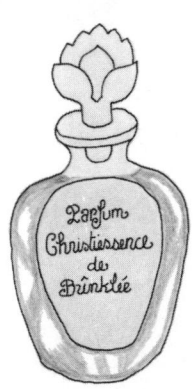

SUMMER SCENTS

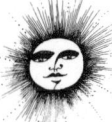 We know now that perfume is a sunbathing no-no. It attracts insects and can make your skin photosensitive and give you a splotchy burn. Of course you'll want to wear perfume other times in the summer. But there is something you should know: Heat and humidity make perfume more powerful, sweeter, and longer lasting. Here are three ways to adjust to summer scents:

Change to a lighter, fresher scent for summer.

Switch to a lighter version of your current scent—perhaps cologne instead of perfume.

Apply the perfume in different "cooler" spots. Instead of behind the ears and at your throat, dab a bit behind your knees. The scent will drift upward and be less powerful but still delightful.

HOT-WEATHER THREATS

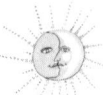

Holidays can be hazardous to your health! In addition to good, old familiar sunburn, there are other dangers that threaten when the weather is hot and you're unprepared.

Prickly Heat

While working on a job in the Caribbean, one free afternoon the other models and I got a game of volleyball going. We played in the heat all afternoon and by nightfall I began to get tiny itchy bumps all over my cheeks, chin, and neck. I thought it must have been caused by insects or perhaps an allergy to some tropical plant. I covered it with cream and hoped for the best, but the next day there was no improvement. I went to the doctor and it turned out that I had a case of prickly heat. The doctor gave me some medicated powder and now, whenever I travel to a tropical island, I bring the powder along and at the first sign of itching or redness I dust myself with it. I've never gotten it again. (Knock wood!)

Prickly heat or heat rash is an eruption of tiny bumps that itch and sometimes burn. It's caused when the body's sweat ducts get clogged. Often a heavy cream or suntan lotion can cause the problem. The cream I used just made things worse.

To get rid of prickly heat you need to stay cool and dry; lots of heavy sweating will just aggravate the situation. You should shower or wash the affected area. If an infection develops, see a doctor, who may prescribe an antibiotic ointment or medicated powder. Calamine lotion will also help dry out the area and relieve the itching.

Heat Cramps

Heat cramps are painful muscle spasms that occur because the body has lost too much salt due to heavy sweating. They strike people who are doing strenuous physical activity in a very hot environment. Firefighters sometimes get heat cramps and so do football players who are working out in their helmets and pads in late August weather.

The remedy for heat cramps is salt water. If you just drink plain water you'll make things worse by diluting the body's already diminished supply of salt. So the victim should sip ½ teaspoon of table or sea salt dissolved in half a glass of water (not ocean water!) every 15 minutes and rest until a doctor can be summoned. Heat cramps do require medical attention.

Heat Exhaustion

My first bout with heat exhaustion occurred in the Caribbean and I should have seen it coming. I was there for a shooting. It was a terribly hot, humid day and we were working very hard. There were lots and lots of clothes to photograph and by the time we were finished I was exhausted. Just as we thought the session was at last over, the client appeared with some knit sweaters to be photographed. I pulled on the first sweater and began posing, and almost immediately began to feel shaky, nauseated, and light-headed. I was pale beneath my makeup and sweating heavily. Someone helped me into the shade and after a large glass of water I felt much better. I realized that I hadn't had much to drink that day and I assumed that's why I'd gotten so weak. I was right!

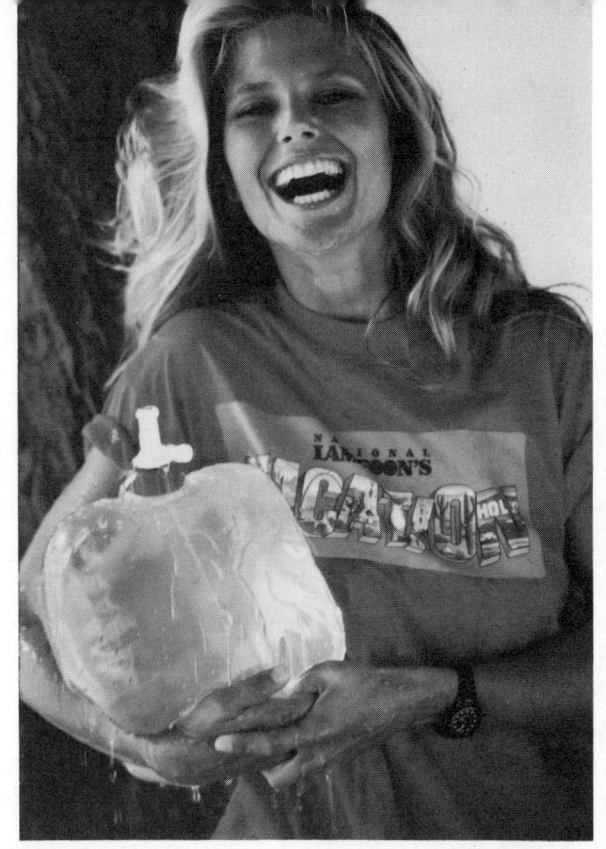

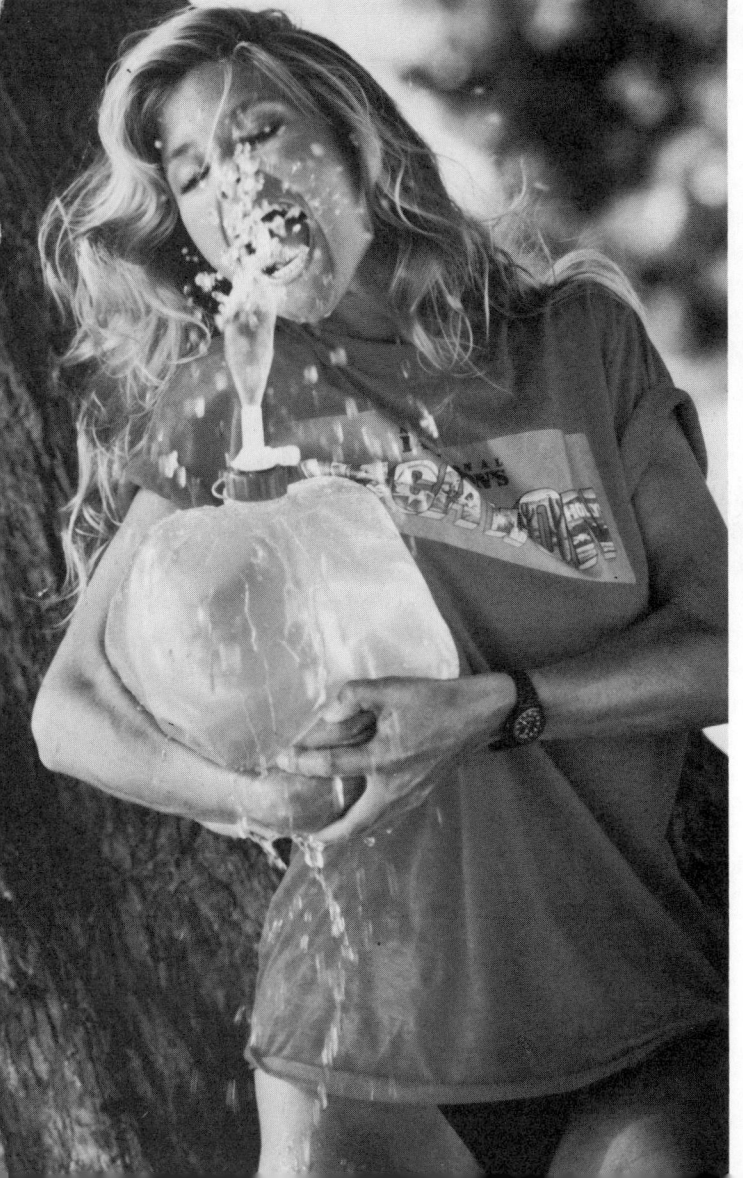

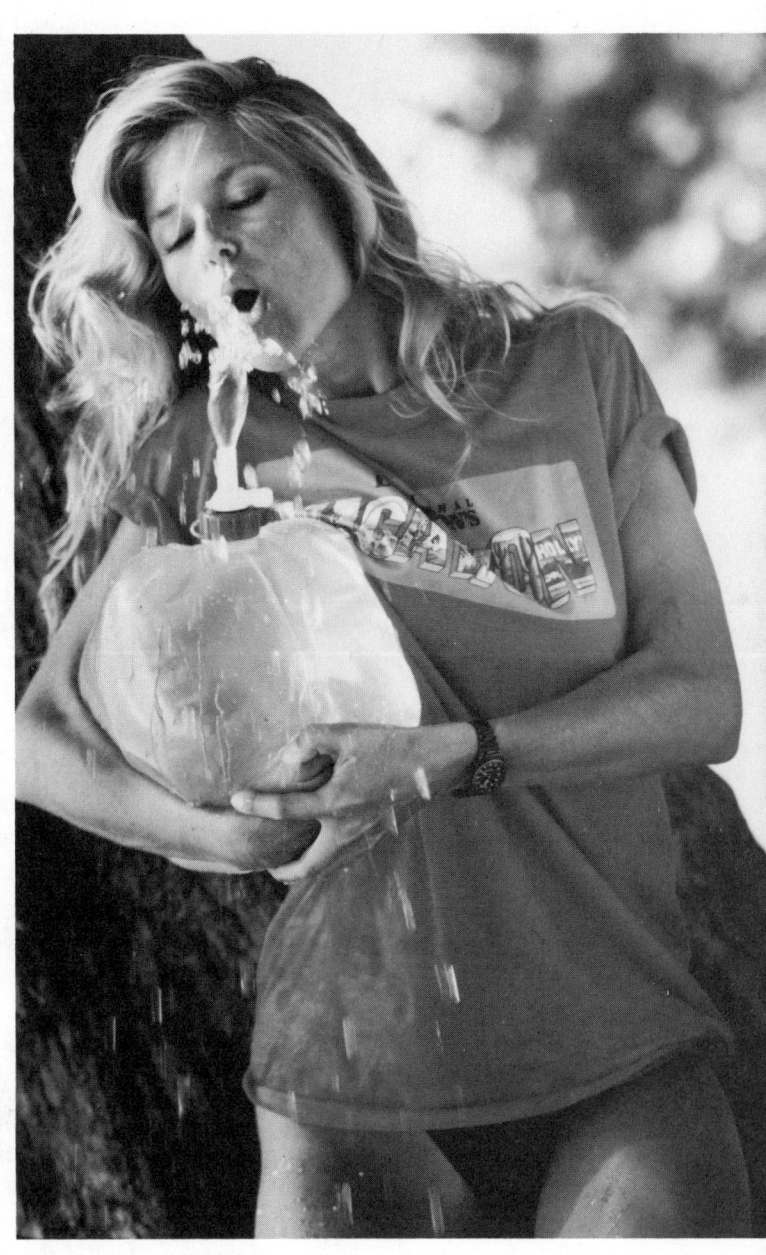

Heat exhaustion, or heat prostration, occurs when your body loses too much fluid and salt. It can happen to a jogger who runs in very hot weather, a visitor to a hot country who hasn't had time to get acclimated, or even a model wearing a sweater on a hot Caribbean beach! The symptoms are weakness, dizziness, nausea, and palpitations. The skin becomes clammy and you sweat profusely. This is important because it's the main difference between heat exhaustion and heatstroke (which is far more dangerous).

The remedy for heat exhaustion is fluids. If you're at the beach, guard against getting terribly overheated. Drink plenty of fluids and it doesn't hurt to munch on a salty snack occasionally. (At last, something good about potato chips!)

Heatstroke

Sunstroke or heatstroke is far more dangerous than heat exhaustion. It occurs when the body is very overheated either through overexposure to the sun or confinement in a very hot place. Heatstroke is what can kill your pet if you leave it in a hot car with the windows rolled up. Elderly people and the very young are most vulnerable to heatstroke, but it's the number two cause of death among high-school athletes, so you can see that even strong bodies in good shape can be victims.

The symptoms include headache, nausea, dizziness, and fever (as much as 105°F or even higher). Muscle cramps may occur. Fainting, coma, and convulsions may follow. The heatstroke victim's body is no longer able to sweat and so the skin becomes hot and dry.

The treatment of heatstroke is to cool the body as quickly as possible either with a cold bath or cold compresses. Aspirin, two tablets by mouth, can help.

Rectal temperature should be taken every 10 minutes until temperature falls to 101 or 102 degrees—not lower, or it may continue to fall below normal.

Medical attention should be obtained as quickly as possible.

Scars and the Sun

If you have a scar anywhere on your body you must take care never to expose it to the sun without some kind of sunscreen protection. A scar has lost melanin and so is unable to protect itself. If you do expose a scar to too much sun, three things can happen. It can become hyperpigmented, which means it gets very dark and never fades back to your normal skin color. It can become spotted with some dark and some light places. Worse and most important of all, because it's so vulnerable to sun damage, a scar can develop skin cancer.

So if you do have a cut that hasn't quite healed, a surgical scar, or any other kind of scar, keep it protected from the sun with a high SPF-factored sunscreen. And if you ever notice any changes in the color or appearance of the scar, check with your doctor.

Those Mysterious Little White Spots

From time to time I have been mystified by tiny, round, flaky white spots that I occasionally get when I tan. They would appear on my chest, upper arms, or back and they would drive me crazy because I didn't know what caused them or how to get rid of them. Creams and lotions had no effect. The only good thing about them was that many models seem to get them and discussing them and our home remedies was always a good ice-breaker in dressing rooms all over the world.

At last, my quest is over. Those little white spots are called *tinea versicolor*. They are a fungal infection that shows up, especially in the summer, when you get tanned and the little infected spots stay white. My doctor prescribed an antifungal lotion which does the trick. So if you find dime-sized white spots on your chest or shoulders in the summer, you'll know what they are and you'll be able to explain to your doctor and get an antifungal treatment. But be sure to wash all the sheets, towels, and clothes you used while a fungus host or you'll catch it all over again!

Those *Large* White Spots

In my search for the cause of my small white spots I learned about vitiligo. Vitiligo is a not-very-common skin condition that is really the opposite of freckling. It's caused by a lack of melanin in the skin in certain areas of the body, and becomes especially obvious in the summer when a tan makes surrounding skin darker. The skin affected with vitiligo will remain completely white or burn red in the sun. Therefore, someone with vitiligo should do what their skin can't do itself: Use sunblocks on the affected areas and avoid excessive exposure to the sun.

Herpes and Skin Cancer: The Real Threat

Unfortunately beauty isn't the only consideration when we examine the long-term effects of the sun. The sun can also be a health menace. Overexposure to the sun has been linked to cancer and herpes.

In order to understand how a simple sunburn can eventually do such drastic damage, it helps to remember that the skin is the largest organ of the body. At any given time as much as 10% of your blood is in your skin. So whatever effect the sun is having on your skin, it's also affecting the rest of your body via the blood that is constantly circulating. Scientists are just beginning to understand this but they think the worst effect of the sun is that it can damage the immune system of the body which is our natural defense against disease. This may explain why overexposure to the sun is connected to skin cancer—the sun has altered the body's ability to fight the cancer. It may also explain why when you get a sunburn you'll often get a cold sore a few days later. The sun has altered your immune system's ability to fight off the herpes virus.

The encouraging news about the bad effects of the sun on the skin is that many scientists are now discovering that they are largely reversible. They're not exactly sure how, but it seems that if you stop overexposing your skin to the sun and start protecting it, the aging effects may begin to be diminished. So even if you've spent 20 summers baking like a turkey, so to speak, it's not too late to learn some "sun sense" and start protecting your skin.

MIDWINTER VACATIONS

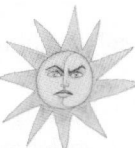

Heading for the tropics in January? Lucky you! But remember that going from a very cold to a very hot climate can be a real stress on your body. Here's how to make the transition safely:

Move more slowly. You're on vacation after all! And your body is working hard to adjust to the higher temperature—your blood actually gets *thinner* as your body gets ready for all that perspiration. So take it easy.

Change your diet. Cut down on high-protein foods. They increase your metabolic heat production *and* water loss. Eat light foods, and if your salt intake is normally very low, increase it a bit.

Listen to your body. If a fast game of volleyball on the beach makes you dizzy, relax! Rest in a shady place for a while and sip a cool drink.

Drink lots of fluids. Remember, you need them to fight heat-related maladies.

(Do I need to tell you this?) Be careful of the sun! So many people have ruined their vacation *the first day* by getting a killer sunburn. Do you want to spend a week in a room reading magazines? Get out that sunblock and don't you dare sunbathe between 10:00 and 2:00! Have a nice cool lunch in the shade instead.

 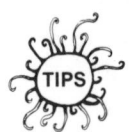

Heading off on vacation? Before you leave, write to the International Association of Medical Assistance to Travelers. For a small contribution, IAMAT will send you a booklet which lists all participating English-speaking doctors, clinics, and hospitals around the world. They'll also include inoculation information and a climate chart. Write to them at: 350 Fifth Avenue, Room 5620, New York, New York 10001.

If you're going to the Caribbean and want information on any medical dangers you should watch out for, write to The Caribbean Tourism Association, 20 East 46th Street, New York, New York 10017.

YOUR FACE AND THE SUN

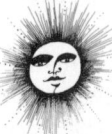

I never, never sit with my unprotected face exposed to the sun! Never. There's no need for it. All those walks on sunny days, those times swimming when your sunscreen wears off, those spontaneous Frisbee games when you didn't get a chance to dab on some sunblock—they all add up. You can't always shield your face from the sun. So eventually it's going to get a bit of color on its own. And the amount it gets in those unguarded moments is enough to give you plenty of color.

Aside from the health reasons for not getting too much sun on the face, I find that makeup doesn't seem to "sit" well on a really tan face. In fact, when I'm modeling for close-ups, the clients always prefer that I have only the slightest hint of natural color in my face.

So take my advice and keep your face out of the sun as much as possible. Use sunblocks and sunscreens on your face at all times. And indulge yourself in hats.

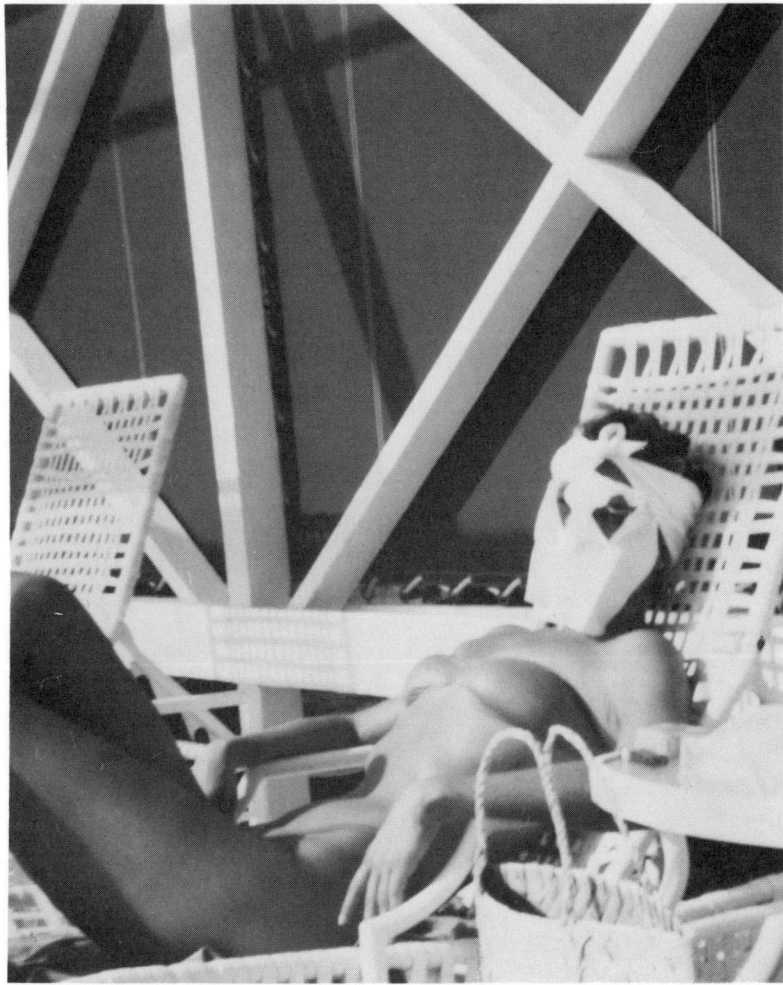

I'll do anything to protect my face!

Hats, Hats, Hats

I love hats! I highly recommend them to all sun lovers! They look great and they've saved my face from a few years' worth of wear and tear.

Beware of synthetic hatbands. The synthetic won't allow the sweat to dry and it begins to irritate the skin. It's like a small case of prickly heat. To combat this, sprinkle the hatband with powder, regular or medicated! Tuck tissues into the hatband to absorb the sweat. Clean the hatband at the end of the day and be sure it's dry when you put it on again. Even though you're wearing a hat, use your sunscreen, and don't forget your chin because it often sticks out from beneath the hat and needs an extra dab of protection.

HATS

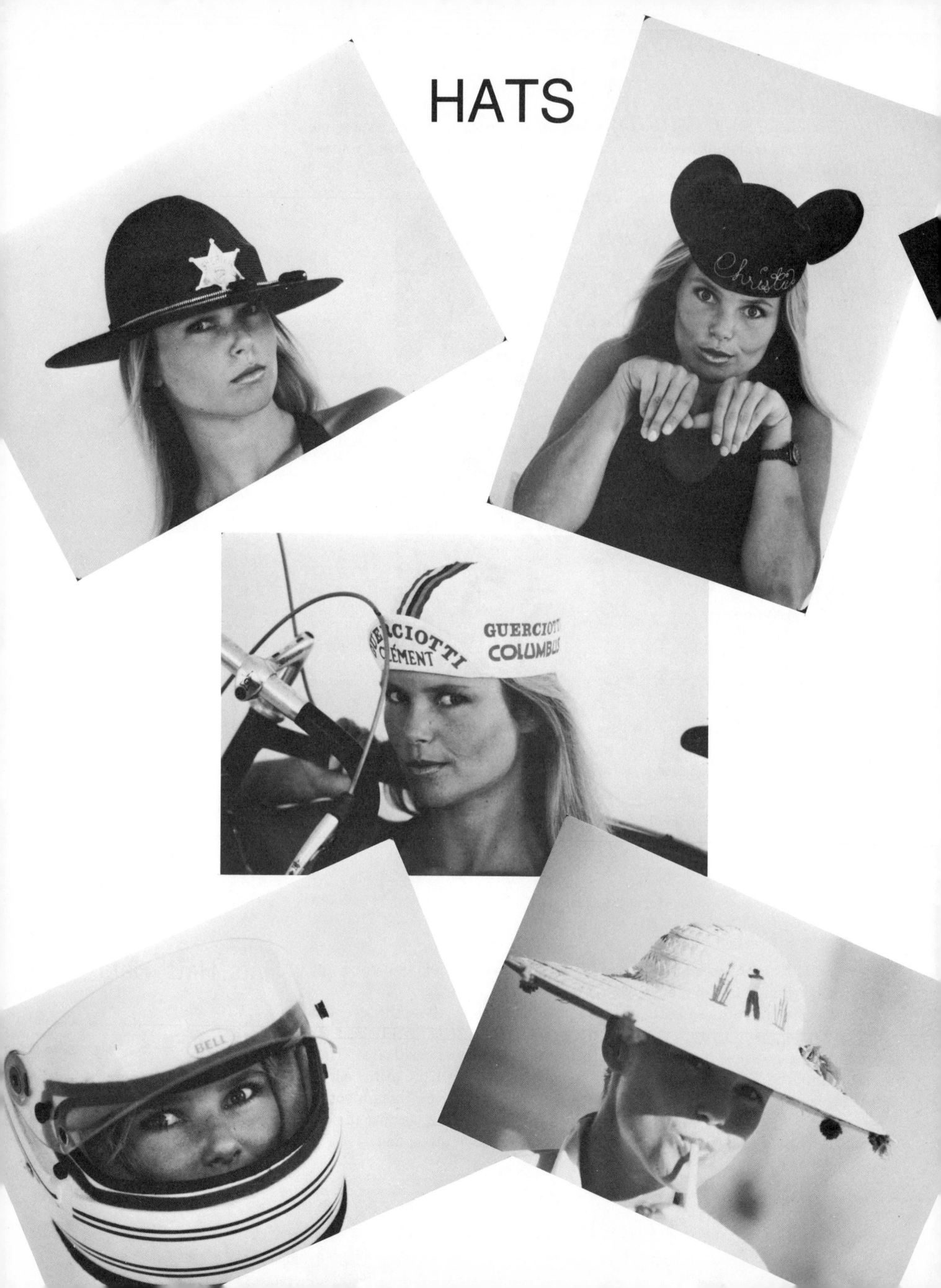

HATS

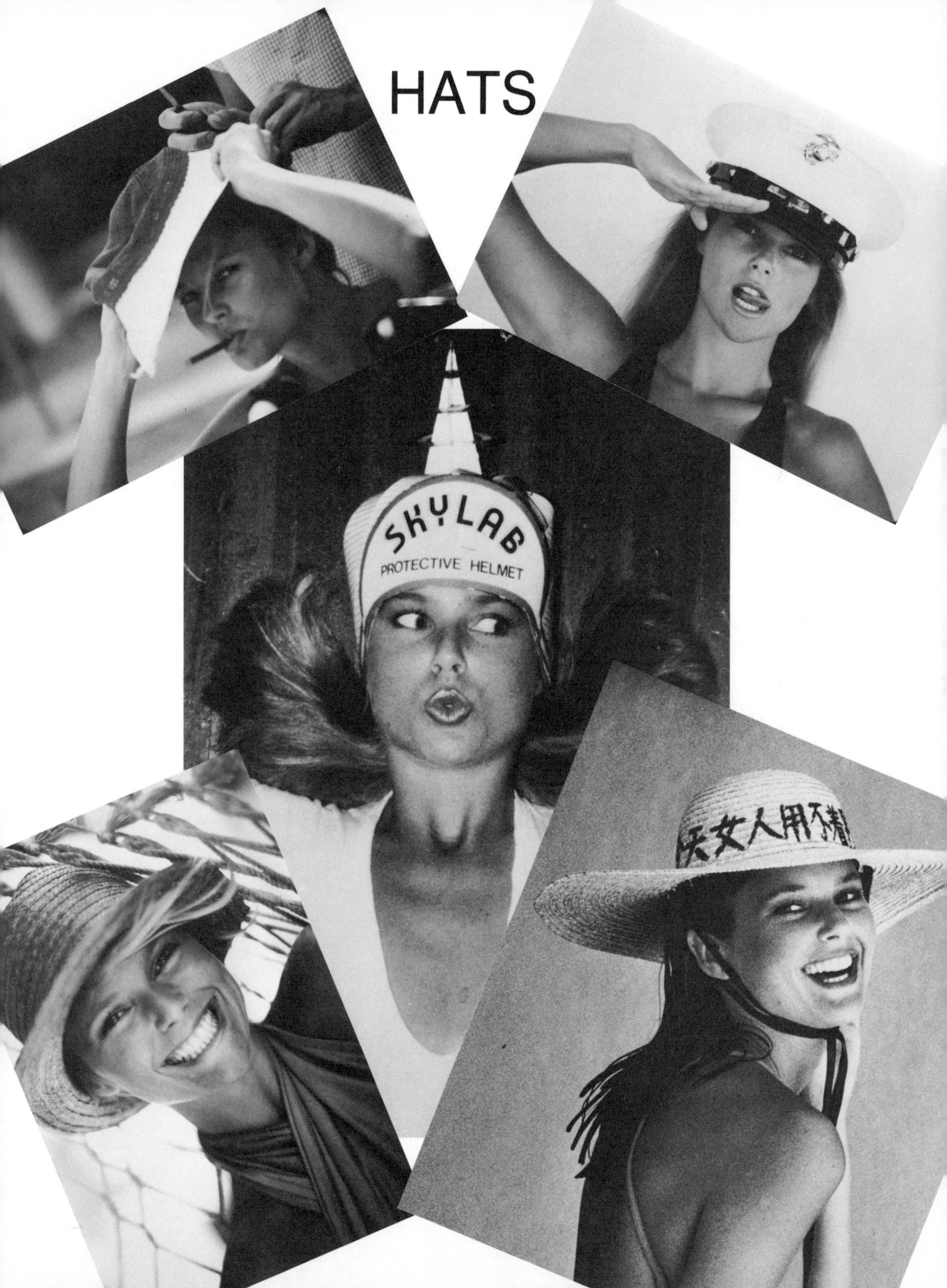

Sunglasses

Crow's feet are my favorite wrinkles! They look happy—like proof of a cheerful past. Sooner or later we're all going to get them—sunglasses are one of the best ways to let it be later. They relax your eyes and prevent squinting. They're glamorous (a little mysterious!), pretty, and practical. But they also tickle my nose so I used to find excuses to "forget" them at home. Until the time I spent a day at the whitest beach you could imagine. There was nothing but sun and sand as far as the eye could see. After a wonderful day at this dazzling beach, I wound up with sunburned eyes! Imagine what it would feel like to have sand under your eyelids. That's what my eyes felt like. They were irritated and itchy and it took a few days for them to get back to normal. Since that experience I've become a sunglasses convert. (And my nose got used to the tickle!)

Sunburned eyes are not very common but you can suffer milder ill effects from going without sunglasses. Sunglasses will help prevent eyestrain that can cause headaches and swollen eyes.

Recently there has been research that shows long-term exposure to the ultraviolet rays of the sun can cause cataracts and other eye problems which usually occur late in life. So anybody who's constantly exposed to strong sunlight like sailors or skiers at high altitudes should think of sunglasses as an investment in their future good vision.

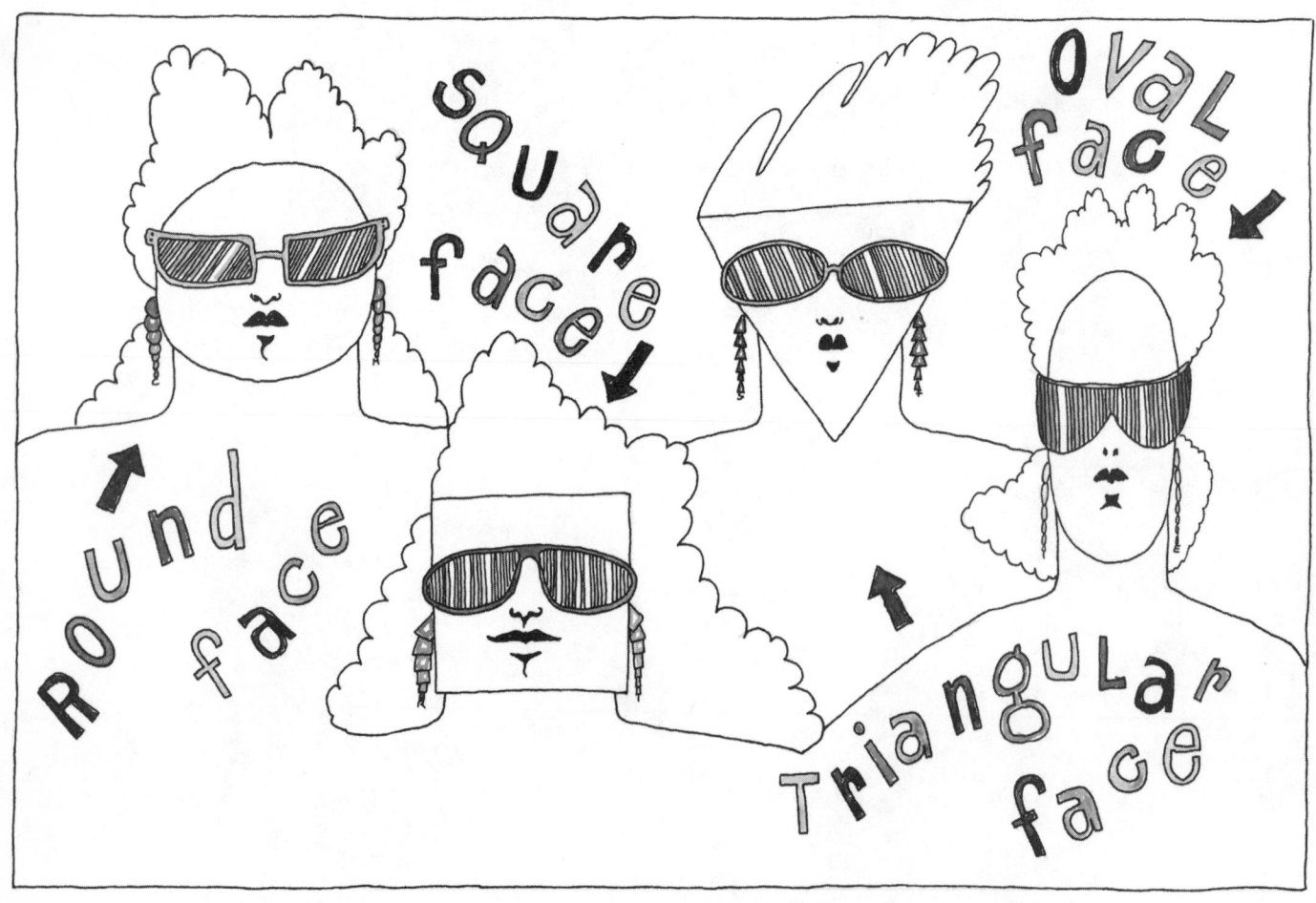

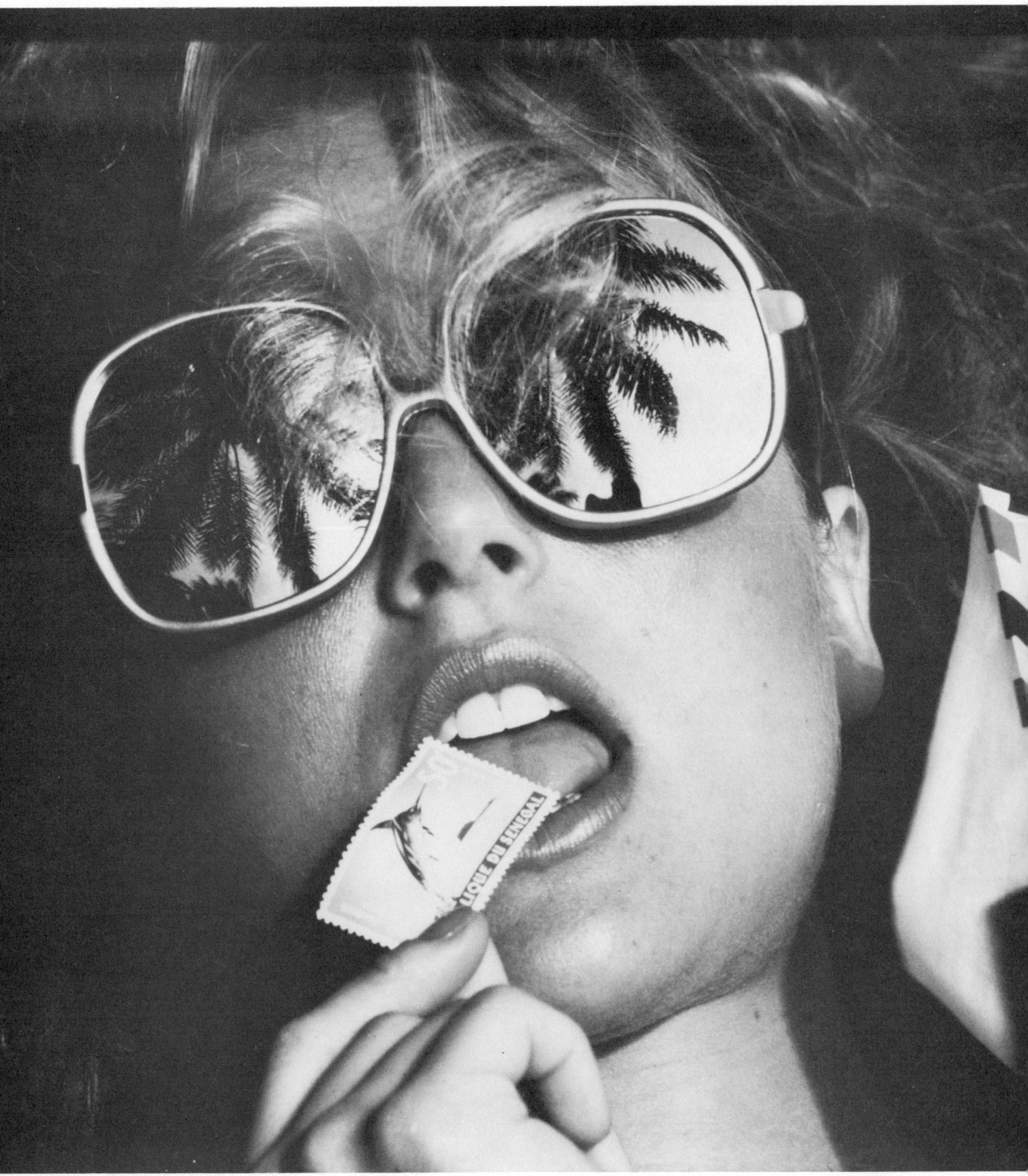

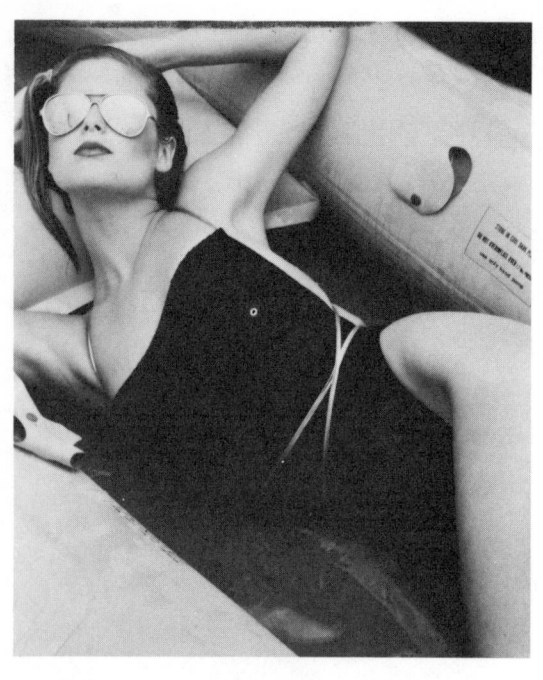

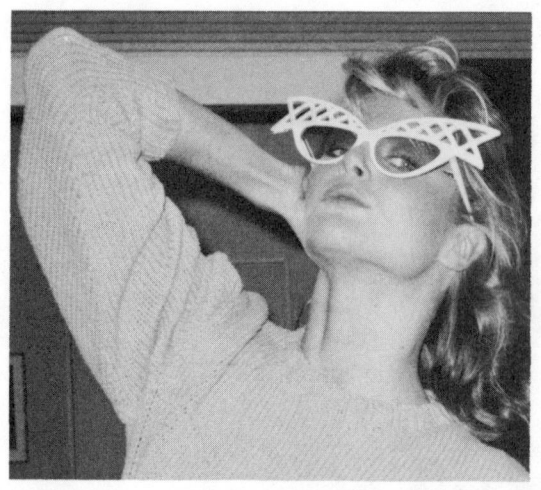

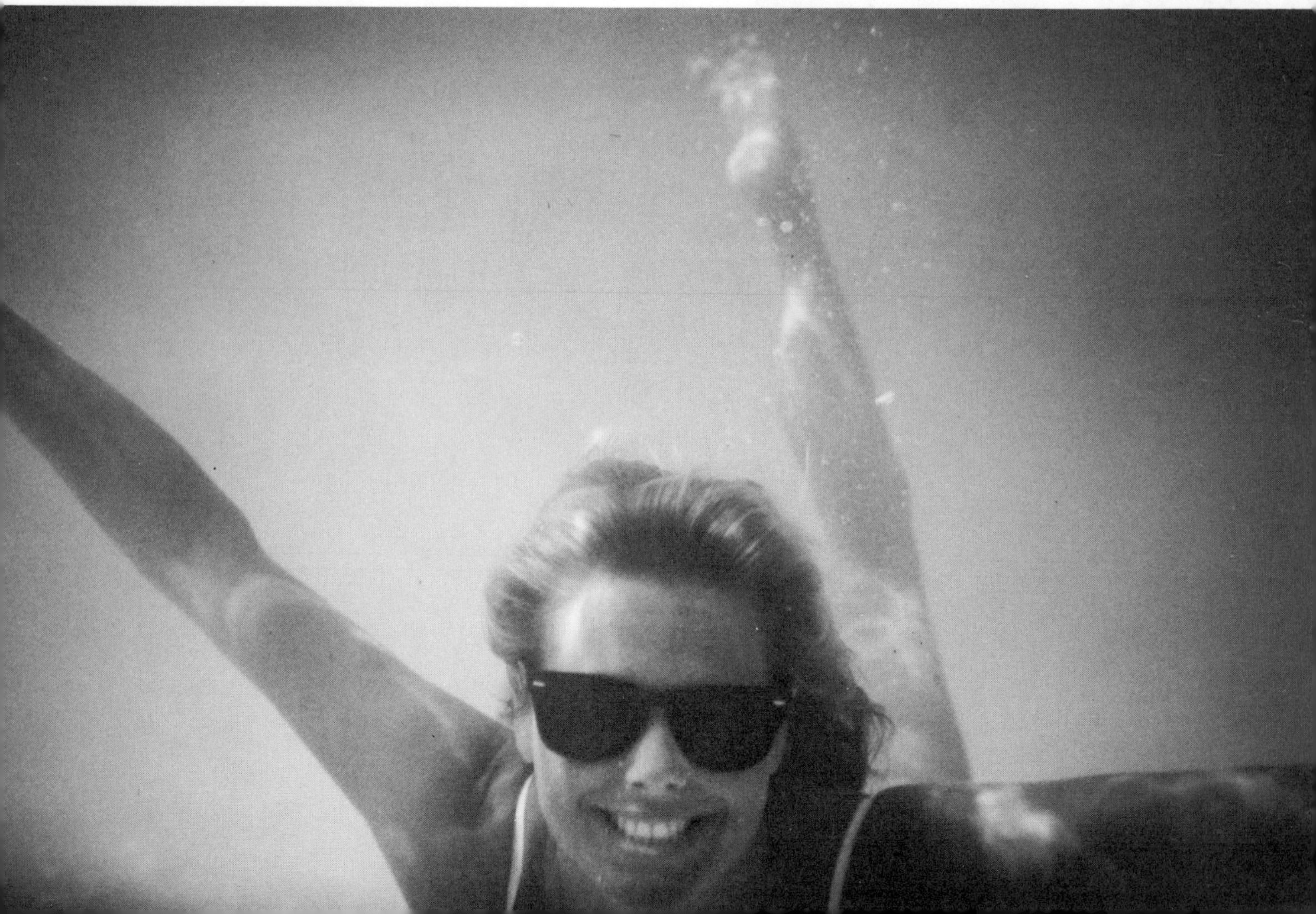

There are three things to consider when you buy sunglasses: the lens color, the lens type, and the frame style.

1. Lens color is important because your goal in wearing sunglasses is to cut down on glare and light. Some colors are better at protecting your eyes than others. Pink, orange, blue, and red are the ones to avoid if you're concerned about protection. They don't really block out enough glare, and blue and purple color lenses transmit too much ultraviolet light to your eyes. Friends of mine who are tennis players tell me that yellow is good for outdoor sports on cloudy days because they increase contrast. I guess every little bit helps. But I know on sunny days, yellow sunglasses are not really strong enough to keep you comfortable.

The best all-round lens color seems to be grey. It cuts rays of light all across the color spectrum and is really efficient in bright sunlight. In fact, airplane pilots favor grey sunglasses over every other color.

2. Lens type. After you've chosen the lens color, you have to decide on the lens type.

Polarized lenses are a good choice for everyday use. They do a fine job of reflecting light and protecting your eyes. They are made of two layers of glass

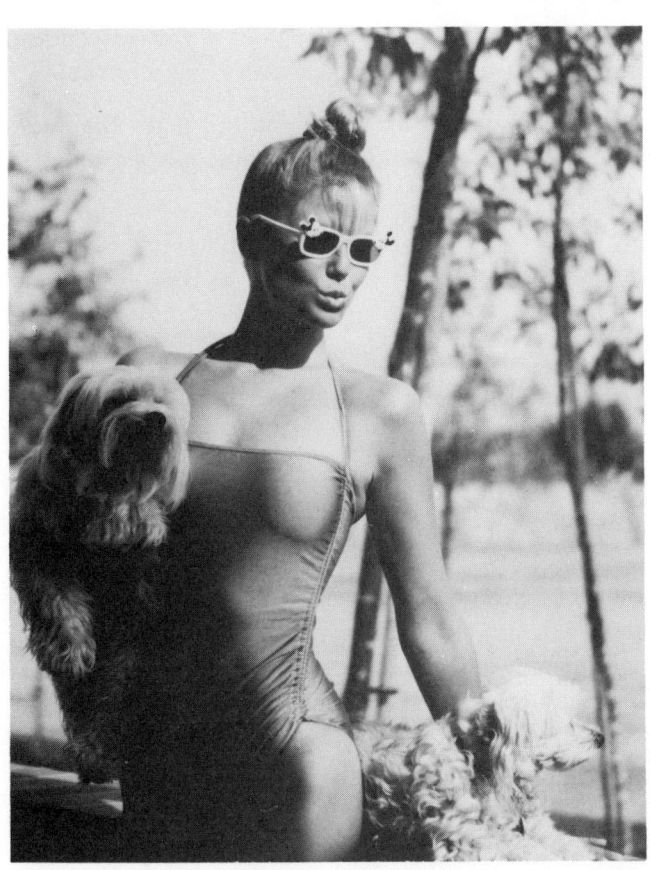

that work to cut both glare and reflection. Polarized lenses can be made up into prescription sunglasses if you require them.

Photochromatic lenses are the kind that change color with the intensity of light: They get darker as the light gets brighter. I prefer them for beach wear because I can sit in the shade wearing them and they're not too dark, but if I'm reading in the sun, they're still effective. One drawback of photochromatic lenses is that it takes them a few minutes to adjust to light changes. So if you're driving from a bright sunny street to a dark underground parking garage you could be temporarily blinded. I think if you're driving, they're not the best choice.

Now that you've selected your lens color and type you can have the fun of choosing your frame style.

3. Frame style. Take your time trying on sunglasses. If you pop them on and off in a second or two just checking frame styles, you won't discover problems that could later make them useless to you.

Be sure the glasses fit properly. If they feel tight at the temples after 30 seconds, you'll be in agony if you try to wear them for 30 minutes. Many stores will fit the glasses to your face in a matter of minutes.

Are they too heavy? Some sunglasses will begin to feel heavy on your face after a few minutes. After an hour you'll probably have a splitting headache.

Will they stay on? This isn't a silly question. Bend down. Do the sunglasses slip to the tip of your nose? Turn your head quickly. Are they still in place?

Are the frames metal? Metal frames can be attractive but if you're spending lots of time in bright sunlight they can also be very hot and uncomfortable.

Are they distortion-free? Hold the glasses up to a light and move them. Do you see bubbles and ripples and waves? If you do, those sunglasses could give you a headache and ruin your tennis game.

Do they block your vision? Some frames are very fashionable but unless you are looking straight ahead they will obstruct your vision, so they aren't very practical. Check your peripheral vision while trying on the sunglasses to be certain it's not blocked.

DARK CIRCLES

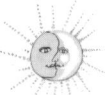

Do you have dark circles under your eyes? The skin there is very thin and allows a lot of sunlight to penetrate, so the melanin builds up, making circles even darker.

Wearing clear prescription glasses in the sun can make things worse by focusing sunlight on the under-eye area.

Prevent those circles by protecting your eyes from the sun: Use a sunscreen (don't get it *in* your eyes) or have your ophthalmologist direct you to special sunglasses that filter the ultraviolet radiation.

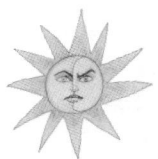 As if my poor hair doesn't suffer enough at work with the blow-drying, curling, teasing, styling, and spraying, it doesn't have much to look forward to when I go on vacation, either. Everything that I love is torture to my hair: the sea and the sun! Yet hairdressers tell me that my hair is in great condition. Knowing about your hair will help you care for it and keep it in great shape.

Getting to Know Your Hair

How old is your hair? Two years old? Six years old?

If that seems like an odd question, look at it this way: hair, like a fingernail, is composed of dead cells. The moment it leaves the little follicle in your scalp, it's dead, and though genetics and general health determine its condition when it first appears on your head, *you* determine its condition as it grows older. If your hair is long, some of those strands may be six, seven, or eight years old. Some of them may have witnessed your first kiss!

If you've been spending much of your hair's life in the sun, then you have to compensate for the damage sun and wind can do. If your hair is long, like mine, or permanented or color-treated, you have to take special care.

Hair and skin are both made up of the same substance. And in many ways they're alike: They're flexible, they need moisture to be in good condition, and they're damaged by sun, wind, and water. In fact, hair and skin both have melanin in them—the protein that determines color. But skin, because it's living tissue, can produce greater amounts of melanin to turn dark and protect itself from the sun. Hair is dead tissue and can't protect itself. When it is overexposed, the melanin is bleached out, making the hair lighter but sometimes also making it brassy and unnatural looking. Just as the color of your hair can be changed by the sun, so can its texture. Again, like skin, it can lose moisture and eventually become dry and damaged. But unlike the skin, your hair is unable to repair itself.

So two things happen to your hair in the sun: It gets dry and it loses color. These two things happen to everybody to a greater or lesser degree, and they can be good or bad depending on the current state of your hair and how you want to look in the future.

Dry Hair

The sun dries your hair by making it more porous and allowing its natural oil to escape. When this happens each individual hair strand becomes brittle. The damage usually shows up first as split ends, but as it gets drier, it begins to break off.

If you do have dry hair, hats and scarves will give you almost total protection from the sun. There are also some new products on the market that are sunscreens for the hair. They're designed to be sprayed on or combed through and they shield your hair from sun damage.

Permanents and Bleach in the Sun

If your hair is processed—either colored or permanented—you must be extremely careful in the sun. If you had a permanent this spring and spend the summer at the beach without protecting your hair, you could begin to look like a steel-wool pad before you know it.

Processed hair is very fragile. The chemicals that are used to color,

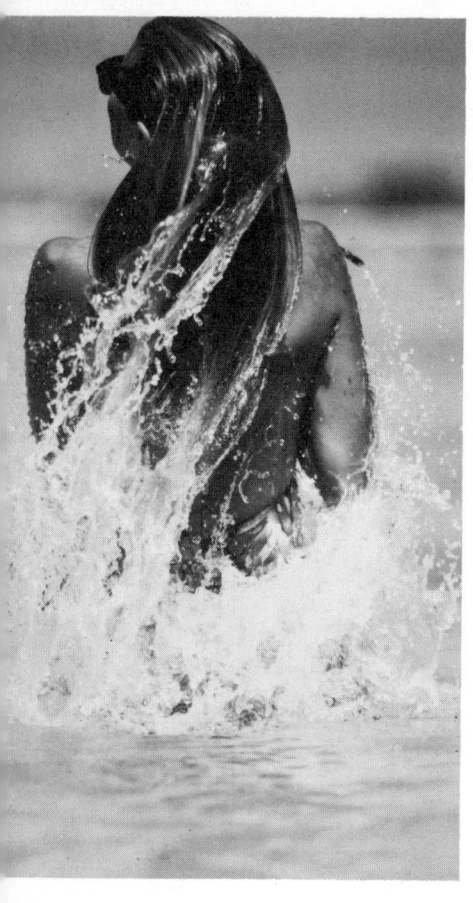

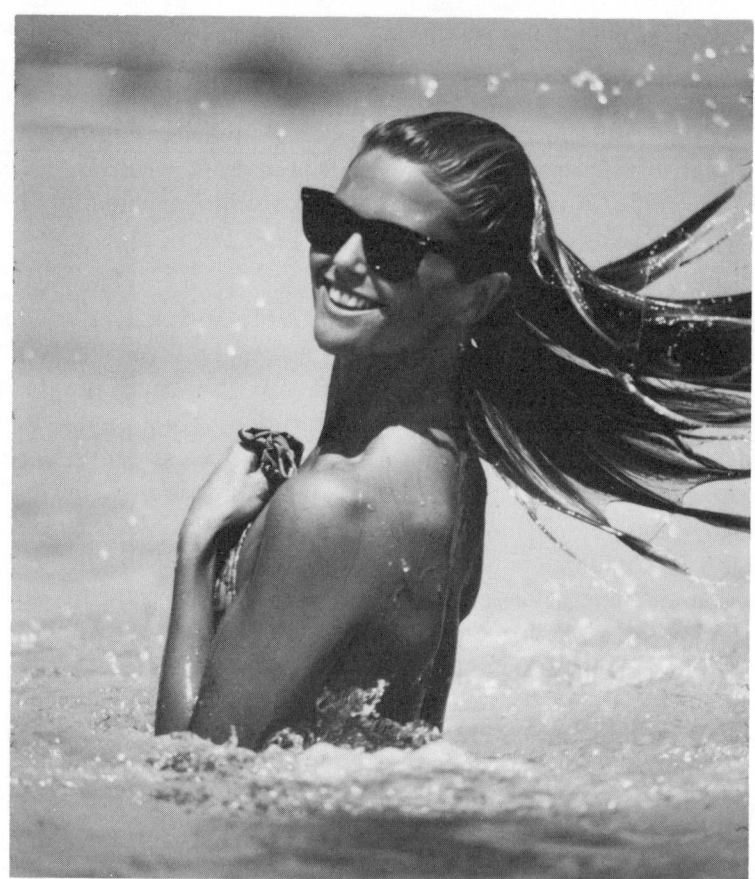

lighten, curl, or straighten your hair change the hair strand permanently. They make it porous and dry. Even the newer, gentle coloring and permanenting methods still change the texture of the hair. The sun increases the dryness and makes your hair brittle and dull.

Besides hats and scarves, you can use sunscreens that are designed especially for processed hair. But before you slather it all over, try it out on a few strands to be sure that it won't damage the color of the hair.

Non-alkaline (or acid) shampoos seem to work best for processed or sun-damaged hair, followed by a cream rinse or conditioners for dry hair.

Be sure not to use dandruff shampoos on processed hair unless the label says the product is safe and you test it first. The chemicals in these shampoos can cause damage and sometimes irritate your scalp.

Highlighting Your Hair with the Sun

My hair is naturally blond but I like it to be even lighter than it is. A good way to do this is with lemon juice at the beach. Just comb the lemon juice through your wet hair. Comb it straight back so the streaks will frame your face when your hair falls naturally. Then to counteract the drying effect of the lemon, pour a very small quantity of oil (sesame is nice) into your palm and rub the ends of your hair between your hands.

One thing to remember is that lemon juice is drying, so use conditioner or a cream rinse when you wash it off at the end of the day.

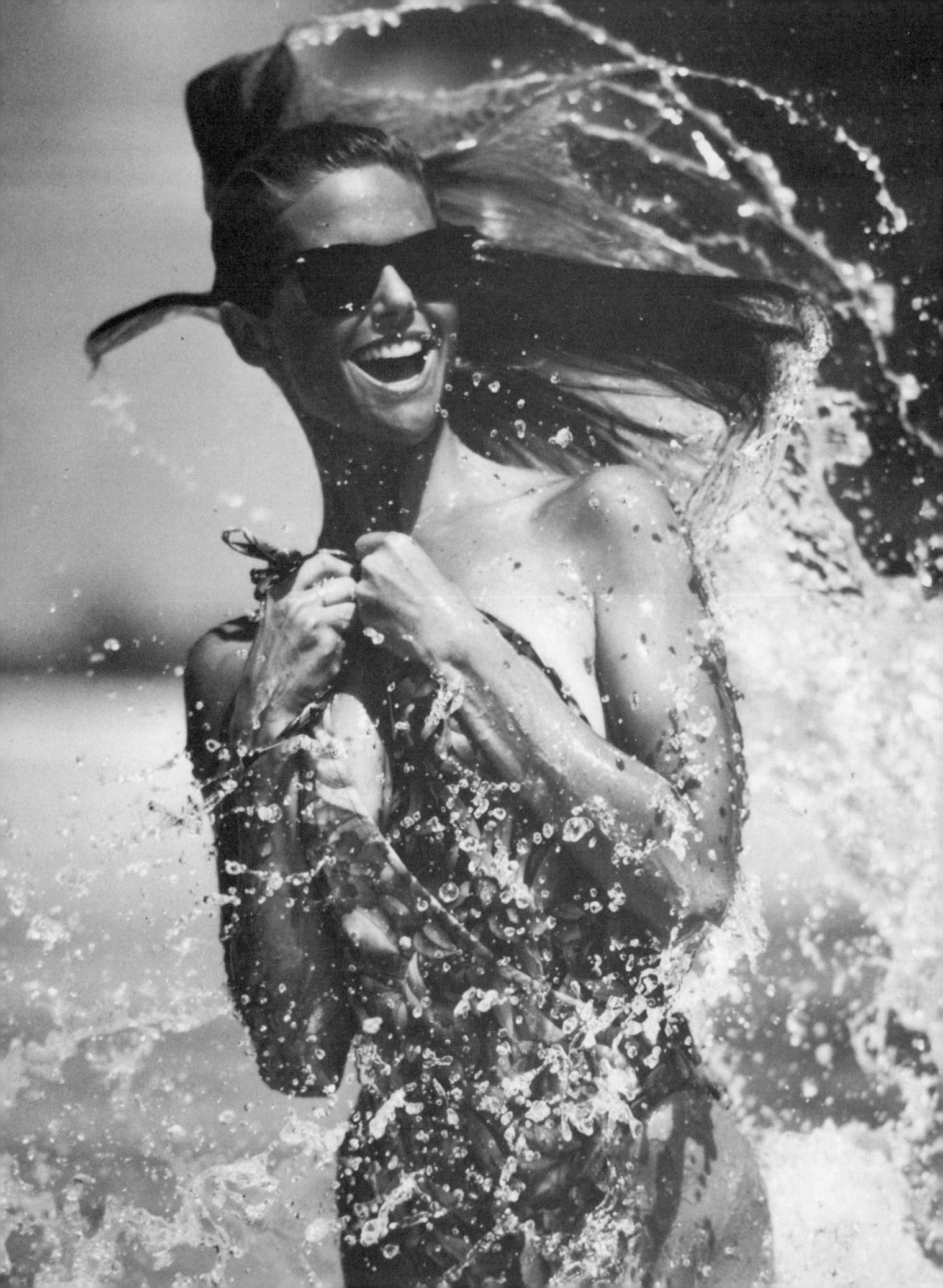

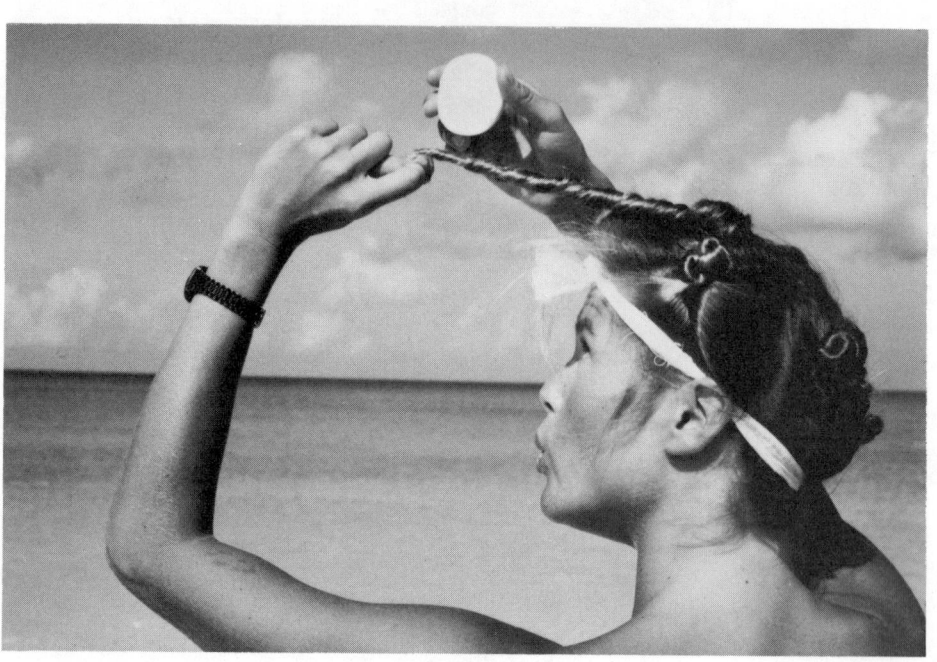

Set and Streak

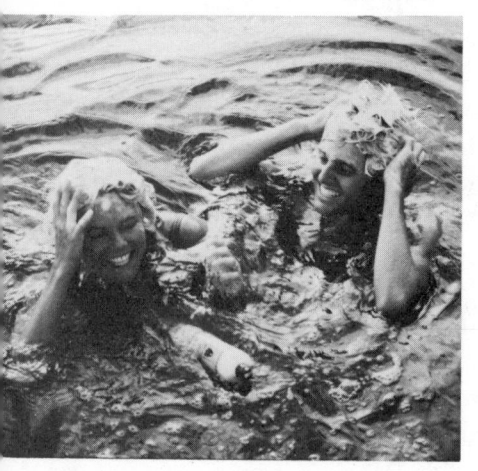

Twist your hair up into little pin curls while you sit in the sun. The heat from the sun bakes the curls in so they really last! (If you're in a humid climate where your hair needs extra hold, dilute a few drops of lemon juice in water; comb on before you twist up your hair. You get highlights *and* hold. Be sure to condition after you wash it out!)

Chamomile oil can also be used to give your hair natural streaks. You buy it at health-food stores. You'll find that it's much stronger than lemon juice so you have to be careful with it. I just use it on swatches of hair; I never comb it through all of my hair at once. It has a nice, natural bleaching effect. For a milder version of this you can use a cup of chamomile tea. Pour it over your head, comb through, and let the sun give you some great highlights!

Once on a sailing trip with my brother, we ran out of shower water on the boat, so each day we would shampoo our hair with chamomile shampoo *in* the ocean. The combination was powerful! By the end of the trip—like it or not—our hair was white! (Luckily, we liked it. *Vive la différence!*)

You don't have to be a blonde to highlight with the sun. Brunettes can get great highlights by using a spritz of strong coffee or tea on their hair. They can also use lemon juice, which will usually bring out reddish highlights. Another way to encourage some red highlights in your hair is to brew some Celestial Seasonings Red Zinger tea. Mix it with just a little bit of lemon juice and comb it through.

The Sunshine Conditioners

One of the best ways I know to deep-condition your hair is to do it with the sun's help. Many deep-conditioning products that are on the market today are formulated to be used with heat. Well, instead of putting a hot towel on your head, use the conditioner at the beach and take advantage of the sun's warmth. Just comb it through your hair and let it work its magic as you bask in the sun. You can wash it out when you get home.

You can also use oils on your hair to deep-condition it in the sun—just be sure to use *light* oils. Once a model told me that olive oil is a wonderful conditioner. It sounded great so I poured nearly a whole bottle on my head and sat in the sun. I figured I was getting a great conditioning and maybe I was. But when I went to shampoo my hair I learned that it's almost impossible to get olive oil out of your hair. It took me about two days before I could get it all out and all that shampooing actually left my hair dried out! If you're going to use an oil on your hair in the sun—apply it only on the ends, not near the scalp, as you could clog pores.

Washing and Drying Summer Hair

I wash my hair once a day to keep it just right for modeling jobs. If you're not used to washing your hair every day, but think you need to in warm weather, here are some techniques you should try.

There's no need to lather your hair more than once. Daily washing is going to keep your hair plenty clean, lathering twice may just dry it out. Of course, if you've been covered in suntan lotion all day, probably a lot of it has ended up in your hair and two latherings may be in order.

If you have really oily hair then you would do well to avoid balsam and protein shampoos. They tend to leave a coating that can make the hair limp and even sticky.

Use a cream rinse (if it doesn't make your hair too soft, as it can with fine hair) or an instant conditioner. If your hair is oily, use the product only on the ends of your hair, which can be dry and brittle even if the roots are oily.

Avoid blow-drying as much as possible. The heat of the blow dryer can be as damaging as too much sun. It's really best to let your hair just air-dry as often as you can, and the heat of summer allows you to do this most of the time. If you must blow-dry, use the cool setting on the dryer and stop just before your hair is completely dry, letting it dry the rest of the way naturally. Those last few minutes with a blow dryer are the worst.

If you must use hot rollers, try one of those conditioning products that can be used along with them. With all the punishment your hair takes in summer, it doesn't need hot rollers used without *some* protection!

If you are using hot rollers, make sure your hair is brushed smooth and rolled up on the roller with the same tension from the ends to the roots so you won't get that creased look.

When drying your hair, either naturally or with a blow dryer, keep turning your head upside down and fluffing your hair away from the scalp, so when it dries it will look fuller and fluffier.

If you're using hot rollers in a humid climate, spray your hair with setting lotion before rolling, but use tissues as end papers: Fold each section into a piece of tissue before rolling it. It will protect your hair and keep the curl smooth.

Wet-Hair Styles

Isn't summer great? You can go to lunch with wet hair! You can jump out of the surf, stick some pretty combs in your hair, comb it out later and have a new hairstyle!

I love the flexibility and freedom of summer hair. Here are some tips on how to handle wet hair so it'll be pretty now *and* later!

Wet hair is very vulnerable to breakage. It's weak and elastic, and rough treatment will break and tear it. It's best to use a wide-tooth comb. If you have long hair as I do, comb it in sections, starting at the bottom and working your way up to the scalp.

If your hair gets tangled at the beach, bring some instant conditioner and spray it on before you comb.

Whenever possible, rinse your hair after you've been in swimming—whether you've been in salt water or a chlorine pool. Both can do damage to your hair. A bottle of club soda makes a great rinse!

Try using combs in your wet hair so it will have extra fullness when it dries. Pull the hair back at the temples and fasten with combs. When it's dry, take out the combs and brush. For extra fullness, spray setting lotion on hair by your temples before clipping back.

If you usually blow-dry to straighten curly hair, try grabbing the head of hair and making a twist on top. Pull it up into one big knot or back into a French twist or any large knot that's flattering to your face. That should smooth out the hair. (But to tell the truth, if I had curly hair, I'd just let it dry naturally without even brushing it—and go!)

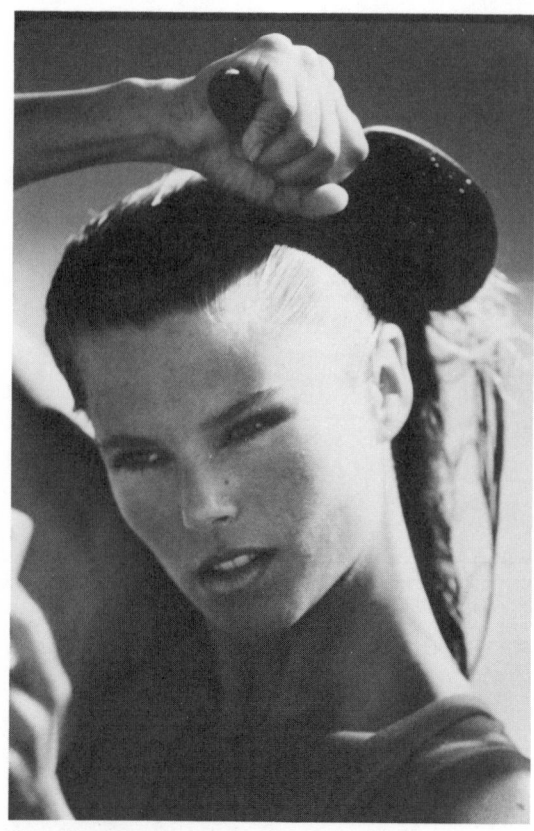

Never brush wet hair *unless* it's full of conditioners, like mine.

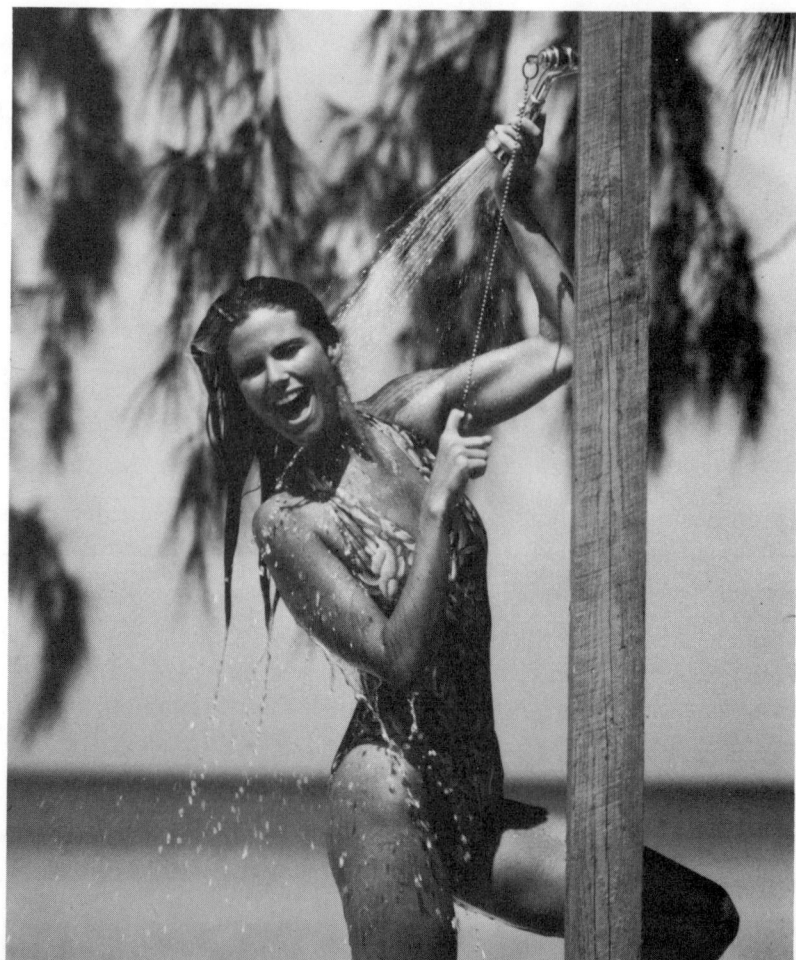

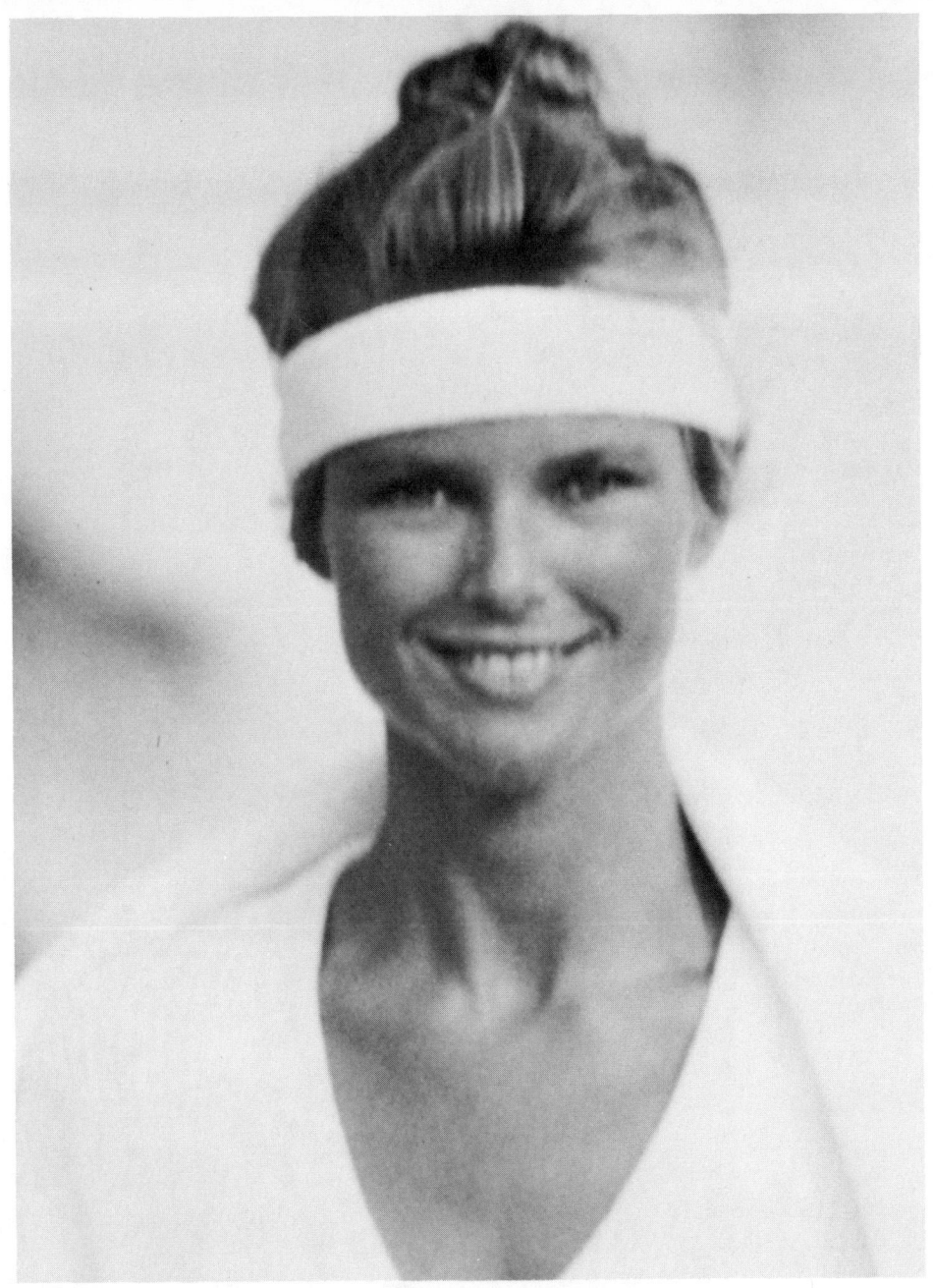

If you have fine or limp hair, setting lotion can be a big help by giving your hair more body and "grip." Put it on your damp hair and massage it into your scalp vigorously while holding your head upside down. Then you can put combs into it, put it into a knot, or just let it dry naturally. When it's dry, comb it out and you'll have lots of body.

Try twisting your wet hair into curls. It's easier on your hair than regular rollers. Hold each section of hair at the end and keep twisting it till it "collapses" into one curl. Then pin it to your head. When it's dry, it'll look like lots of natural waves.

For softer, natural-looking wavy curls, take sections of your hair and twist them (spray with lotion if your hair needs body) and roll the sections onto sponge rollers. The tighter the twist, the wavier the set.

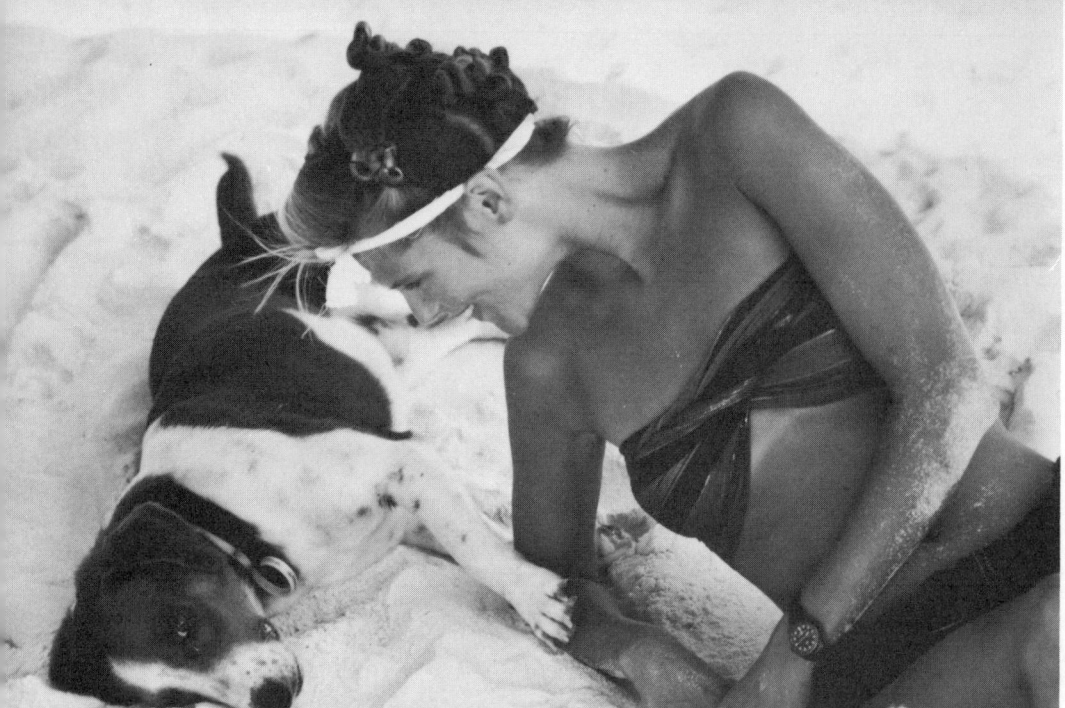

Sponge roller set and sponge roller comb-out

Twist set

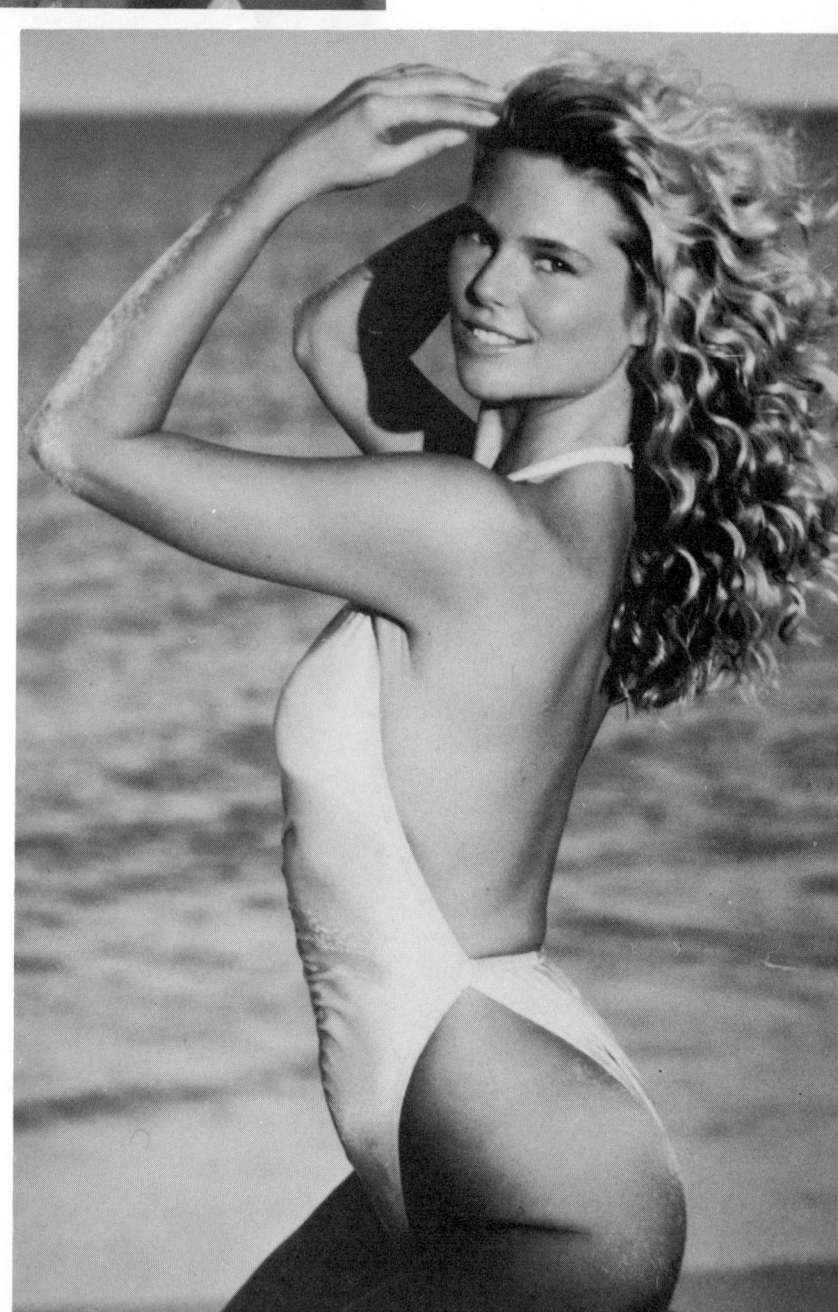

Twist set comb-out

146

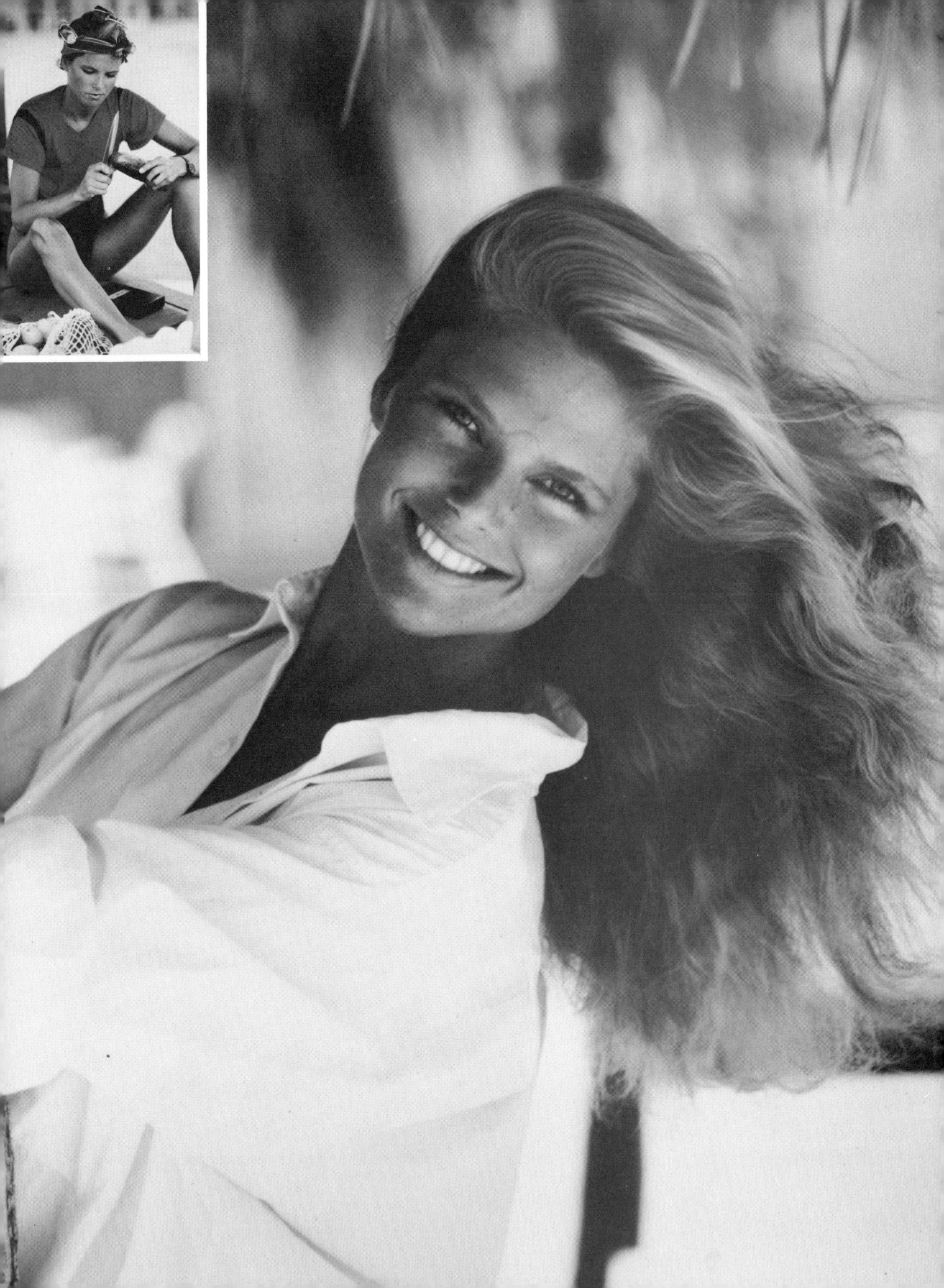

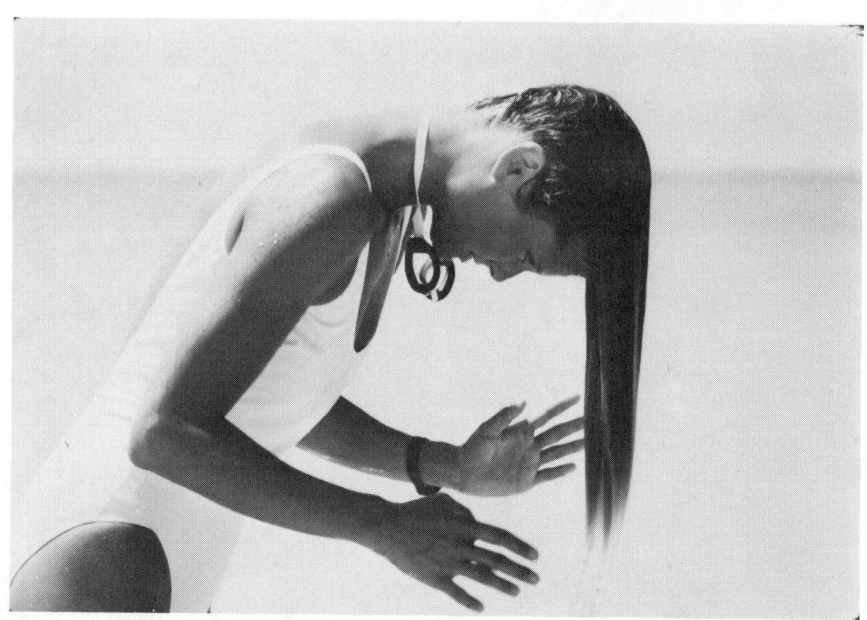

Dunk head upside down in water.

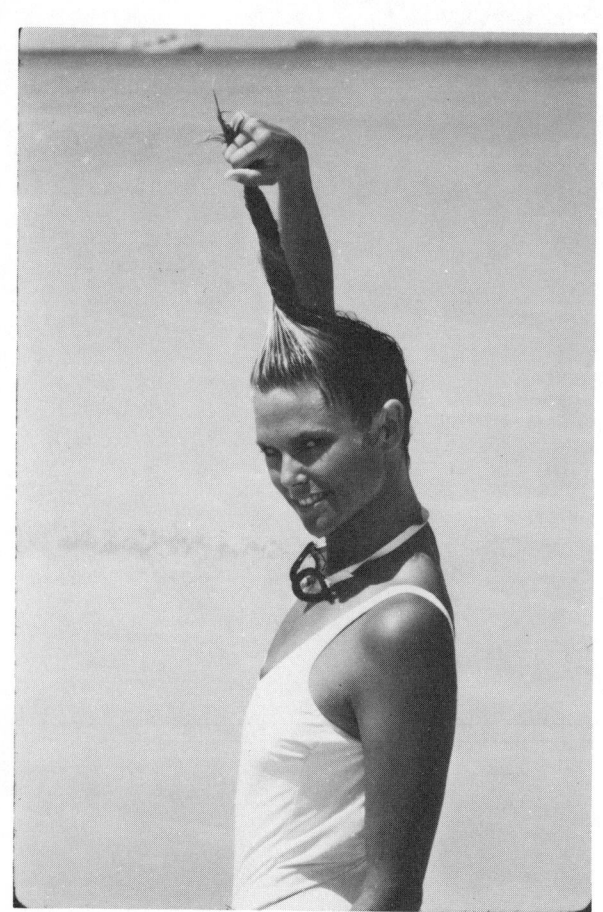

Grab hold of it and twist.

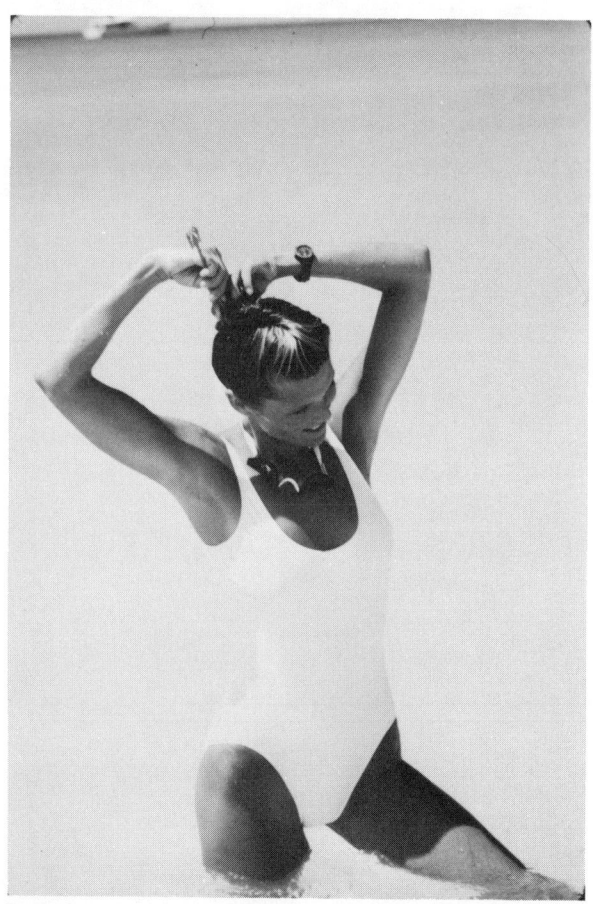

Fasten with swizzle sticks or chopsticks (or even a twig from a tree).

I bet you thought setting lotion was only used to give extra hold when using rollers. But lately, every time I walk into a photographer's studio, a hairdresser is using setting lotion in a different way. If you've never used it, now's the time to give it a try. Experiment with a few different brands until you find one that works well on your hair.

The three main uses for setting lotion are: as a texturizer, a controller, and as a set.

As a Texturizer

Take your favorite setting lotion and dilute it with water to half strength. (If you have extra-fine hair, you might want it a little stronger.) Put the diluted lotion into a spray bottle. Start with damp hair and spray the lotion on your head, concentrating on the roots. Now hang your head upside down and, using your hair dryer, dry your hair. Keep moving your fingers through your hair as you dry it. "Hair is like soufflé," one hairdresser told me. It's got to have plenty of air.

The lotion, combined with an upside-down drying, will encourage your hair to dry with a body and fullness that's great. And much longer-lasting than you could ever get without the lotion.

But remember, you want to concentrate the lotion on the roots of your hair. If you have fine or very dry hair, the combination of heat and lotion on the ends could be damaging.

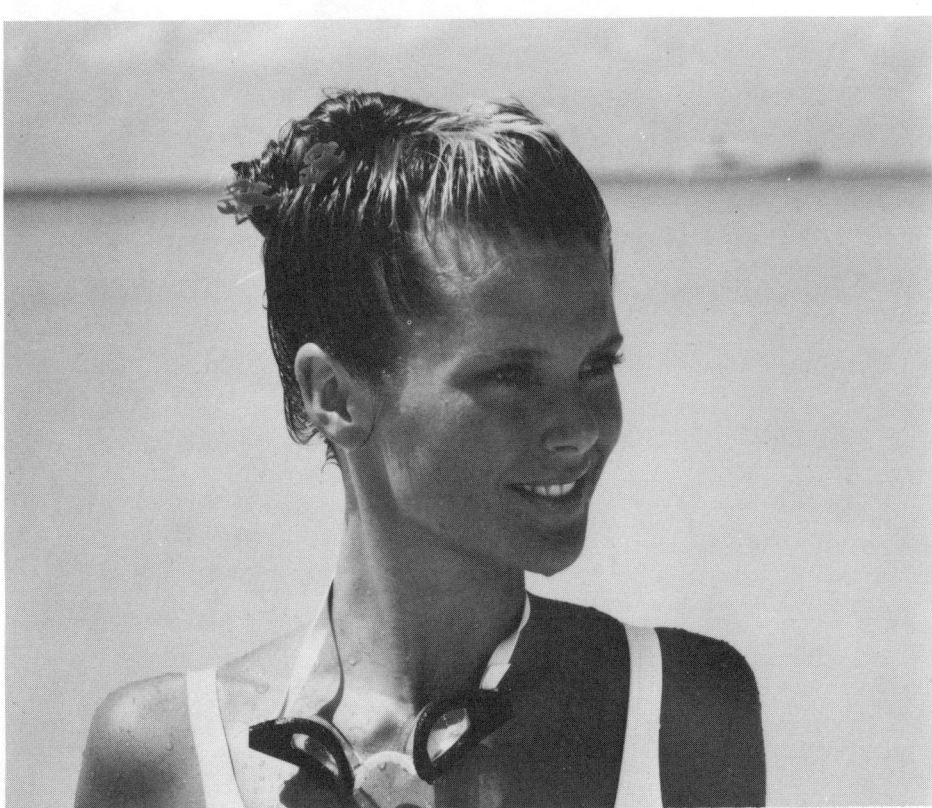

Finished look

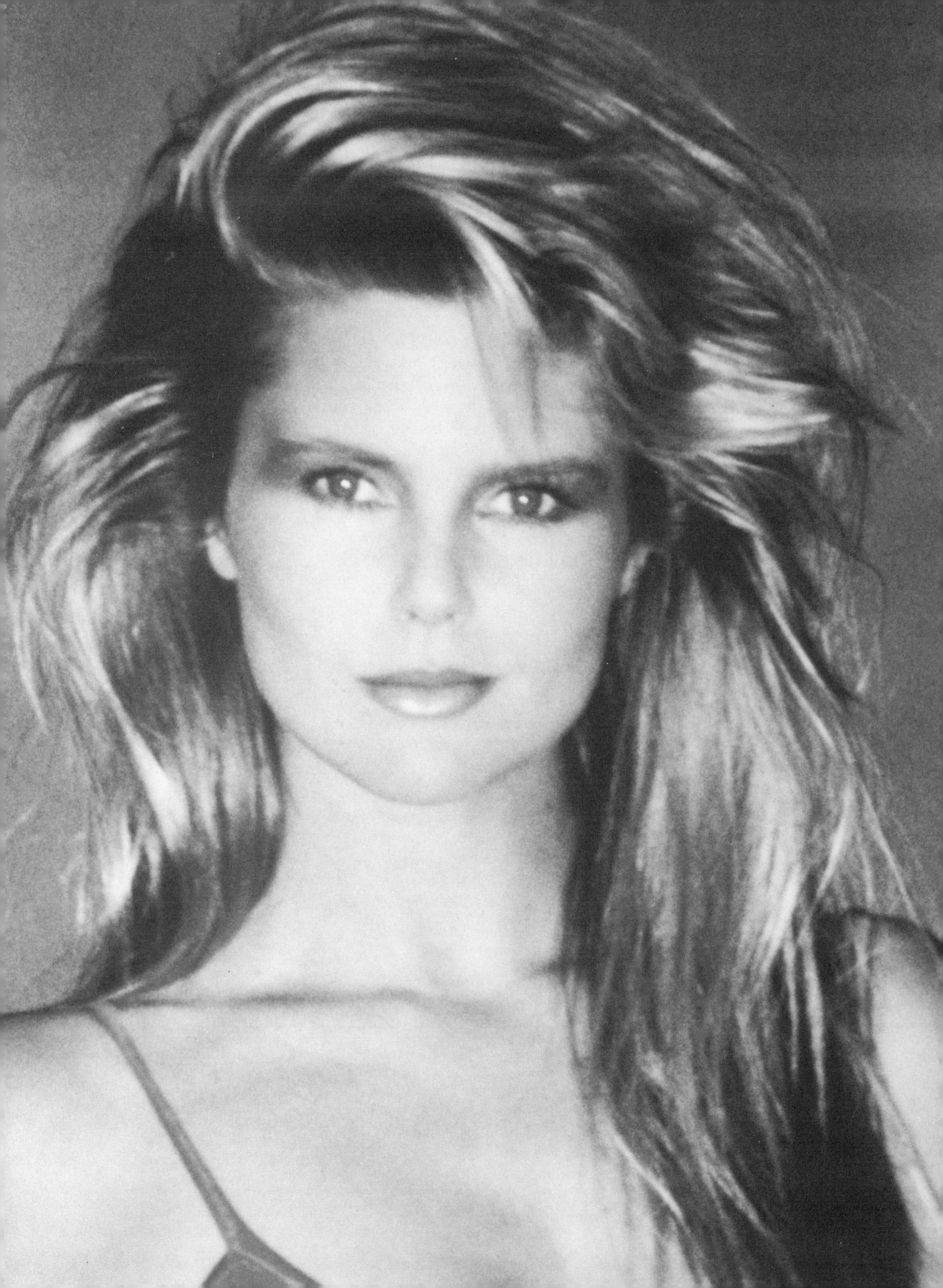

If you want an even more dramatic, wild, evening look, when you've finished drying your hair, back-brush it by lightly brushing sections from mid-hair length toward the scalp. Start at the crown and work toward the forehead. After brushing, smooth hair with your fingertips. The setting lotion gives the hair better "grip" and you can get real fullness without a teased look.

As a Control

Setting lotion is a great way to control hair, whether it's straight, curly, long or short. You can get a severe tuxedo look, a boyish look, or a spiky look. You just apply the lotion, style your hair, and let it dry.

Setting lotion will also give you extra control when you want to keep your bangs brushed back or keep all your hair in a sleek non-wispy ponytail or twist. Just dab it on where you need to tame some strands.

As a Set

Setting lotion will give your set staying power. And you can always use it half strength for a milder hold. Just spray it on each section before rolling. And when your whole head is set, spray all the rollers again. You'll have more hold when it dries.

The tuxedo look

The ponytail tamer

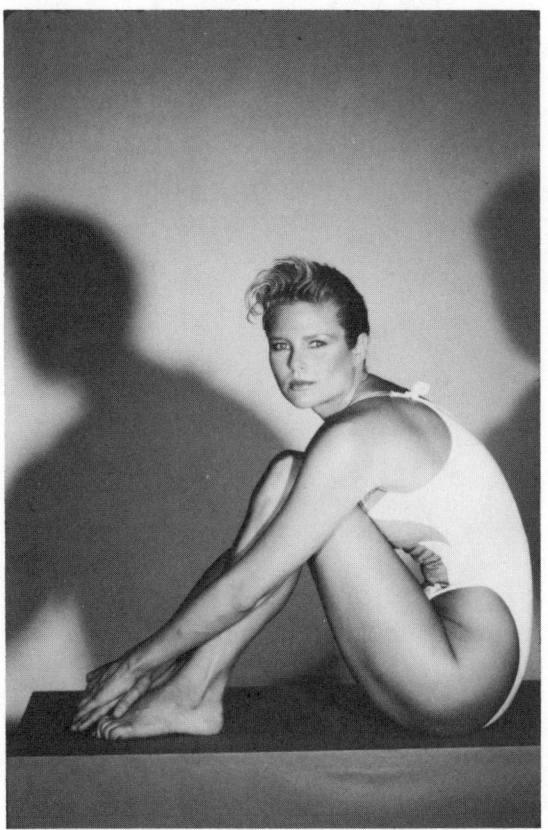

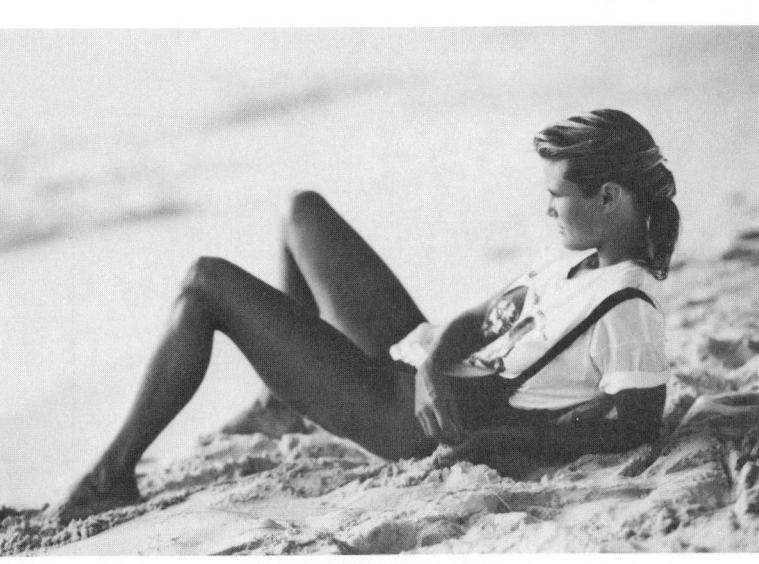

The dramatic evening look

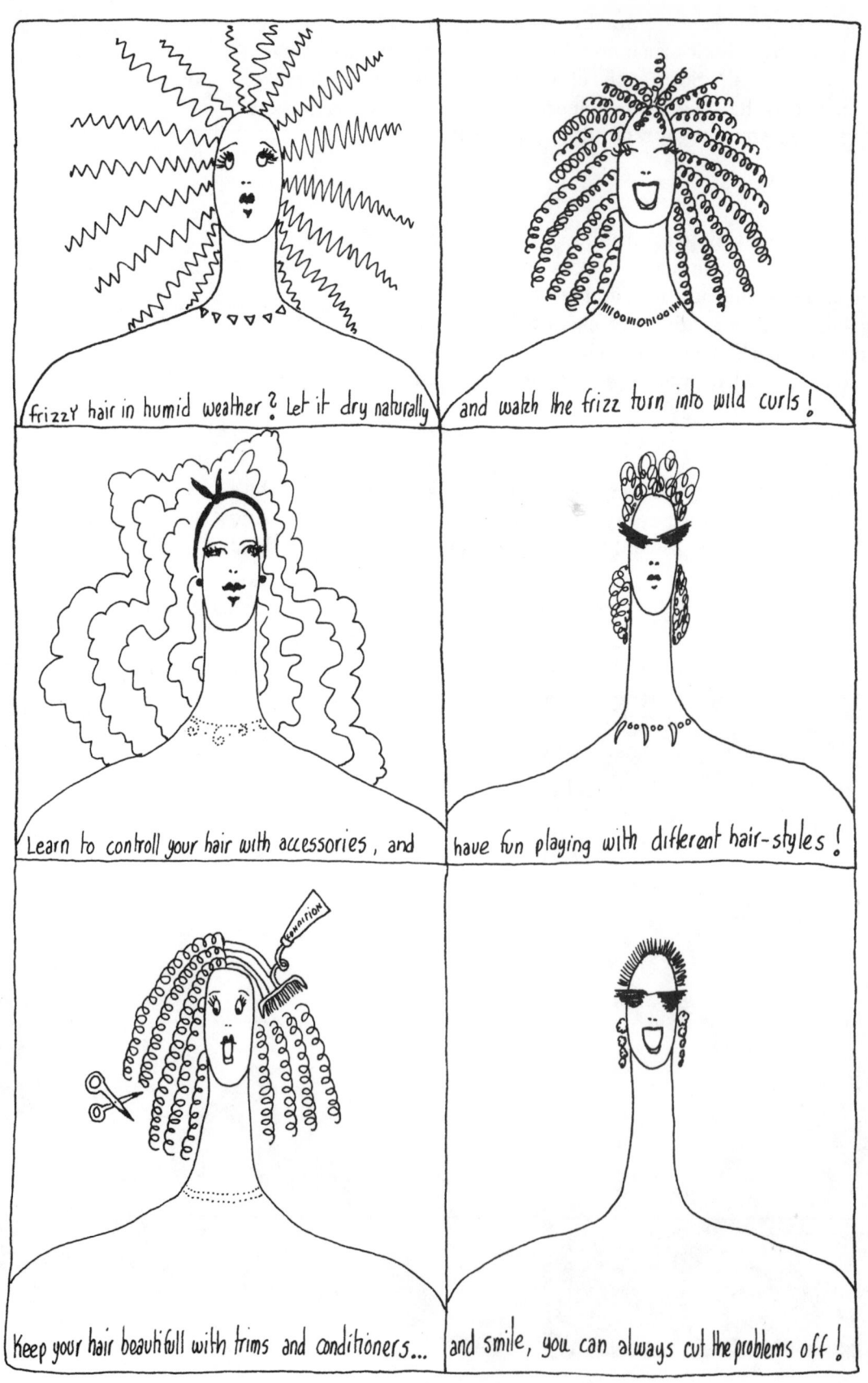

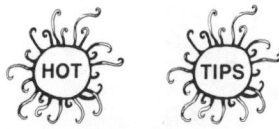

If you're a blonde and you're thinking about having your hair cut, get it done at the beginning of the summer. It looks darker after cutting and an early cut means that you have the whole summer to let it lighten in the sun!

Lemon juice—if you're using it for highlighting—will dry hard on your hair, as if you had poured a bottle of setting lotion on it. So have fun combing your hair into different shapes.

If you have very hard water and your hair is oily, by all means avoid using an acid shampoo —one with a low pH. The acid reacts with the hard water and somehow makes it very difficult to rinse the oils and dirt out of your hair. Even just after shampooing, your hair can look dirty and stringy.

If your hair turns green from the chlorine in a swimming pool, mash six aspirin into warm water and comb it through your wet hair. Let it sit a few minutes and when you rinse it out you'll rinse out the green, too!

Don't overexpose your face to the sun while trying to highlight your hair. A visor is the answer. The hair is exposed and the face is shaded.

Beach party over? Take that half can of flat beer and comb it through your hair. It acts like a setting lotion. When it's dry, comb it out for lots of body and shape. (And I promise you won't smell like a brewery!)

Flat champagne poured over blond hair and then rinsed out will give wonderful highlights!

Here's a great natural hair conditioner that'll keep you pretty on a desert island. Mix about a teaspoon of avocado with coconut milk. Comb it through your hair and leave on for about 5 minutes. Rinse and shine!

If you've brought a lemon to the beach for hair lightening, after you've cut it in half and used it on your hair, put the halves of the lemon on your elbows (or ankles, knees, or fingernails!). Prop yourself up and watch the world go by. After 10 or 15 minutes your elbows will be bleached white and won't have that dingy look.

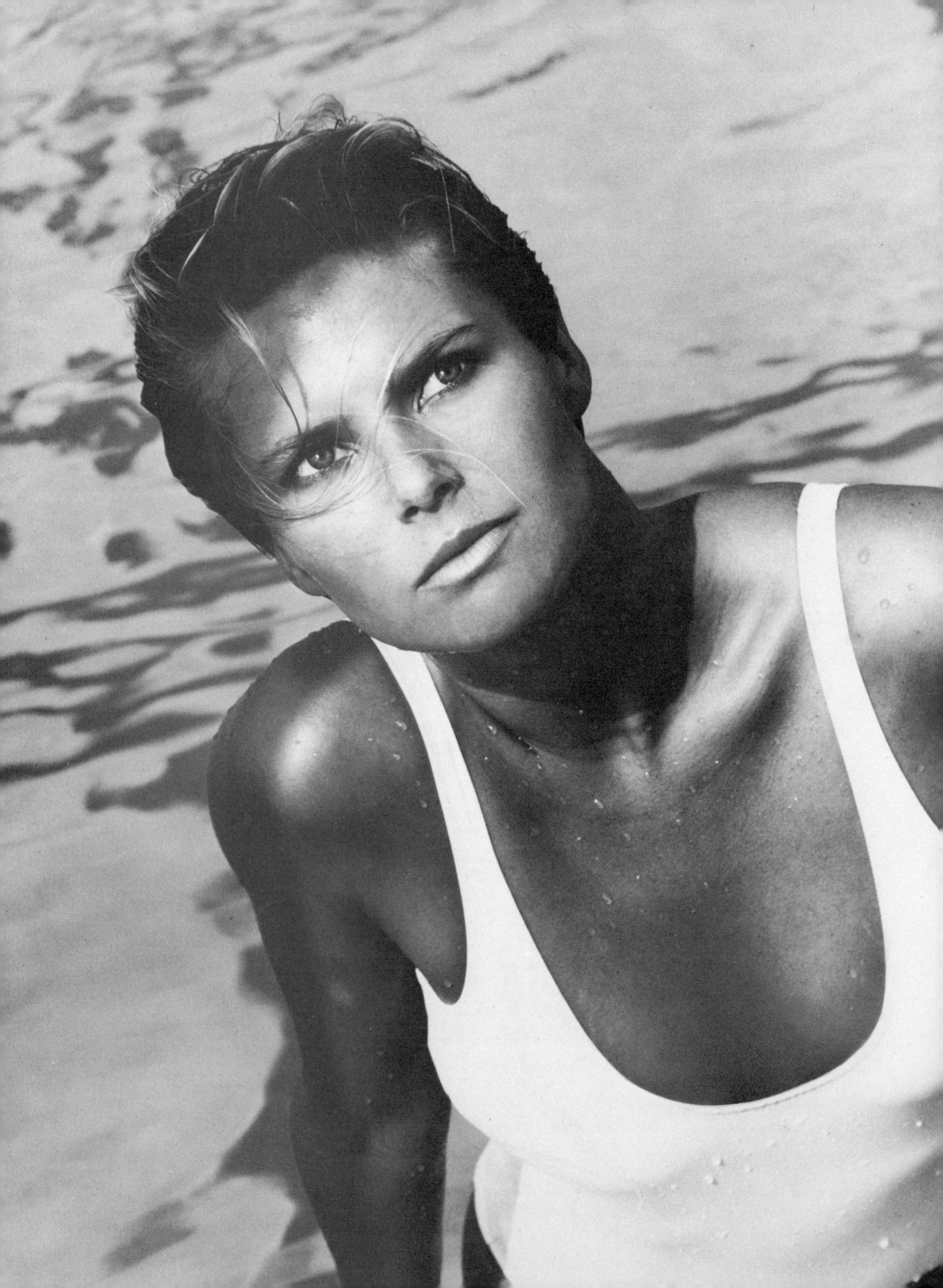

THE SEA

I love swimming! And swimming in the ocean is about my all-time favorite activity. It's great exercise but doesn't seem like work at all. In fact, swimming is the best exercise there is. It's aerobic—it gets your heart pumping and your blood circulating. It trims and firms almost every muscle in your body, but because the water is supporting you, you're not likely to strain the muscles as you work them.

I'm a good swimmer and I like to give myself a workout by doing the crawl or the breaststroke. It takes about twenty minutes of this to really get my heart pumping and my muscles warmed up. Sometimes I use one of those kickboards for exercising my hips and thighs, which I suppose are everybody's major swimsuit figure problem. The little kickboard is handy because it helps you keep your head above water and I find I do a lot more leg exercising with it than I would do if I had to concentrate on keeping my face above water at the same time.

SWIMMING

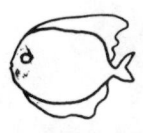

Bodysurfing is great fun and great exercise! It combines swimming and running, and while you're running you're usually moving through the resistance of the water, which makes it that much more strenuous and good for you. I especially like to bodysurf because it's like a game—you versus the sea. Of course you need the sea for this one; bodysurfing in a concrete pool is too much of a challenge even for me.

BODYSURFING

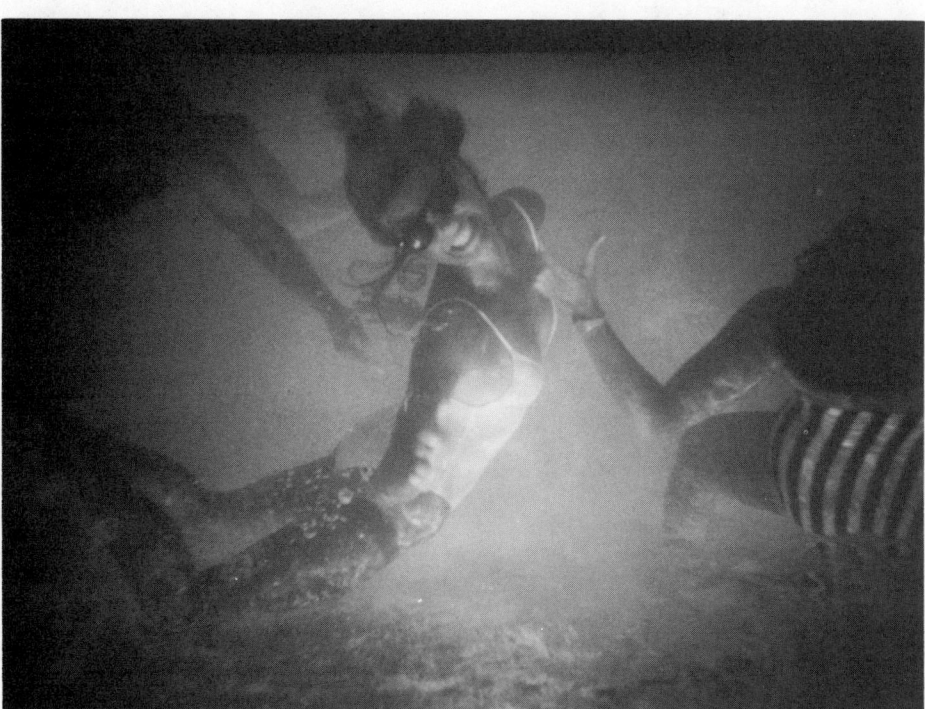

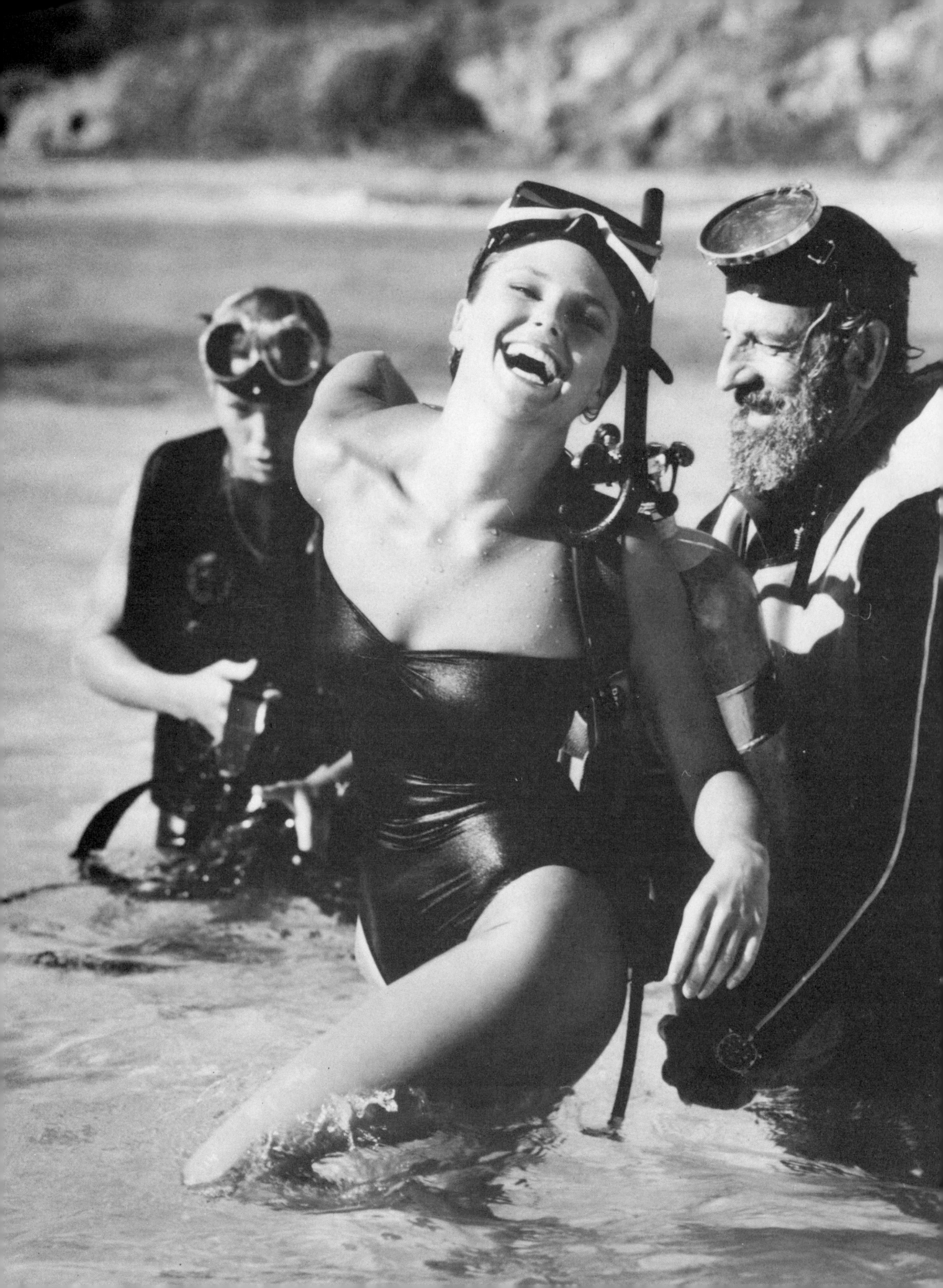

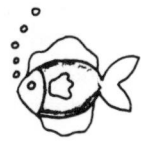 Scuba diving is another of my favorite water sports. When you're under water with all those beautiful fish and exotic coral and plant life, it's like flying through another world. I never think of scuba diving as exercise but in fact, it's a terrific body conditioner. It does wonderful things for your legs. Those big flippers really give your thighs and calves a workout. And having the weight of the tank on your back, which increases as you move toward the surface, gives your muscles even greater resistance. It has the same effect as working out with weights but it's lots more fun.

SCUBA DIVING

 Snorkeling is also a good exercise for the legs. But watch out for your back! Many people get so involved watching the amazing sea life they forget about the sun being magnified on their backs and end up with a bad burn!

SNORKELING

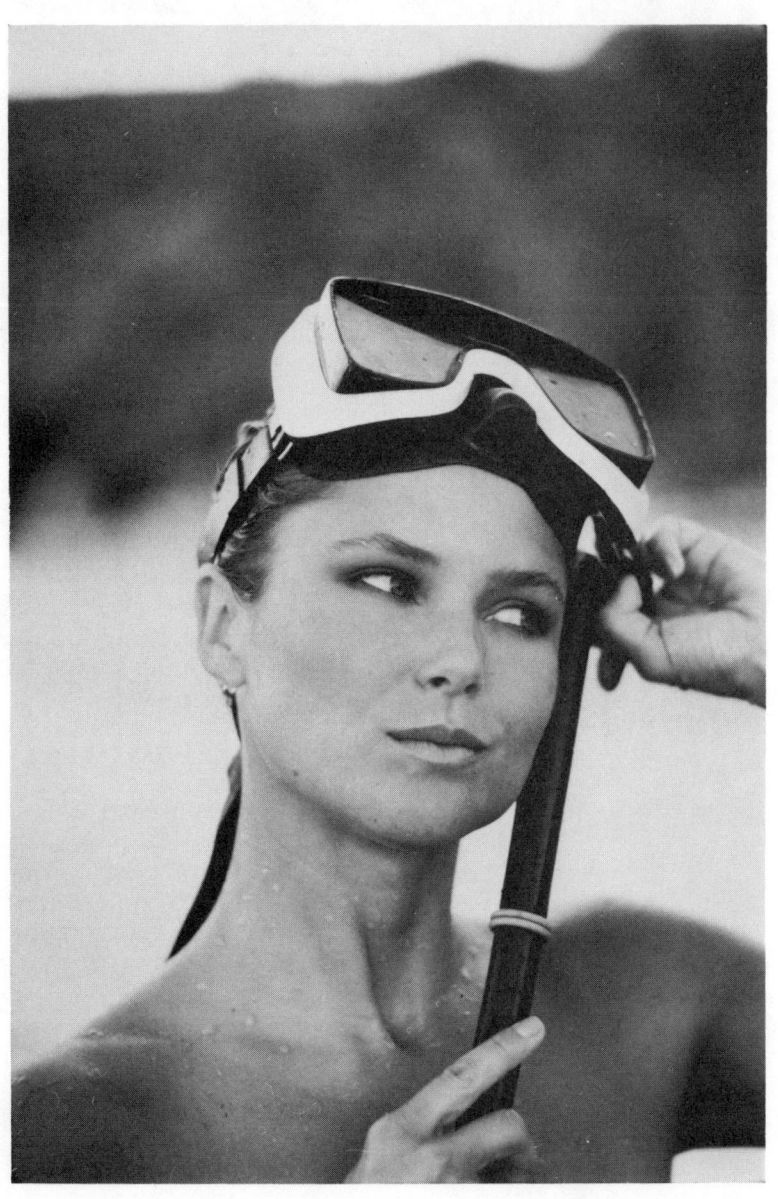

SAILING

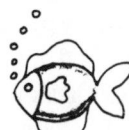

Sailing is a fabulous sport because you can do it at any age and any level of activity. I find that sailing a small boat single-handed gives your body the best workout. You're moving from one side of the boat to the other, bracing your legs, shifting your weight, and really working out your arms and shoulders as you trim the sheets. Windsurfing, which uses about the smallest sailboat around, is fabulous exercise because you're in constant motion and you're using almost every muscle in your body. If you're lucky enough to be on a large sailboat you'll surely have a great time, but you'll probably do more chatting and eating and drinking than exercising. In that case, I advise getting off the boat for a vigorous swim.

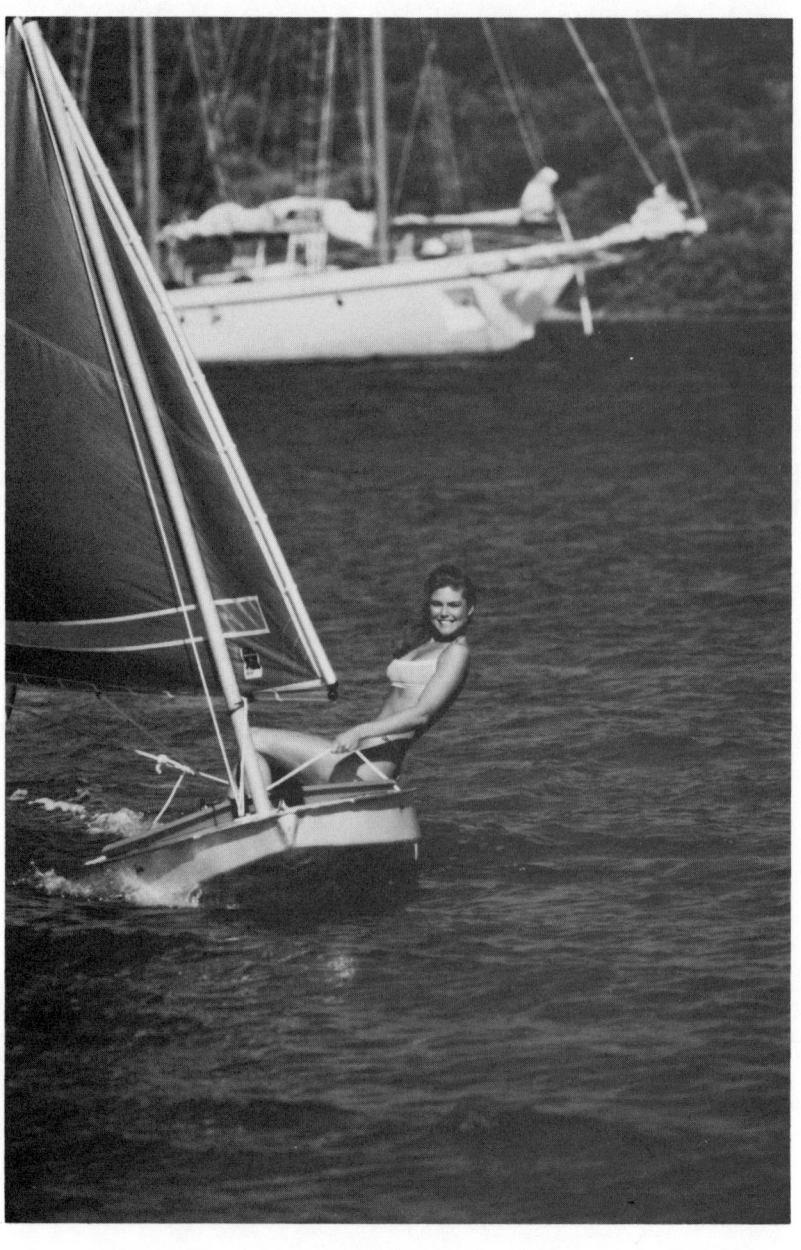

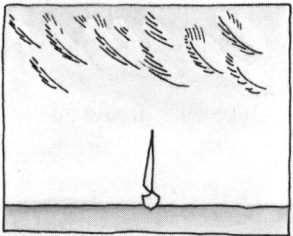

CIRRUS

HIGH WISPY clouds resembling feathers. Early warning of bad weather if followed by cloud build-up. Cirrus dissolving means improving conditions.

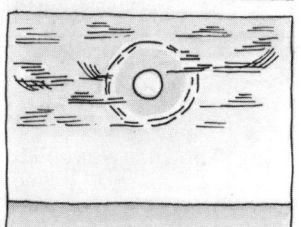

CIRROSTRATUS

WITH SOLAR halo_foul weather indicated, especially following cirrus clouds. The larger the halo, the sooner the onset of bad weather.

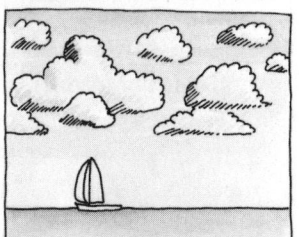

CUMULUS

Small fluffy clouds signal fair weather, but watch out if they grow larger_ you can expect bad weather with thundery showers.

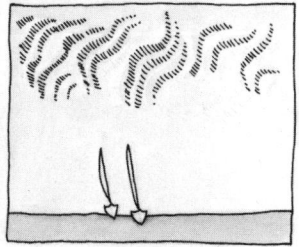

CIRRO-CUMULUS

or "mackerel sky". Formation resembles fish scales and indicates a change in the weather. as the sailors say, "mackerel sky, mackerel sky, not long wet, not long dry."

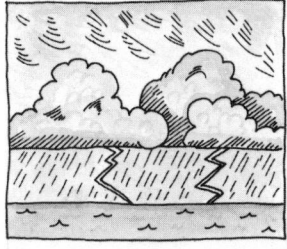

CUMULO-NIMBUS

or "thunder clouds"_ Like cumulus but has "false" cirrus on top. Brings heavy rain and possibly violent squalls. Get out your foul-weather gear!

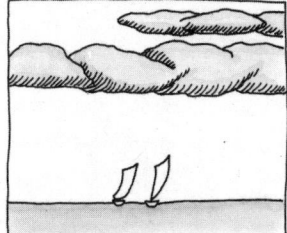

STRATO-CUMULUS

Dark "twisted" shape clouds. Strato-cumulus clouds, despite their coloring, do not bring rain.

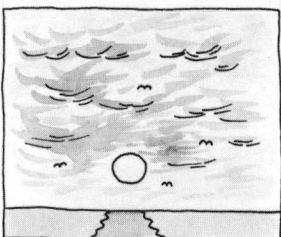

Pink sky at night, sailors' delight.

Pink sky in morning sailors take warning.

WATER EXERCISES

Water is a wonderful medium for exercise. It provides resistance and helps develop muscular strength. It also provides buoyancy and eliminates the stress of gravity on the spine. Because there's very little tension on the muscles, they remain supple and there's less chance that they will cramp. Water exercises are especially good for pregnant women and people with knee injuries as they put absolutely no stress on the body.

I use water as often as I can as my favorite place to exercise. The spray and resistance of the water are marvelously therapeutic. In thalassotherapy, high-pressure jets of water are shot against the body as a form of massage. They say it stimulates, relieves tension, and improves circulation. I've always found that standing in the breaking waves has had that effect on me and exercising in water amplifies it!

All of the above are great reasons to do water exercises, but my favorite reason is that it's fun.

Next time you're at the beach or in a pool, instead of just floating around, try some of the following exercises. Then invent some of your own—whenever a movement in the water causes resistance, simply repeat it a couple of times!

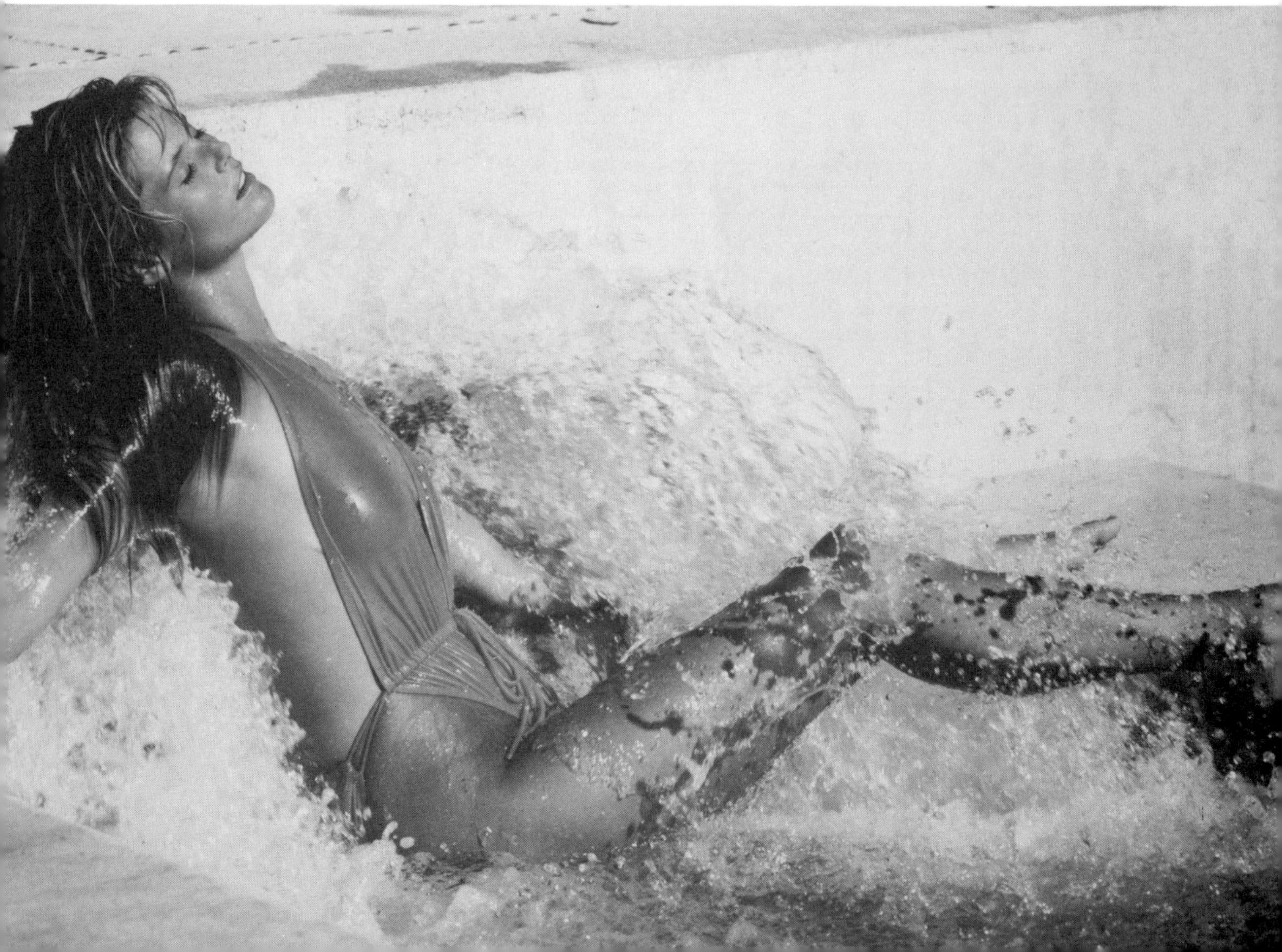

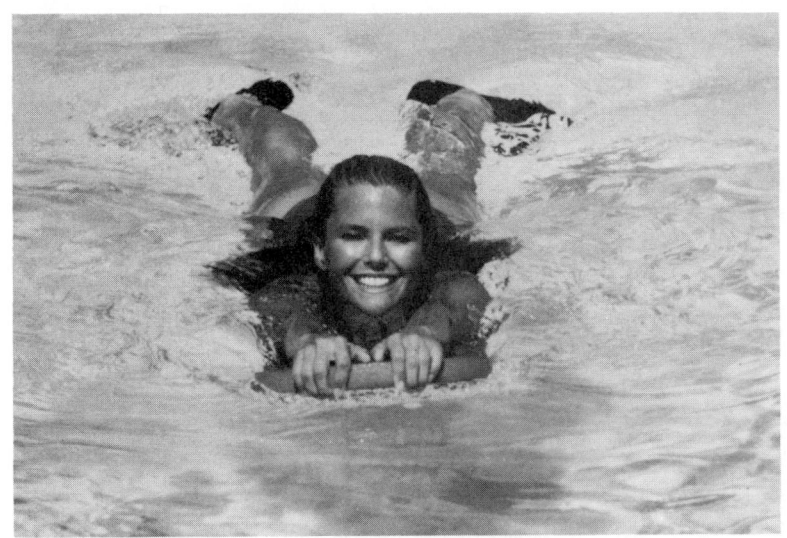

La Grenouille (Translation: The Frog)
This "scissors kick" does a great job on your legs and fanny. Because of the power of the flippers, it's like using an exercise machine. Hold on to the top of a kickboard and extend your legs behind you. Open your legs as wide as you can and pull your body backward through the water. Close your legs and propel yourself forward.

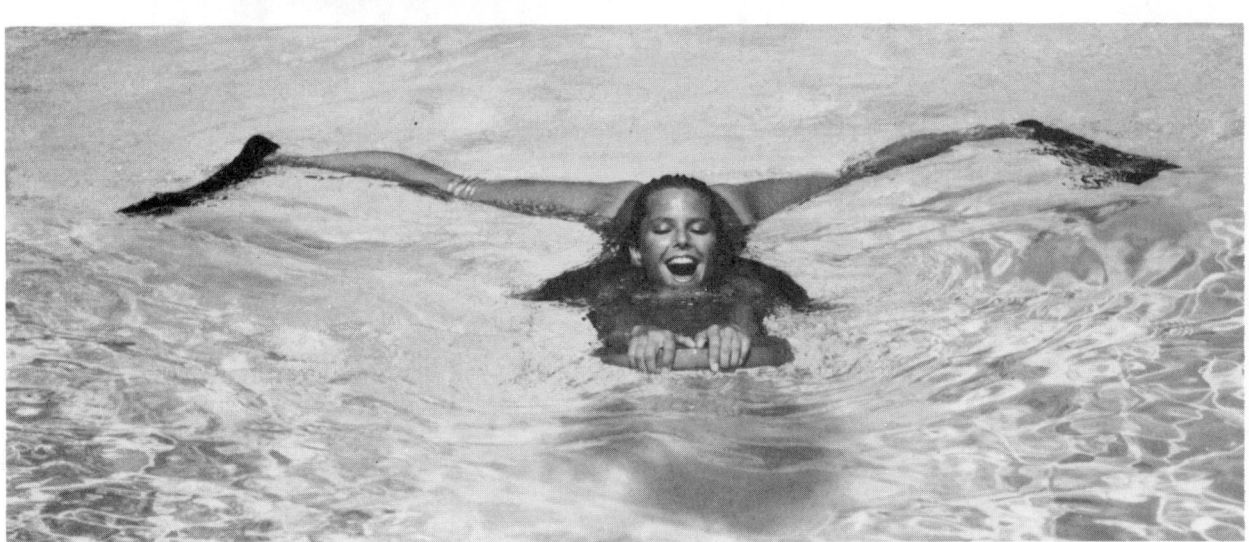

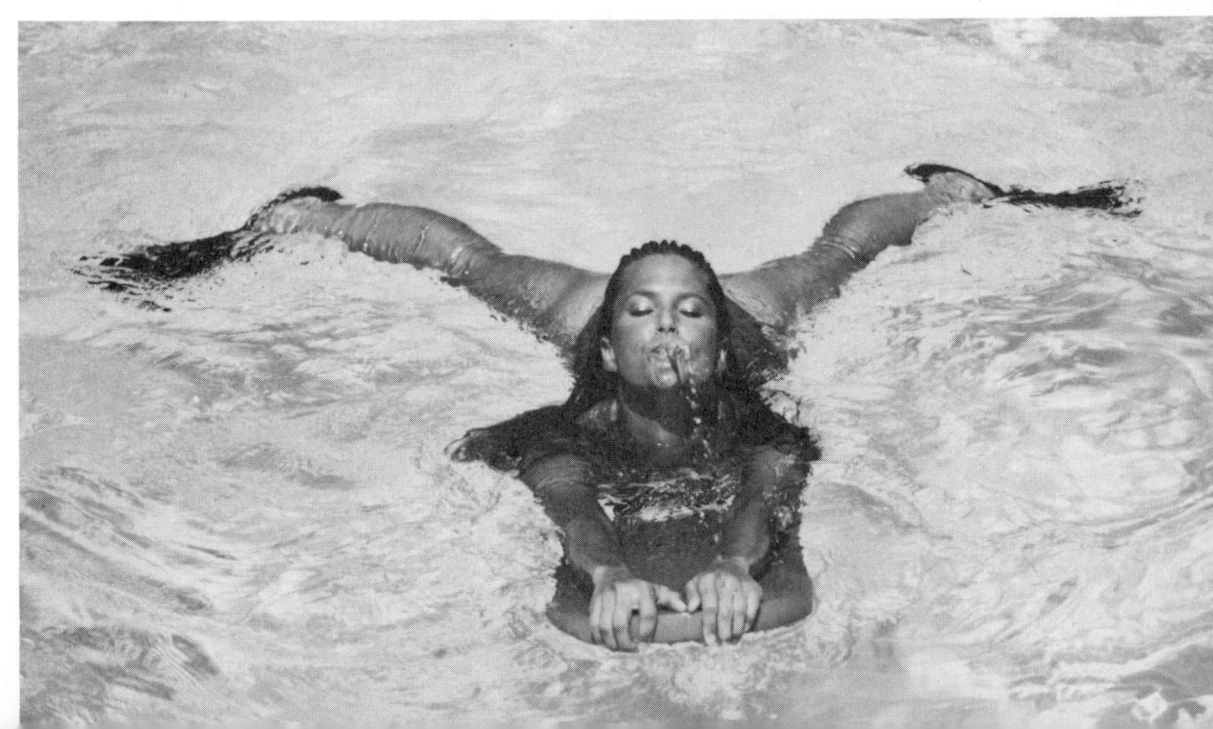

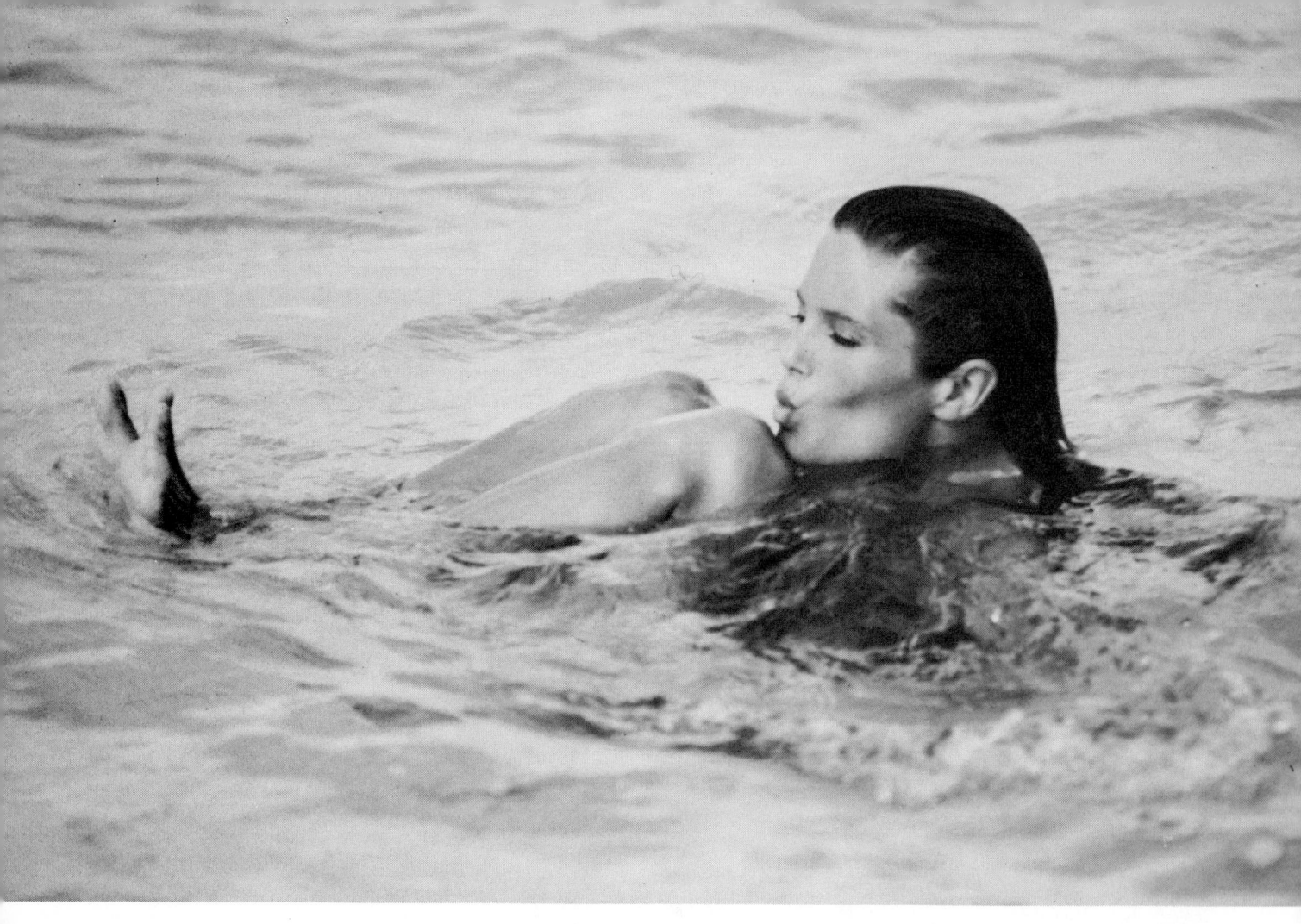

Mama Mia! (My mom's invention)
Tuck yourself into a round ball. Try to keep your knees up to your chin. Point your toes out of the water and paddle your arms. You'll feel this one in your stomach, thighs, and arms. For variety, try racing with a friend!

Scissors Kick

This is good for the legs and stretches the torso as well. It's much like *La Grenouille* except that I don't think it's quite as effective. But you don't need the flippers or kickboard to do this one. Hold the edge of the pool or the pool ladder with your legs extended behind you. Open your legs as wide as you can, feeling the pull on the inside of your thighs. Close legs and repeat.

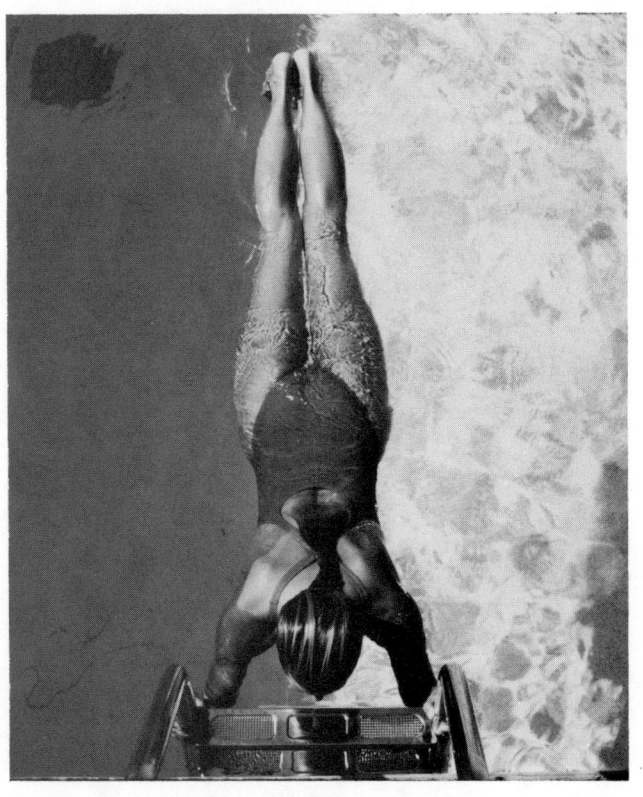

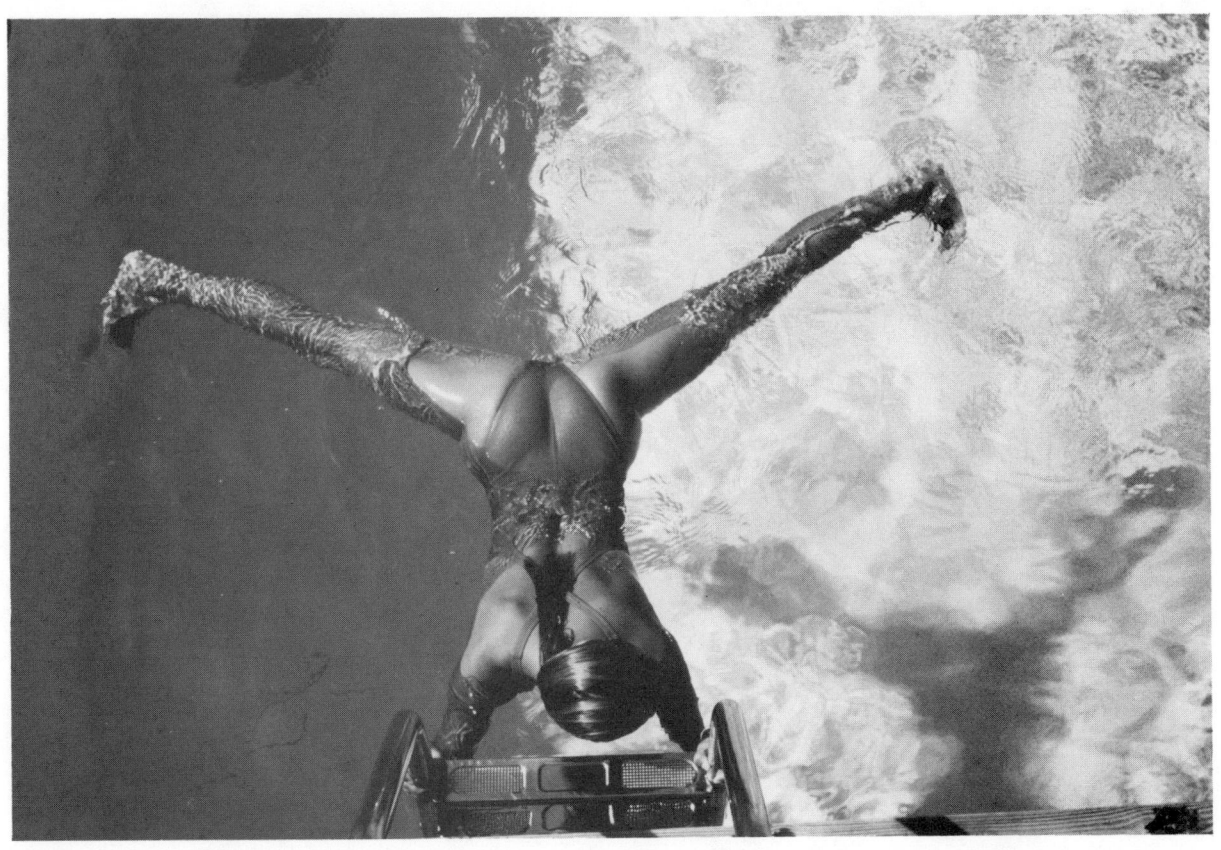

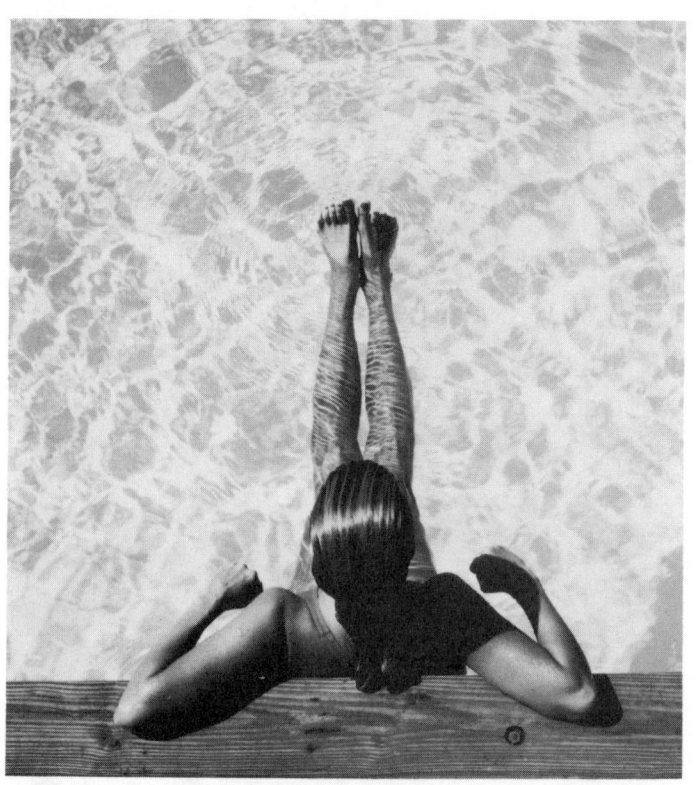

Reverse Scissors Kick

This is good for the thighs (especially the inner thighs) and the stomach. With your back to the edge of the pool, hook your arms over the side of the pool to hold yourself in place. Extend your legs in front of you with your toes pointing up out of the water. Open your legs as wide as possible, holding the extension for a moment or two. Keep your toes out of the water and your feet flexed. Repeat the scissors movement. Maintain a fast rhythm.

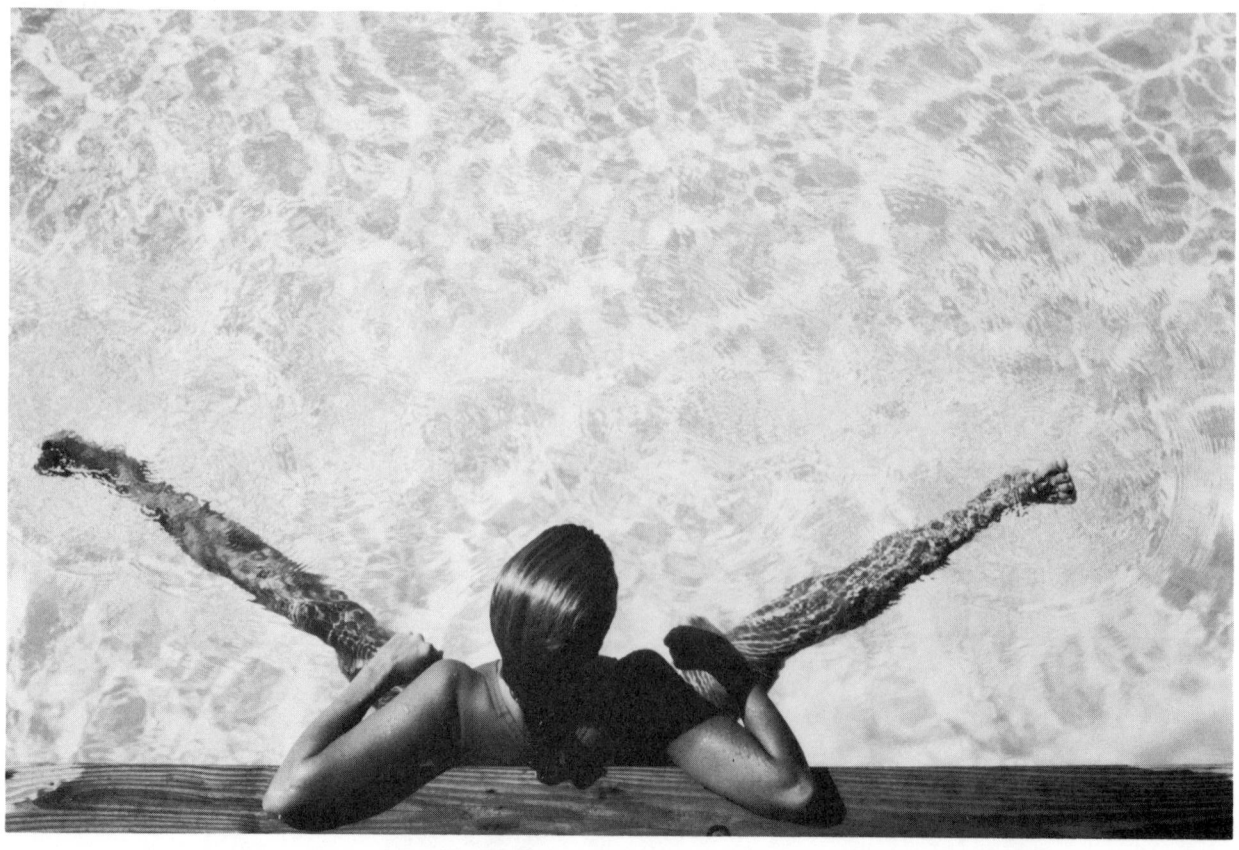

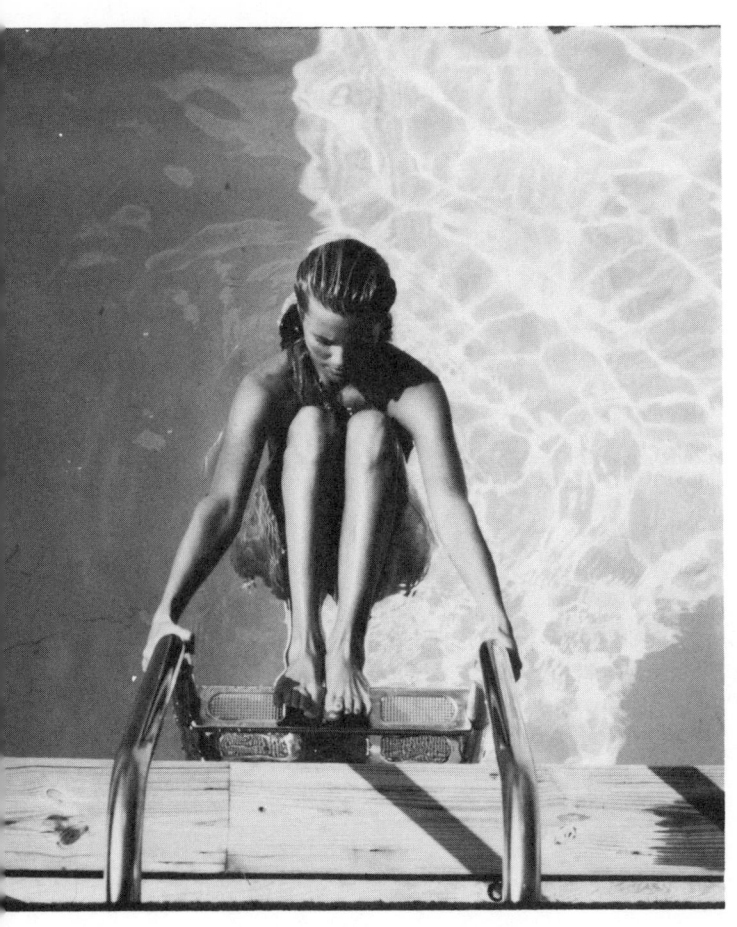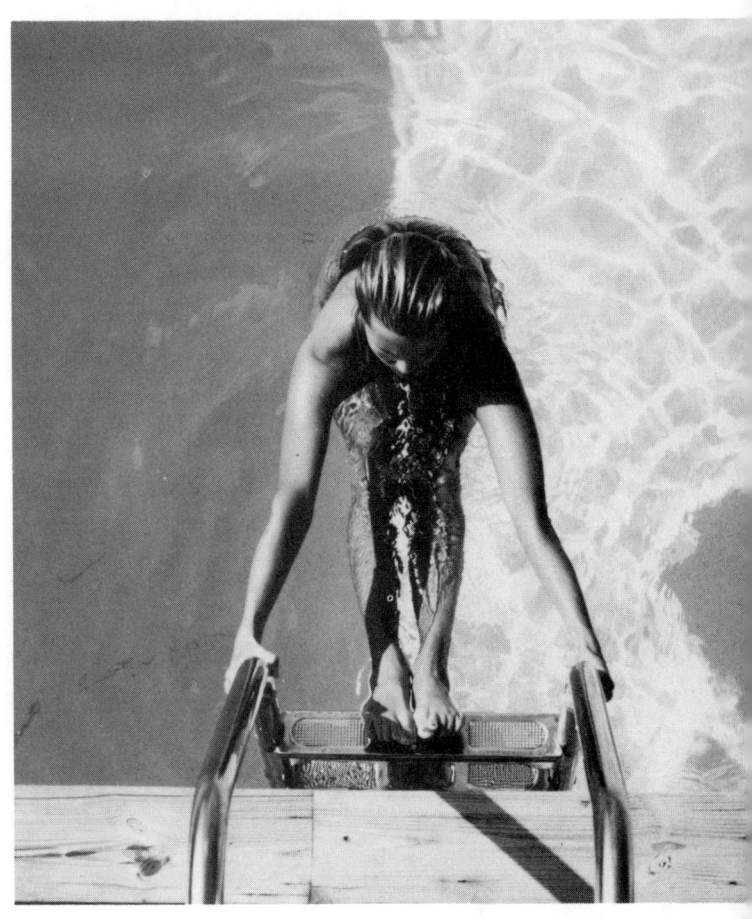

Hamstring Stretch
This stretches the hamstring and limbers up the legs. Hold the ladder at the side of the pool and with your knees bent, place your feet so that your knees almost reach your chin. Slowly straighten your knees until they are completely straight. If you're more advanced, lower your chest to your knees.

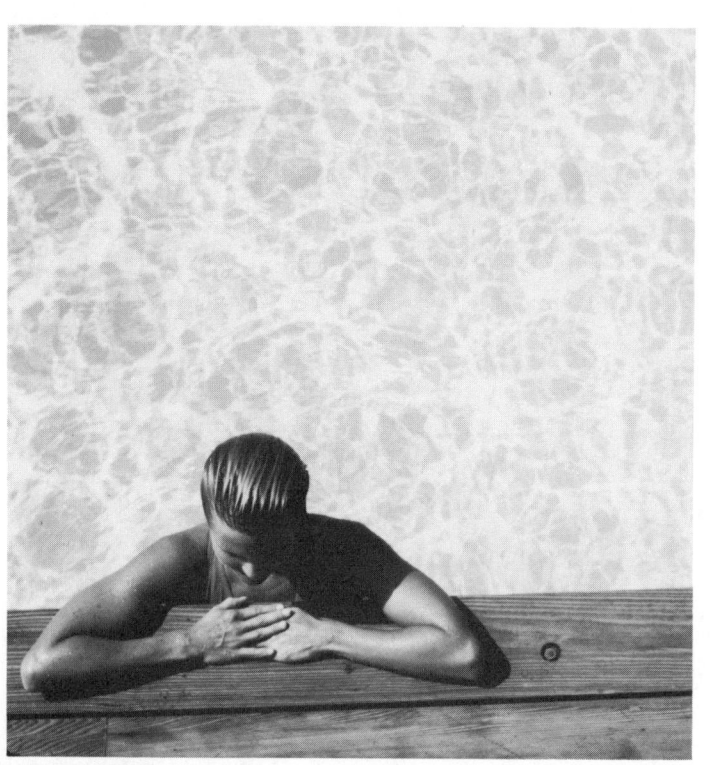

The Pendulum

This is a fine waist-trimmer. Hold your body in a straight line against the wall of a pool, gripping edges, your back to the water. Keeping your feet together, swing both legs at once to the side. Bring them to the surface of the water if you can. Reverse to the other side and repeat.

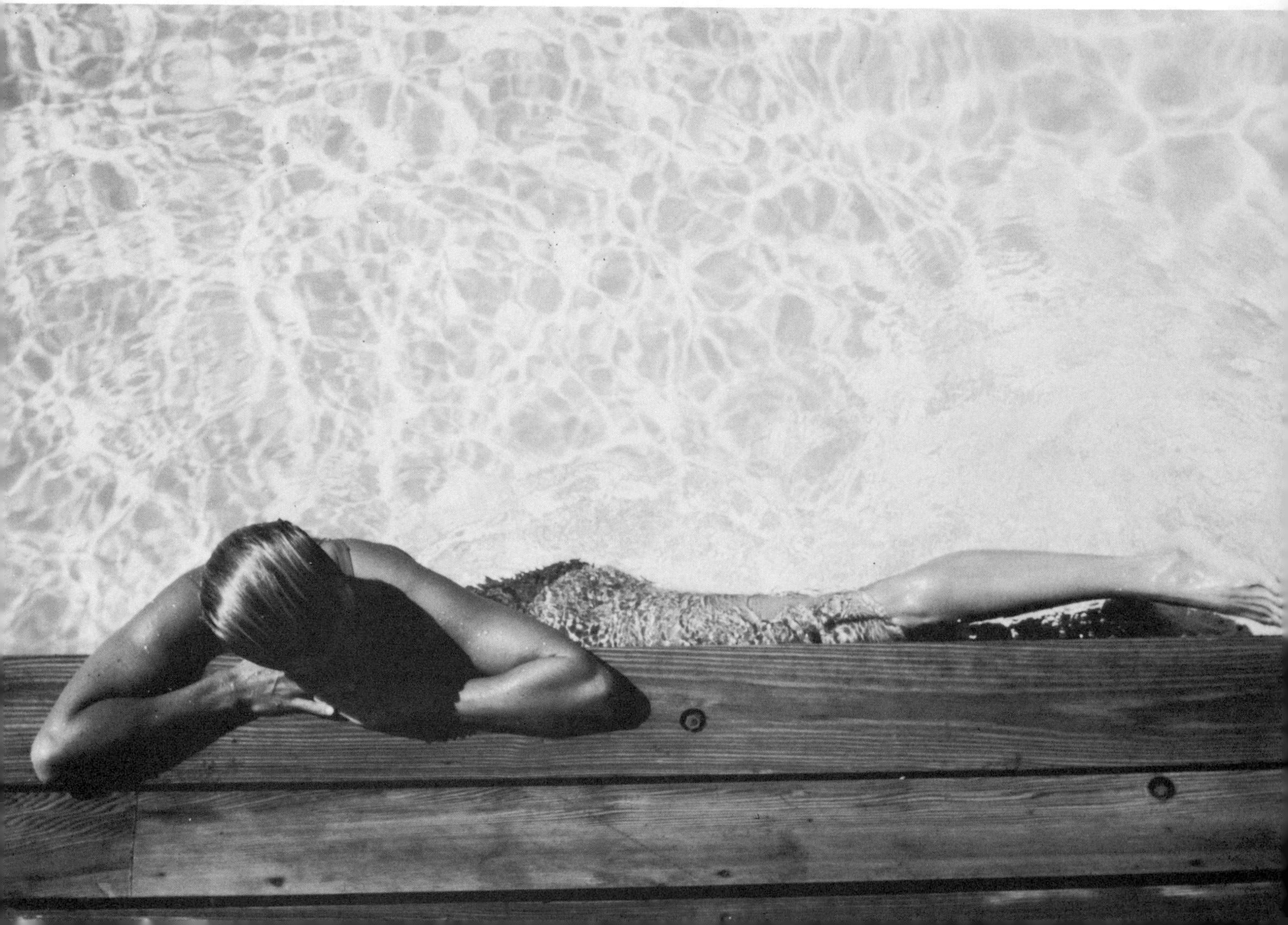

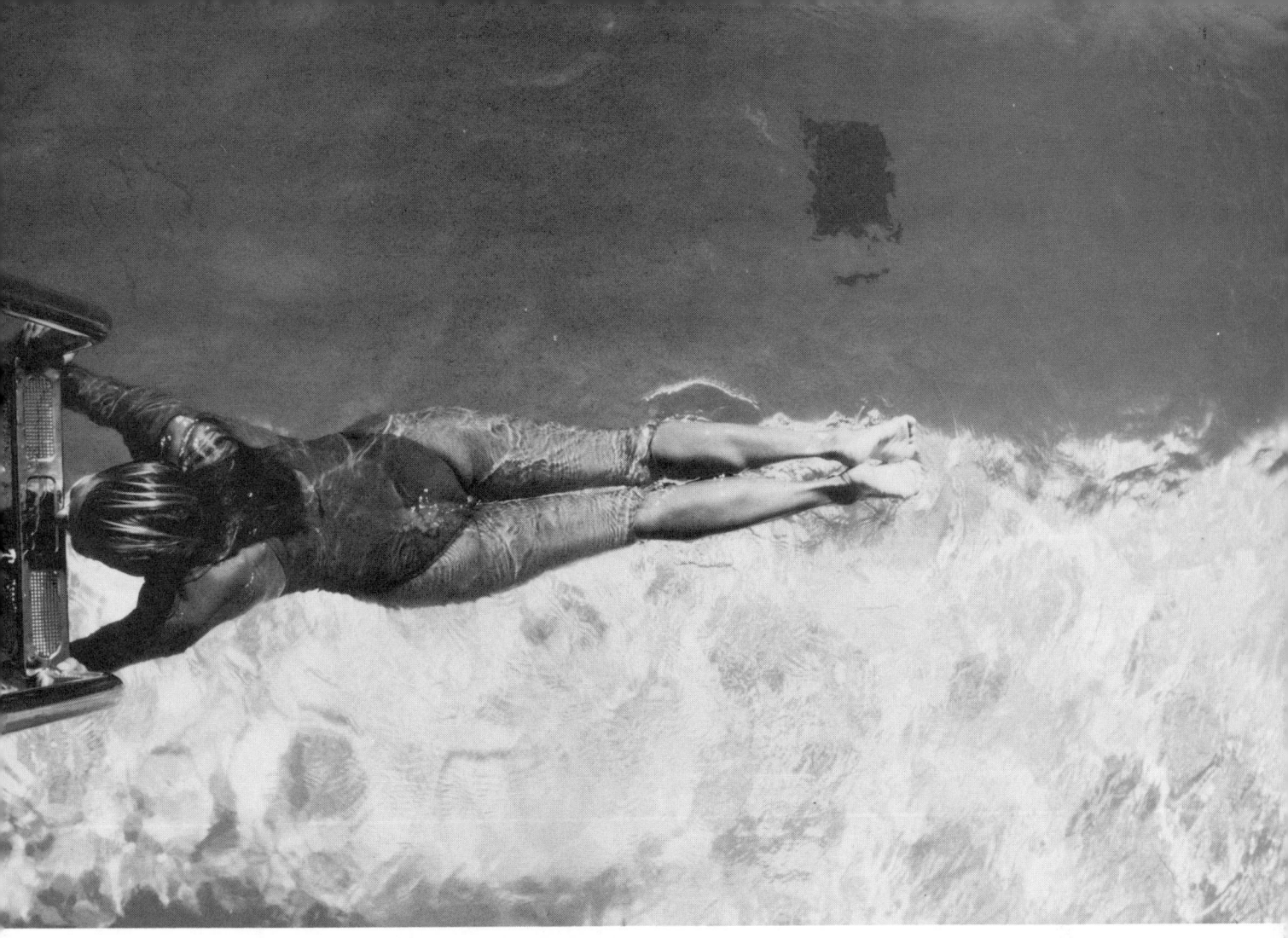

Leg Lift
This is a good workout for the lower back. Hold the side of the pool with your legs stretched out behind you near the surface. Keeping legs straight and body flat, lift your feet out of the water behind you. Ouch!

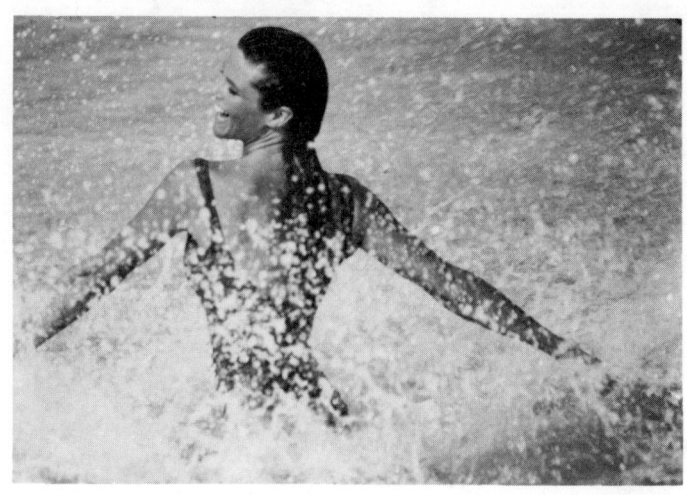

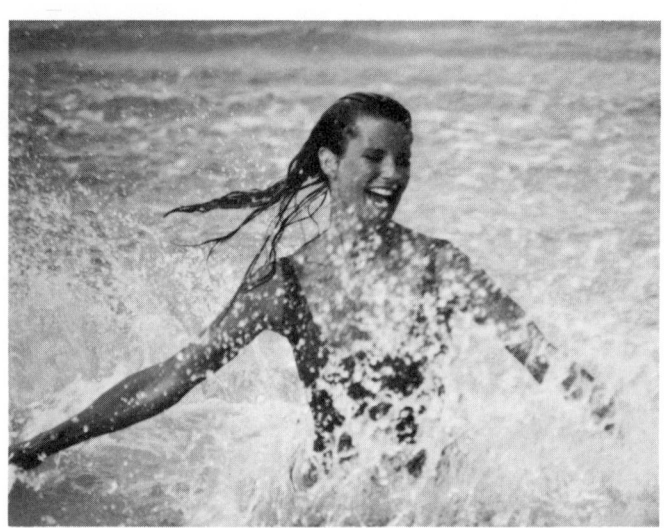

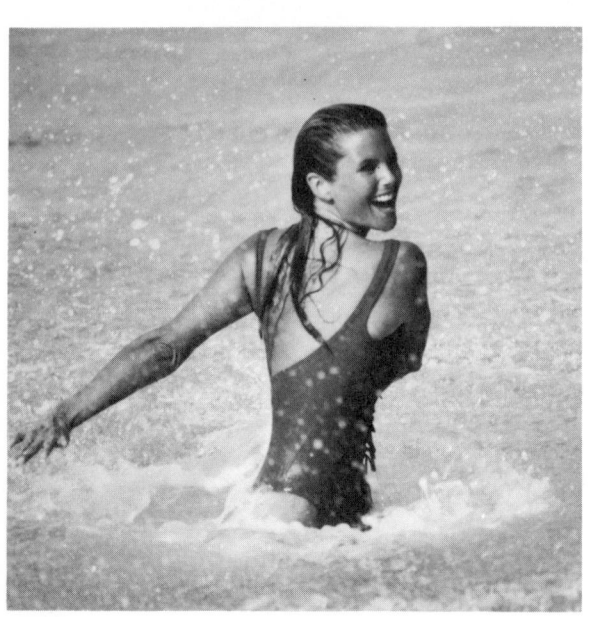

Splash Twists
This is good for the whole upper body —especially the waist. It's also fun to do! Stand in water that's about waist deep. Keep your feet apart for balance. Cup your hands and dip them into the water. The deeper your hands, the more difficult the exercise. Twist from the waist, keeping your hands below the surface of the water for resistance. Twist as far as you can to the right and then reverse and twist to the left. See why it's called the "Splash Twist"?

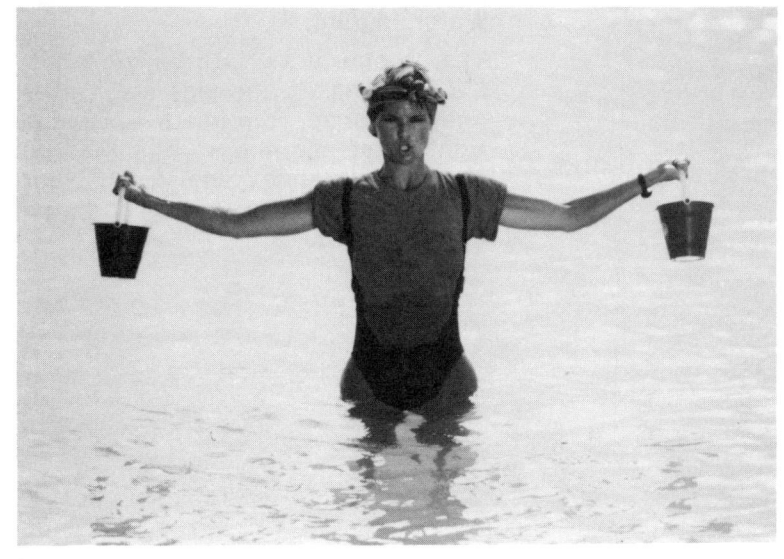

1

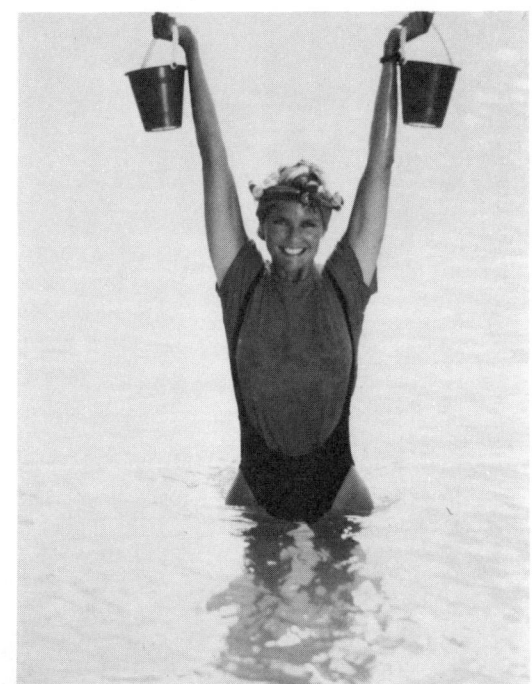

2

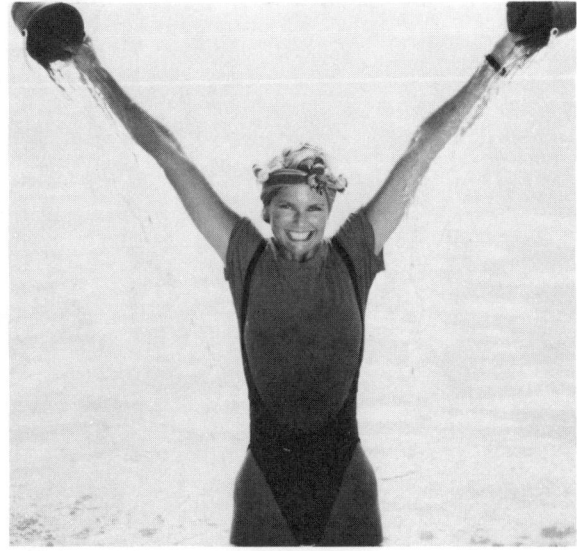

3

Sand Buckets

Be inventive at the beach. Just for fun, I used sand buckets as weights to reach new muscles in my arms—wet towels would work, too!

This is good for the arms, back, and chest. And there are lots of variations. You can let your imagination run wild.

Stand in water that's about waist deep. Hold a bucket in each hand. You can fill them with water or with wet sand. Make them heavy enough to give yourself a little resistance. Here are three movements that I like to do with sand buckets:

1. Open arms wide and as far to the back as you can, then bring hands together in front.
2. Keeping arms at sides, lift as far above head as you can, then lower to water's surface.
3. Windmill your arms in circles. Make sure your companions don't mind getting hit with flying sand or water!
4. Swing buckets, with arms extended to the sides, in small circles.

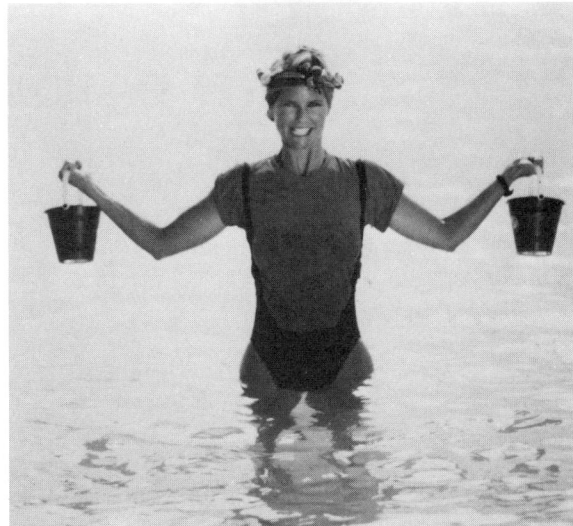

4

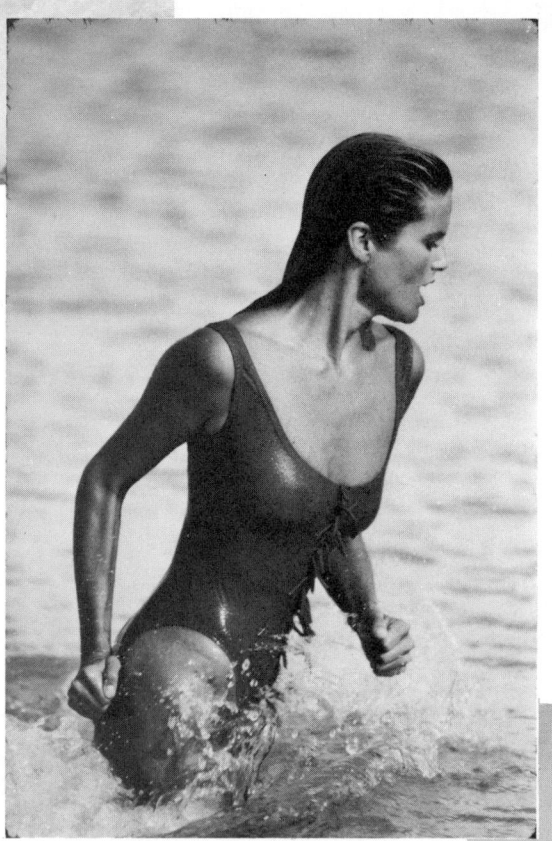

Water Jogging

This is one of my favorite exercises. It's fabulous for the legs and thighs and, of course, your heart. To get the right resistance, the water should be above your knees and below your waist. Jog as far as you can and then go another 100 yards.

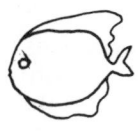 I suppose because I grew up by the sea, I've always felt very comfortable with it. I love a big surf and I relish a stormy day on the beach. But I also have a great respect for the sea and I'm very aware of the dangers she holds for people who are ignorant or foolhardy.

HAZARDS BY THE SEA

The Waves

A Set of Waves

I've seen people jump out of their cars, throw their towels onto the sand, and run right into the sea. In the 30 seconds they spent looking at the water it seemed quite calm, and when suddenly a huge wall of water appears they're quite unprepared for it. These hasty folks find themselves tossed about by the surf and sometimes scraped by rocks and sand.

What they don't know is that waves come in regular sets. Usually there are three or four waves in a set. If there's a surf (there *are* days when the ocean is just calm all day with no waves at all), you'll notice that there's a calm interval between sets of waves. The unfortunates who leaped from their car into the sea didn't know that they were between sets; they didn't expect any waves at all.

The great thing about sets of waves is that they create an ideal time to enter the water without encountering the "washing-machine" effect. You just observe the time between sets of waves so you know how much time you have to get into the calm water. Then, just as one set is finished, you take advantage of the calm to move out beyond the breakers and into quiet water.

Beyond the Breakers

Not so long ago I was having a meeting at the beach with my attorney, Arthur Kleinman, who is also a friend, and we decided to go for a swim. We waded into the surf together and started to swim out beyond the waves. I thought Arthur was just behind me, but he'd slowed down right in the break line to catch his breath. That's when the set came up—a monstrous series of waves that I'd been planning on, but which took him totally by surprise. I realized he wasn't a strong enough swimmer to move beyond the breakers in time, so I started to swim back to him. He was panicked. I noticed how terrified he was, which didn't require any great perceptiveness on my part, as he was saying "I'm going to die" over and over again with the vehemence of a true believer. I yelled "Dive deep! Dive! Dive!" but he thought I was saying "*Die! Die!*" As that was exactly what he planned to do, he didn't respond at all. (He should have known I wasn't saying that; I'd be *lost* without my attorney!) The wave crashed over him and when I pulled him out of the foam he was still talking about his final hours and was totally disoriented. Of course, he was unprepared for the next wave. We were swamped by three waves before I could get him beyond the line of breaking surf. Swimming in the line of surf was like trying to swim in a washing machine. But calm and manageable waters were just a few feet away and had been all along.

The lesson in my story is that if you know how to handle ocean waves, you should never be frightened by them. The second thing to know is what my

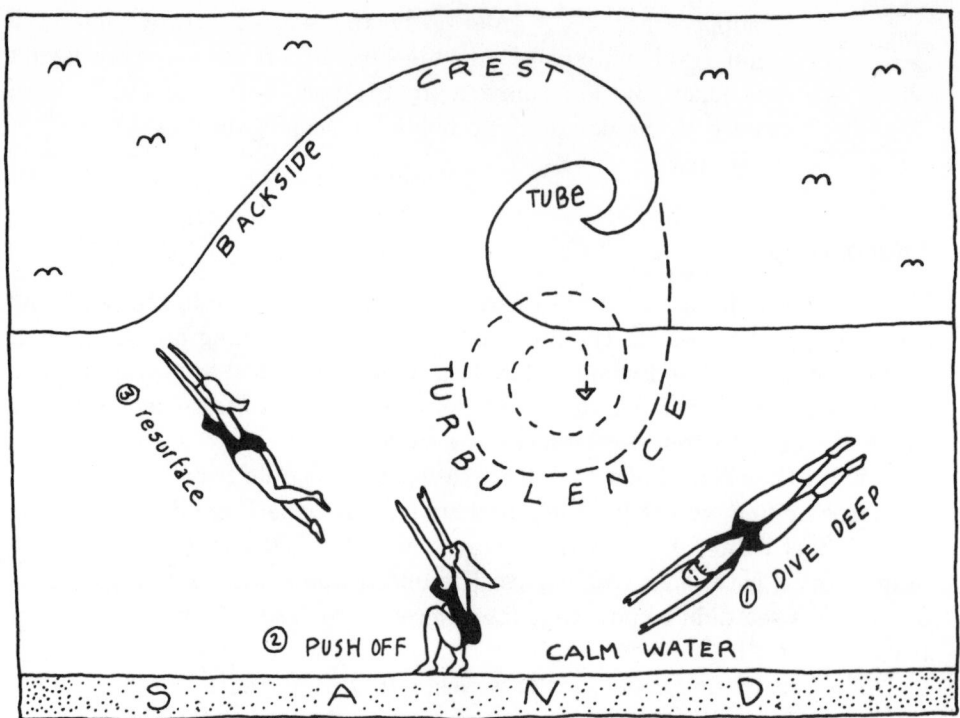

friend didn't: There is a line of breaking surf where the water is turbulent. It couldn't be easier to spot: It's where the waves crest, break, and turn to white water. Behind that line of surf the water is calm, though there may be swells. The trick, if you want to do some real swimming, is to get beyond the line of surf.

Dive Deep

In the story of my friend who was pounded by a full set of waves before I could drag him to safety, you'll remember that I yelled "Dive deep" to him. Diving deep, below the turbulence of the breaking wave, is how you avoid being tossed about like a sock in the spin cycle.

As the wave is building, just as it begins to break (that moment when, in a big surf, you feel at least a little bit afraid), you take a deep breath and dive beneath the wave, projecting your body beyond the turbulent waters.

If the wave comes up very suddenly and you don't quite have time to dive, you can still take a deep breath and try to *sink* beneath the breaking wave. Then, as soon as you can, get a toehold on the bottom and push yourself through the wave and into calm water.

Wave Lifts

I've noticed people at the beach jumping up with a wave as it crests to wave to their friends on the beach and show them how high the wave has lifted them. This is an exhilarating feeling—being bounced by all those tons of water—but you have to know what you're doing or you can be sucked back into the wave as it breaks. Again, you'll be tossed about and possibly hurt and, because you're not expecting it, it can be a traumatic experience. If you're

MY TRAVEL SCRAPBOOK

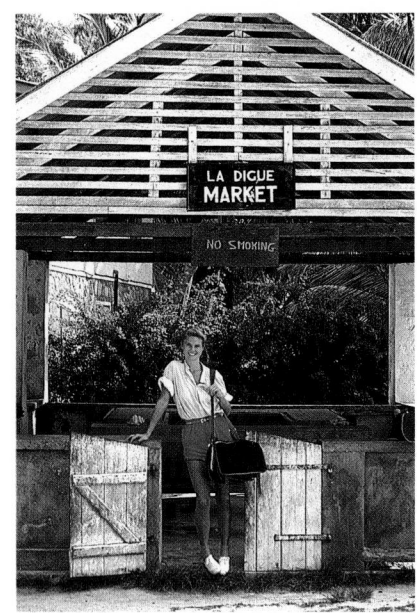

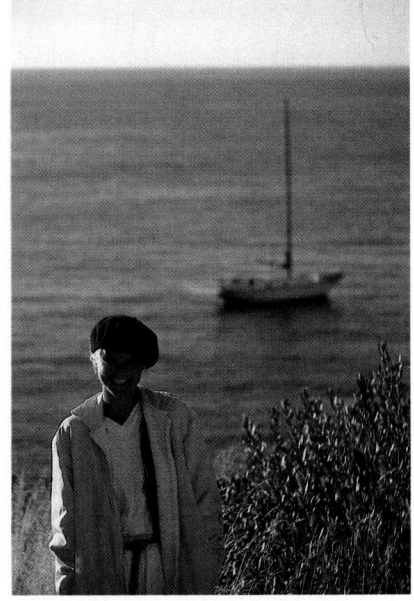

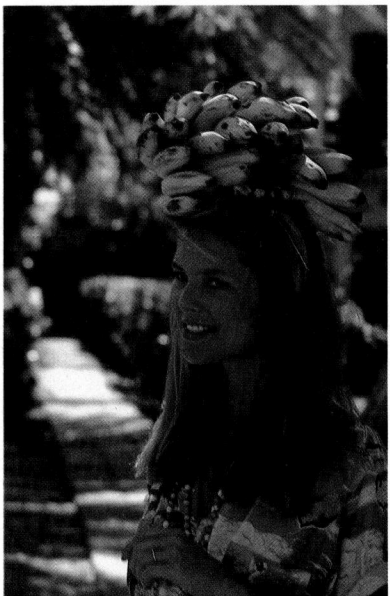

La Digue, Seychelles Islands
A Walter Ioos, Jr., snapshot

Catalina Island, California
Photograph by Greg Brinkley —
''nutritionist,'' ''actor,''
''production assistant,''
''best brother in the world''

Malibu, California
Olivier Chandon

St. Bart's, West Indies
Olivier Chandon

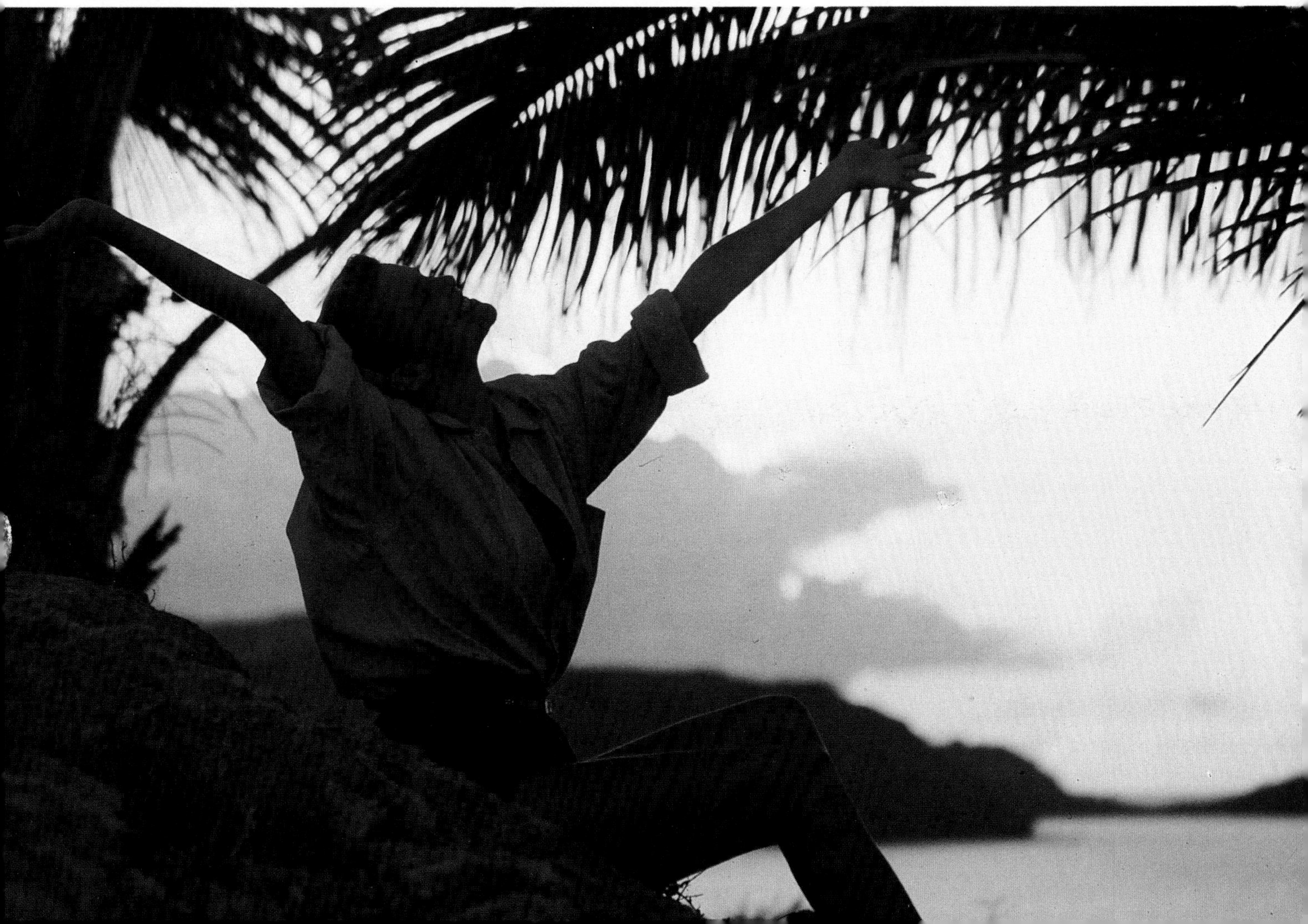

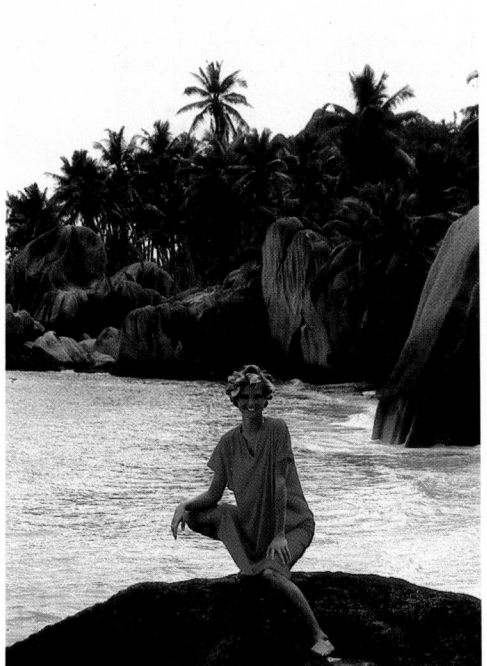

Seychelles Islands
A friend

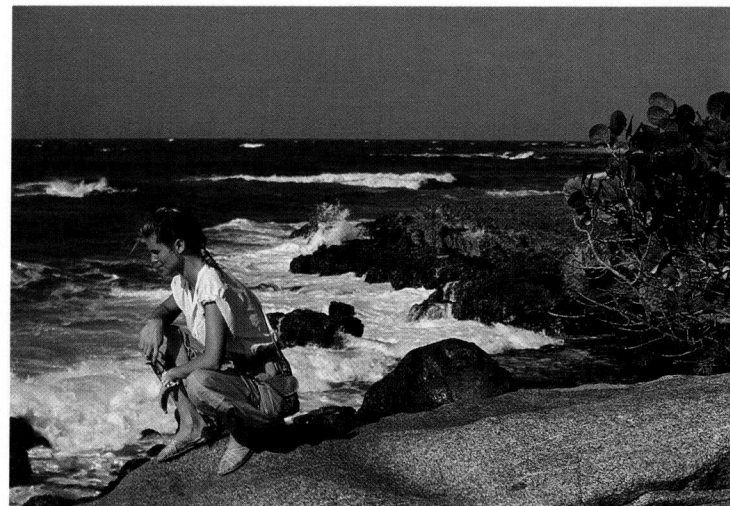

Aruba
Jean-François Allaux

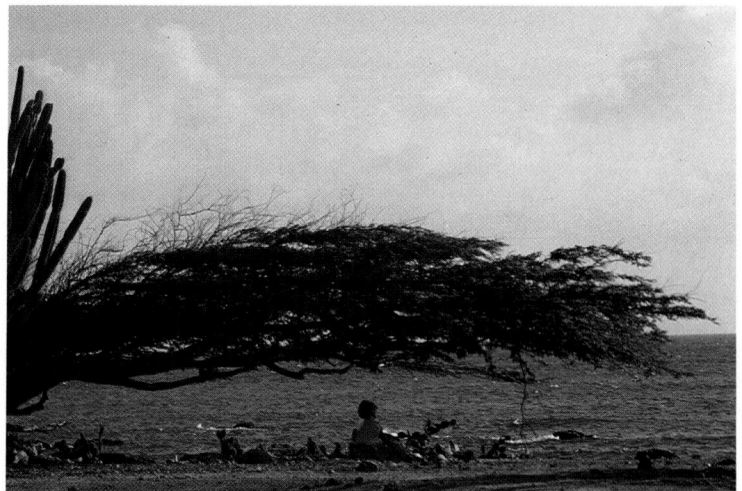

Under a divi-divi tree in Aruba
Felicia

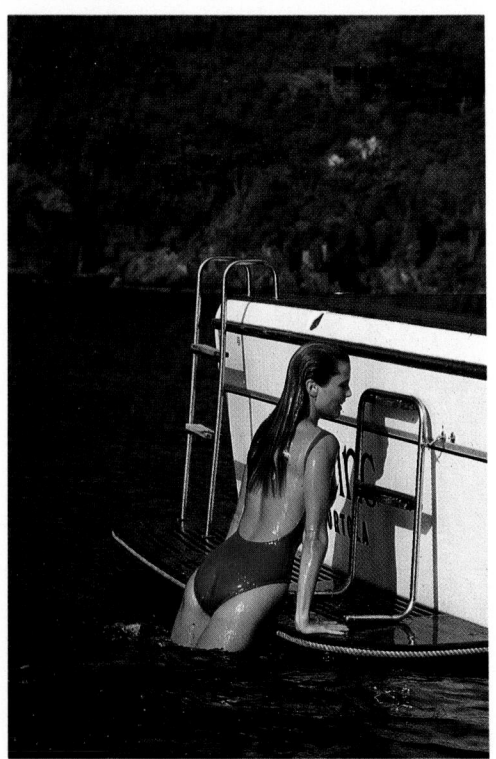

Carreyes, Mexico
Patrick Demarchelier

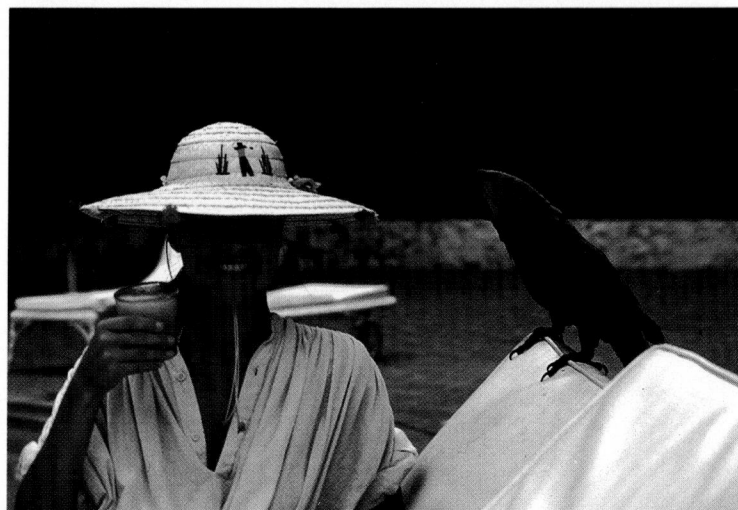

Puerto Vallarta, Mexico
My mom

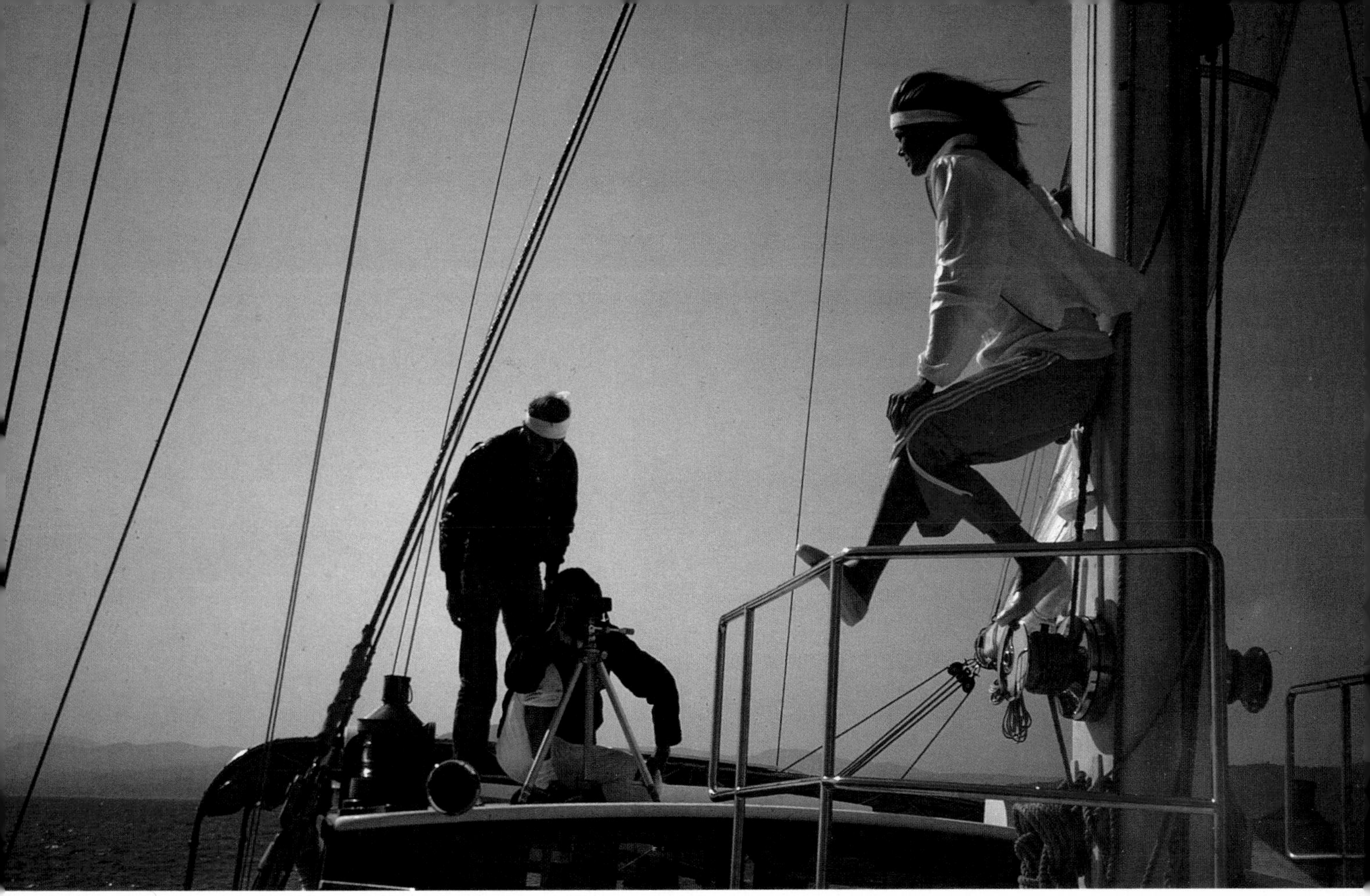

St. Tropez, France
A friend

Concha di Marini, Italy
Olivier Chandon

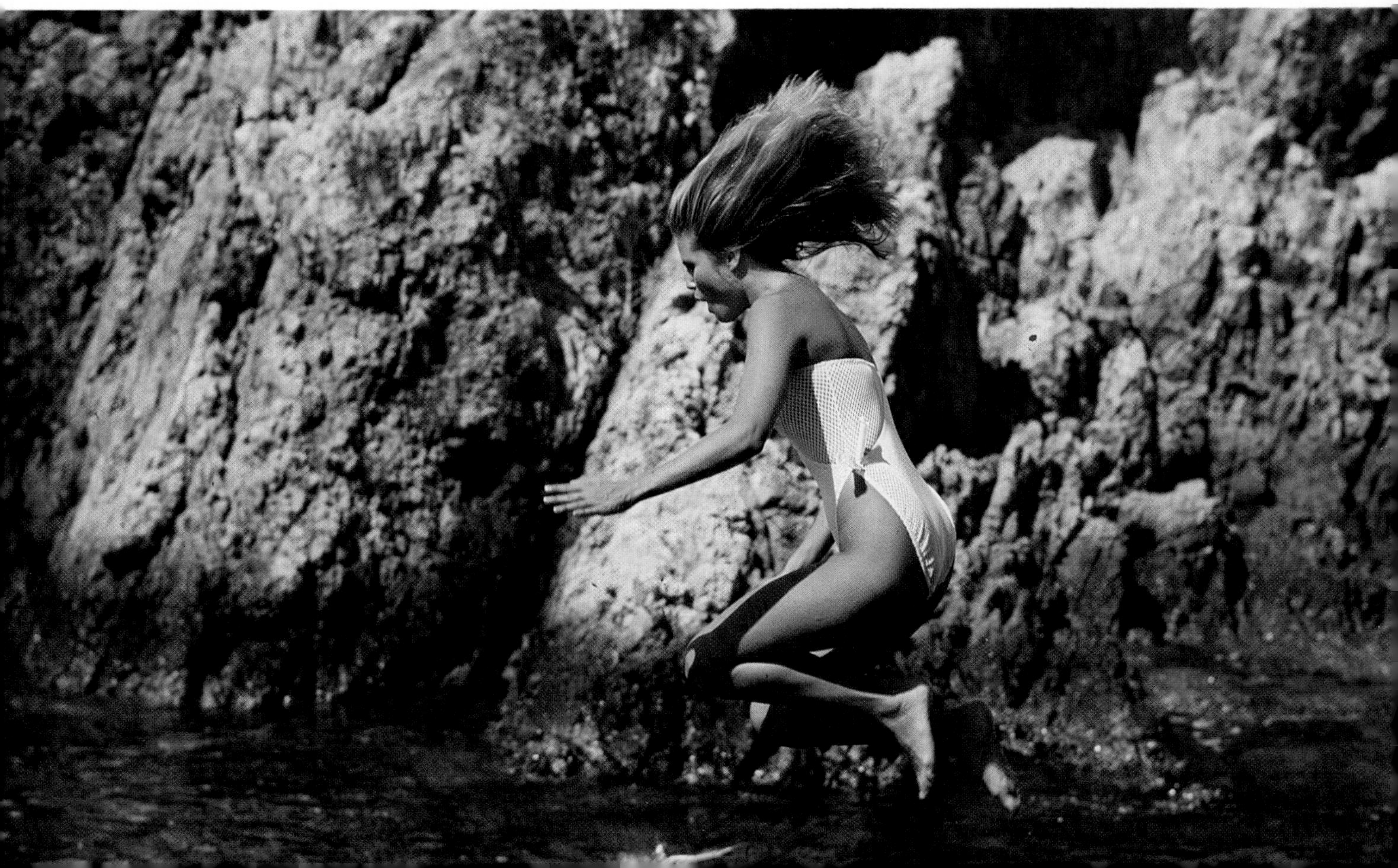

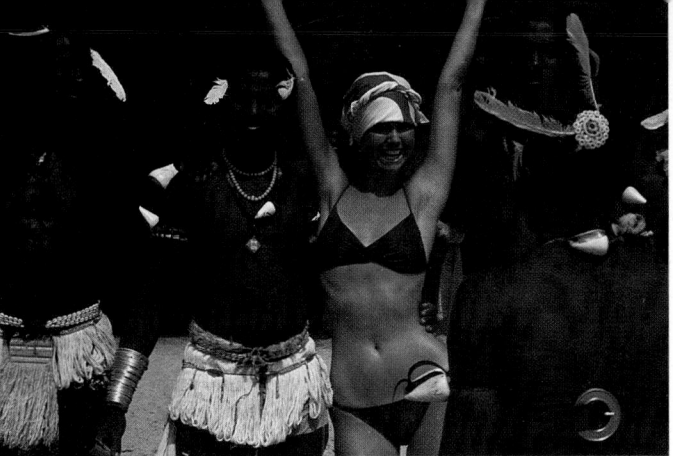

Senegal, Africa
François Ilnseher's nephew

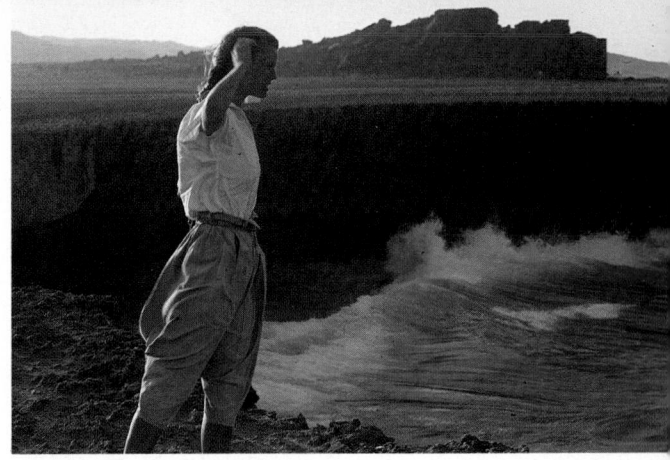

Aruba
Jean-François Allaux

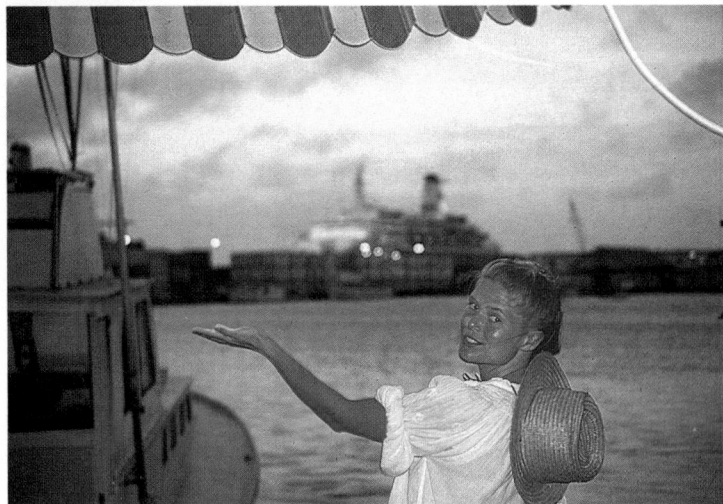

Curaçao
Maury ''Hops'' Hopson

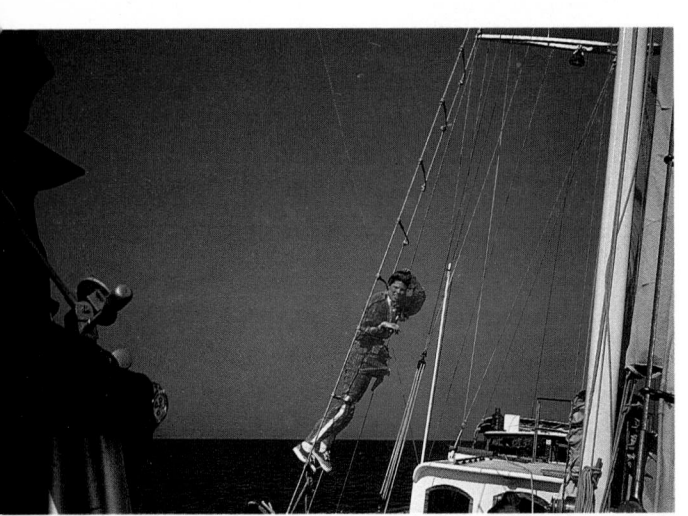

St. Tropez, France
Bruno

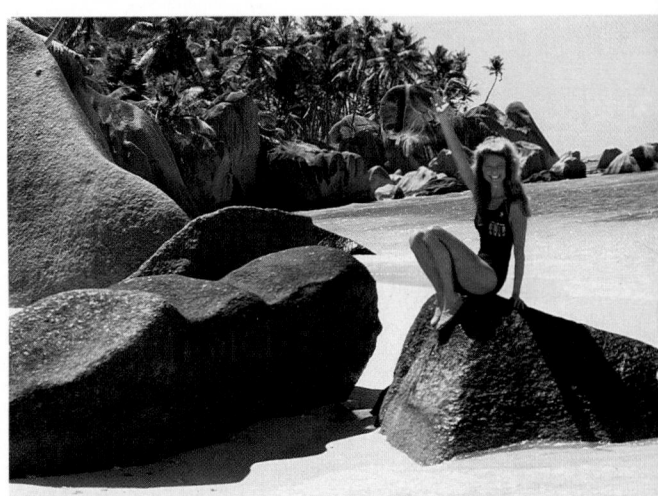

La Digue, Seychelles Islands
Jule Campbell

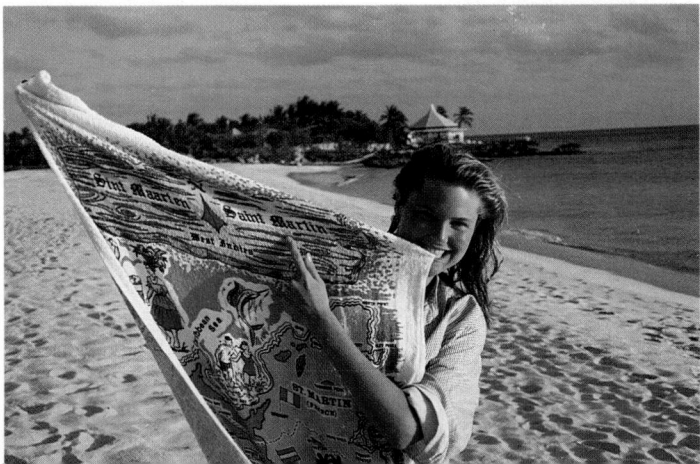

St. Martin, West Indies
A friend

leaping up with the waves, make sure you're not doing it near the line of surf but are farther out in the water.

The Currents

Once when I was on a modeling job in Greece, I was sunning myself on a little island. I saw another island across a glistening bit of sea and I decided to swim out to it and explore. The swim across was fine and I was delighted with my adventure, that is, until I got close to the other island. Suddenly there were currents that swept around the edge of the island and out to sea. Even though I am a strong swimmer, it was very difficult for me to make my way to the beach. When I finally climbed ashore I had that sinking feeling that my "adventure" was pretty foolhardy. The distance was greater than I had anticipated. The current was strong. And I was really tired.

I sat on that tiny island, wondering if I would ever make it back to the olives and feta cheese. Luckily a fishing boat full of friendly Greeks came by. I'm forever grateful to them for the ride back.

The point is there are invisible dangers you should be aware of. So if you're swimming in a strange place, ask the locals about water conditions before you plunge into the surf.

Also, unless there are lots of capable people on shore or you are completely familiar with the area, don't try a solo swim. I know I sound very girl-scoutish, but I've learned so much about the dangers of swimming in strange waters that it's a rule I never break.

I hope I'm not scaring you out of the water! But once you know about these hidden dangers you'll be able to avoid them and that will make each trip to the sea safe and happy.

Riptides

Riptides are like fast-flowing rivers of water that are moving against the regular tide. Often they're running parallel to the shoreline. On either side of the flow of a riptide is an eddy of water that swings back to shore. If you're caught in a riptide, never try to fight it! You can't win. Instead, swim diagonally across it until you reach the bordering eddy. Then you'll be out of the riptide and can safely swim to shore.

Undertows and Backwashes

An undertow or a backwash can be terribly frightening. I know they're responsible for the two or three grey hairs on Mom and Dad. You can be standing in knee-deep water and yet the undertow can be pulling you out to sea with such power that you panic. The undertow is really the water that's retreating from the shore after being carried in by the waves. Sometimes it's just a slight tug but other times it's fierce. If you're in deep water and get pulled out by an undertow, there's one important thing to know: The undertow travels in two directions on two different levels. The upper portion of the water is moving inward while the lower portion of the water is going out to sea. So you have to push off the bottom and swim along the top surface of the water back to shore with the waves. Stay calm and you'll be fine.

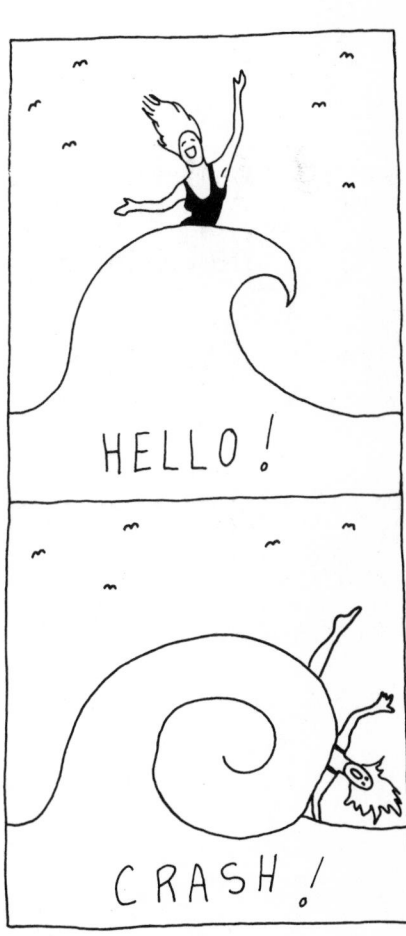

HELLO!

CRASH!

Rescue at Sea

It's a sad fact that every year 7,000 people in the U.S. will drown. Here are some tips in case you're ever on the scene at a water emergency:

Never, never try to swim out and save someone unless you are a strong and experienced swimmer. Better to alert someone else who can help or try an alternative method.

Try throwing a rope with a ring buoy or a flotation device, if one is available, to the victim.

Try extending a branch, a pole, or even your own leg (if you have something to hang onto) to the victim so he can pull himself to safety.

If a boat or surfboard or raft is at hand, use it to reach the victim and carry him to safety.

A drowning person will almost certainly need mouth-to-mouth resuscitation if he is not breathing. You must act quickly.

Position the victim face up. Tilt his head far back, chin pointing up. Lift with one hand under the neck. Press down with the other hand on the forehead. Pinch the nostrils shut with thumb and forefinger of the same hand. Take a deep breath and begin:

Step 1. Open your mouth wide and seal it over the victim's mouth. Blow into his mouth to fill up his lungs. Look to see that his chest rises.

Step 2. Remove your mouth. Take a deep breath. Look to see that the victim's chest falls as the air escapes.

Repeat steps 1 and 2 every five seconds for an adult, every three seconds for a child.

Make sure someone has gone for help.

The Coral Reef

Magical, mysterious, breathtakingly beautiful—you're so lucky if you're visiting an island with coral reefs! To dive around one is an unforgettable experience, but there are a few things to beware of. Most coral is very sharp and can give you a bad cut. Also, because of the irregular shape of the coral, the cut it gives is often ragged and takes a long time to heal. Also, some coral is poisonous and can give you a bad infection.

In addition to regular coral, there also exists something known as stinging coral or fire coral. Its rosy spiny formations that look like large feathers are so pretty that scuba divers or snorkelers are tempted to break off pieces to bring home. And that's when they learn about stinging coral and how it got its name. This isn't really a coral at all, but rather a collection of tiny organisms that cling together for mutual protection. As soon as something touches them they retaliate with a sting that causes a searing white-hot pain. They can also give a nasty wound with their razor-sharp edges.

Rocks and coral reefs beneath the waves can be dangerous if you're out for a swim. In clear tropical waters you can usually see such things, but in northern waters you can be taken unawares. Be sure to ask locals or other folk on the beach about any obstructions. Often you can tell that there are rocks or reefs beneath the sea because you'll notice that the waves are breaking in an unusual pattern just above them.

There are other reasons not to touch coral, although, because of its beauty, it can be tempting. But how it saddens me to see a magnificent and integral part of nature displayed on someone's coffee table! Please don't be selfish and thoughtless: Leave the natural beauty for others to enjoy where it belongs—in the sea!

The Tide Pool

Tide pools are fun to explore because they're tiny microcosms of the ocean. For that same reason, they can also be dangerous. Wear your protective shoes and watch your step. Sea life of every kind can get trapped in a tide pool. Eels, some of which are poisonous, love to snuggle along the rocks lining a tide pool. Sea urchins with their painful needles can tuck in along the rocks. Even sharks have been known to be caught in tide pools and you can imagine that they wouldn't be in a good mood after a few hours in a small, shallow pool!

Jellyfish

Jellyfish can be a menace if they're the stinging kind. I've been told a rather odd, but apparently effective method of relieving a jellyfish sting: You pee on it! There's something in urine, perhaps the uric acid, that diminishes the pain of a jellyfish sting. Don't laugh! One of these days you may find yourself miles from a doctor but pain-free because of this tip! Vinegar is good, too.

Sharks

If you're going to be swimming in areas known for sharks, buy a good book about them to read on your trip. Sharks are truly fascinating creatures, many of which, like the nurse shark, are completely harmless! More divers are hurt through their own panic at spotting one than by the shark itself. Information is always your best friend, so read as much as possible!

Giant Clams and Other Scary Creatures

There are lots of other things to watch out for beneath the waves, including the "Killer Clam" which grows to 6 feet across and weighs 500 pounds or more. (That's some chowder!) But if you spend a lot of time diving, you'll learn about these beasts elsewhere, hopefully in a book. Enjoy your swim!

MICRO HAZARDS

 Here are a few things to watch out for if you're a frequent swimmer. They're not especially common but forewarned is forearmed!

Swimmer's Itch

Swimmer's itch is an inflammation of the skin that's caused by a bug called a schistosome. This bug lives in many lakes in the U.S. and it deposits its larvae on people swimming in those lakes. The larvae are frequently deposited on the arms where they cause little red bumps that are terribly itchy. Because there's no effective treatment for swimmer's itch, the best remedy is prevention: If you've been swimming in a lake, rub yourself dry with a towel afterwards, paying special attention to your arms.

Swimmer's Ear

Swimmer's ear is another name for an infected ear canal. It's called "swimmer's ear" because water in the ear is a frequent cause of the disorder. You know you've got it if your ear hurts and the pain intensifies when you pull your earlobe. Once your ear is infected, a doctor will have to treat it. The best prevention is keeping your ears dry either by wearing ear plugs or by using drying ear drops (ask your doctor about this) after swimming.

Schistosomiasis

About to dive into that glistening inland tropical lake? Stop! Many freshwater streams, lakes, and ponds in South America, Africa, Asia, and other tropical places are infected with a parasite which enters the body through the skin. It causes a chronic disease called schistosomiasis. All you need to do to get the disease is to come in contact with water where the parasite lives. So don't swim in fresh water unless a reliable source assures you it is parasite-free. Your best bet is never to take a chance. And, by the way, you don't have to worry about chlorinated pools and salt water in these locations.

Sea Urchins

I was in Barbados once playing Frisbee with some friends by the edge of the water. We were all in high spirits, leaping around and splashing in the surf. Suddenly an agonizing pain shot up my leg.

I thought I had been bitten by a shark and I screamed in pain and terror. My leg felt almost paralyzed but I managed to pull myself up to the shore and my friends dragged me out of the water. When I could bear to look, I saw that my foot was completely full of sea-urchin needles. I hadn't realized that there was a reef covered with sea urchins directly beneath the sand where I was playing Frisbee.

The pain was horrible, but I learned a lesson I'll never forget: Never walk barefoot on any unfamiliar ocean floor. In most resorts you can be sure that the public and hotel beaches are safe, but if you're going to do any exploring bring along a pair of tennis shoes or any kind of flat slip-on shoe to wear in the water.

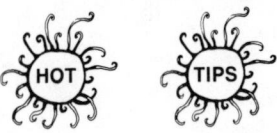

When I had my awful experience in Barbados of a foot full of sea-urchin needles, a waiter at a beach restaurant taught me a remedy. He grabbed a candle and some limes, lit the candle and dripped hot wax over the needles. When he squeezed lime juice over the wax, the pain left my foot instantly. Apparently, as the wax hardens it draws the poison out of the needle.

It's not a good idea to go spearfishing in sharky waters—the speared fish you keep near your body can attract a hungry shark!

Oceanographers rarely agree when it comes to information on the mysterious shark. But I read somewhere that sharks love red bathing suits. So I stick to black and blue suits when I share the sharks' waters!

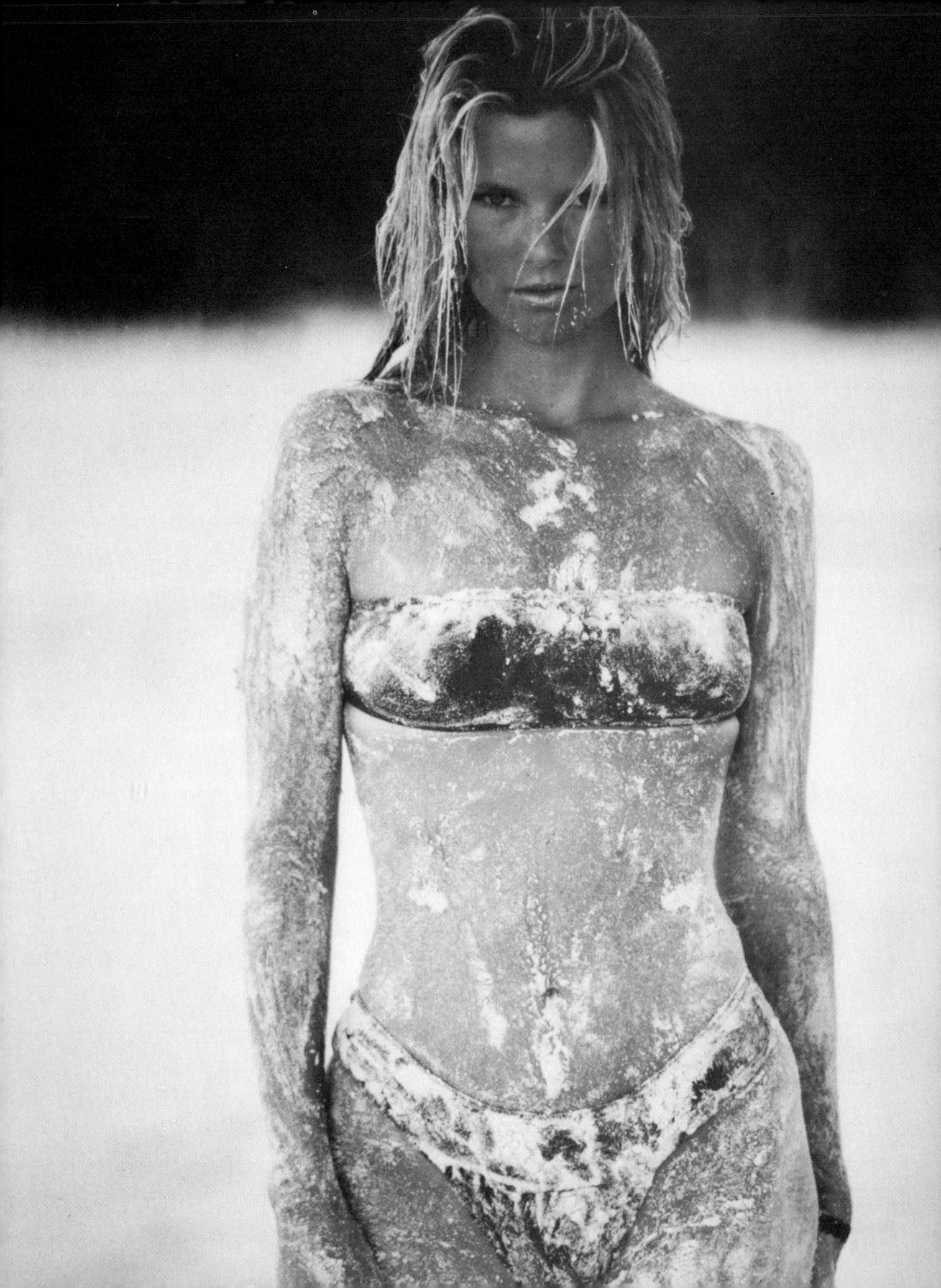

THE SAND

I think the beach is the best natural playground in the world. It's resilient and provides resistance for exercising, friction for body-smoothing, and the most comfortable possible cushion for relaxed sunbathing. And, of course, it's the ideal location for building sand castles! So don't just think of the beach as a place to toss your towel and stick your umbrella. Use your imagination and open your mind to all the possibilities the beach has to offer.

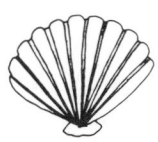

BEACH FEET

Kick off your shoes! Walking barefoot in the sand is just great for your feet and your legs. The sand acts as a natural pumice, softening and removing your calluses. And the effort it takes to walk barefoot in the sand strengthens your calves. But first you have to get your feet into beach shape so you don't have to hide them under the sand. I've read directions on how to give yourself a pedicure that sound as if you have to devote two hours to the job. This is nonsense. A good pedicure takes only a few minutes (except for the time when you're soaking your feet, and you can be reading then or making some phone calls).

Here are five steps to a charming instep:

1. Soak your feet. Dissolve some mild detergent or even a bit of shampoo in a basin and soak your feet for about 15 minutes. This will soften up the skin.

2. Get rid of those calluses with a pumice stone. Keep your feet and the pumice stone wet with the soapy water to speed the process.

3. Push back your cuticles with an orange stick (or a clean pencil eraser or the wrong end of a makeup brush: i.e., whatever you have that will work).

4. Cut those nails. Straight across, please. If you cut the edges to curve down, you irritate the skin and can get ingrown toenails.

5. Buff your nails with a buffer to give them a rosy glow or polish them. That's it! Your feet should now be beautiful.

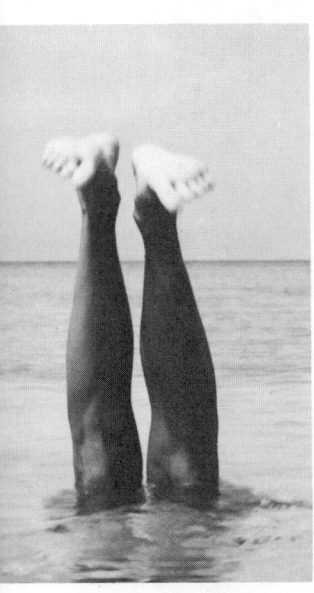
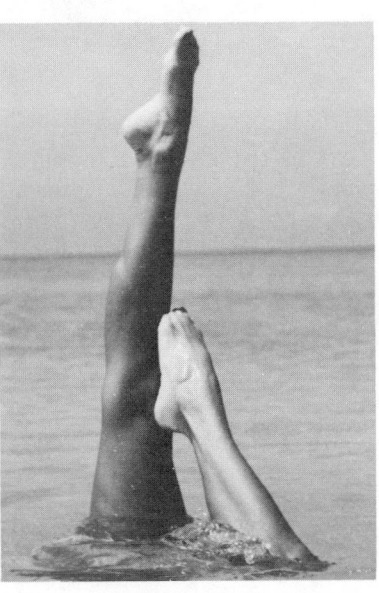
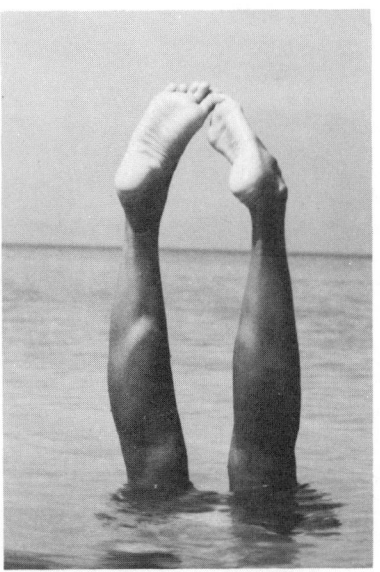
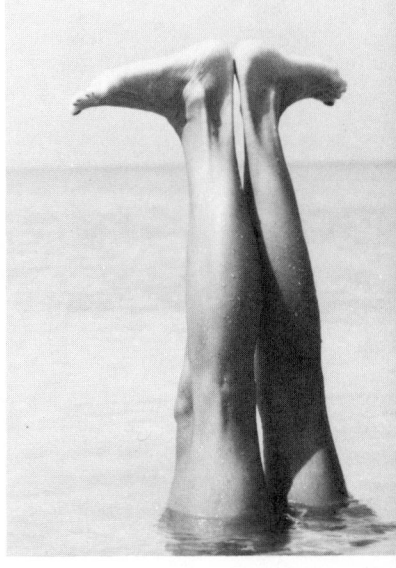

HOT FEET RELIEF

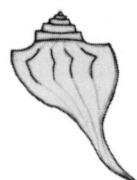

In the summer when your poor feet are trapped in tight shoes for hours on end they often swell. And they often become tired and ache, and sometimes they feel hot and burning. The best relief for this is an apple-cider vinegar rub. You simply wash your feet in warm water and then splash them with cool water. After you dry them, pour some apple-cider vinegar into your palms and massage it into the soles of your feet. (Doesn't that feel good?) After a few minutes of this you'll be ready for anything.

SAND SCRUB

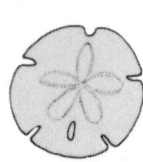

Get off your towel and onto the beach for the best body scrub and softener of all. Take handfuls of wet sand and massage it all over your body. (It's even better when someone else does it for you!) The finer the grain of sand, the harder you can rub. It works like a loofah, removing dead skin cells and stimulating circulation.

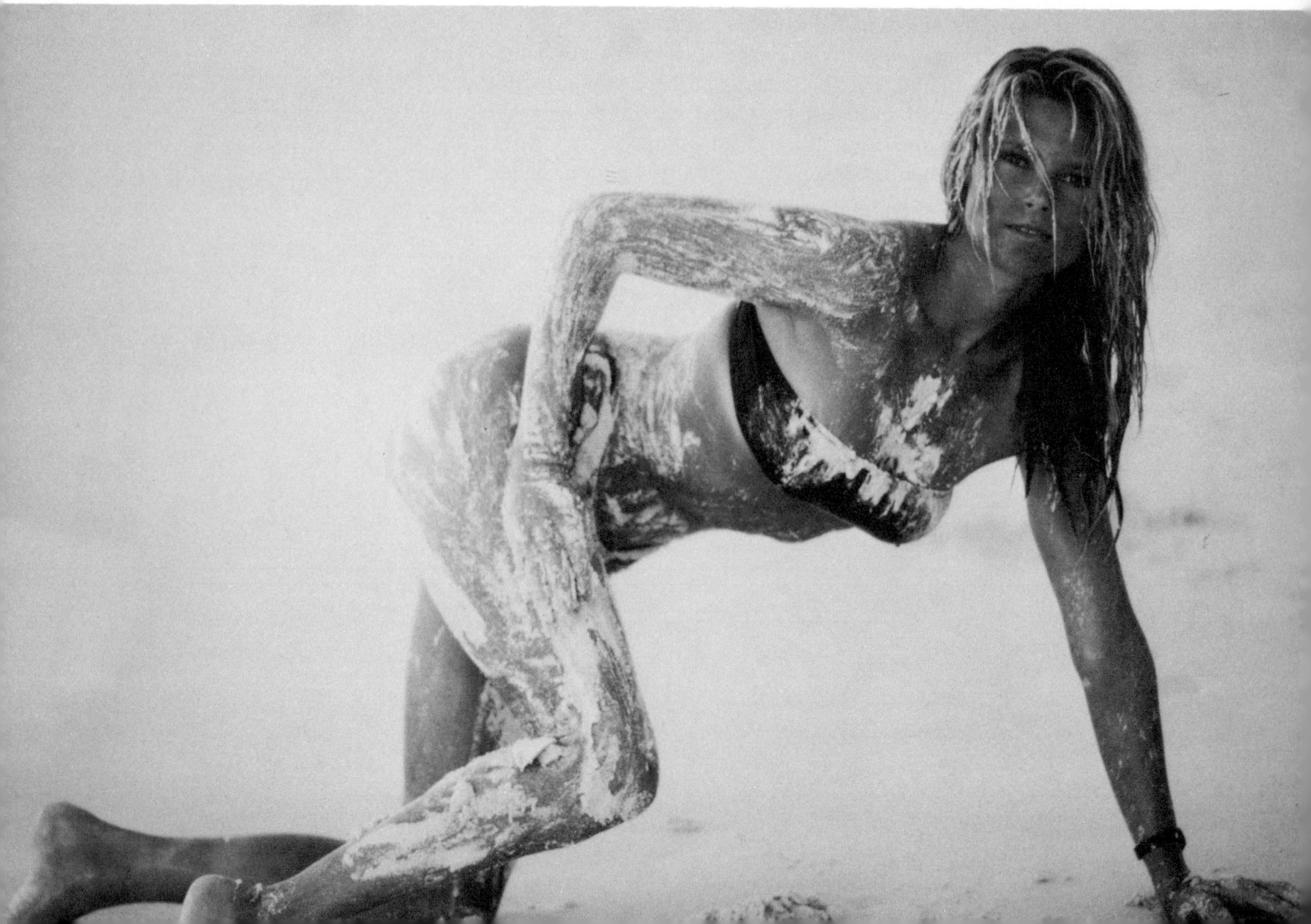

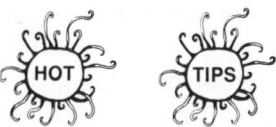

If you polish your toenails and you're going to be walking on a beach, cover your polish with a coat of nail hardener. With the extra protection, your polish will stand up to the abrasiveness of the sand and last much longer.

When I'm on location, I often have to change clothes in a jiffy and there's usually no dressing room. I've developed a solution for this that you might find useful at the beach—an instant changing room. I always bring a long skirt with an elastic waistband, and when it's time to change I pull it up around my neck and switch wardrobes in the privacy underneath!

If you forget your instant changing room, head for the surf and switch suits in the privacy of the sea!

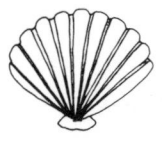

BARE FEET AND ACHING LEGS

Have you ever noticed that if you go barefoot for a few days, your legs begin to ache? High heels are the culprits. Most women wear heels of some sort almost all the time. Even shoes that we think of as being "flats" have some sort of heel, even if it's only a half inch. After a few years of this the tendons in your legs shorten. When you kick off those heels and go barefoot for a few days, the tendons begin to stretch out and can feel uncomfortable.

To avoid this problem, I always try to wear running shoes whenever I can. If you can't manage that, there's an exercise on page 43 that will stretch out your tendons and keep them from shortening.

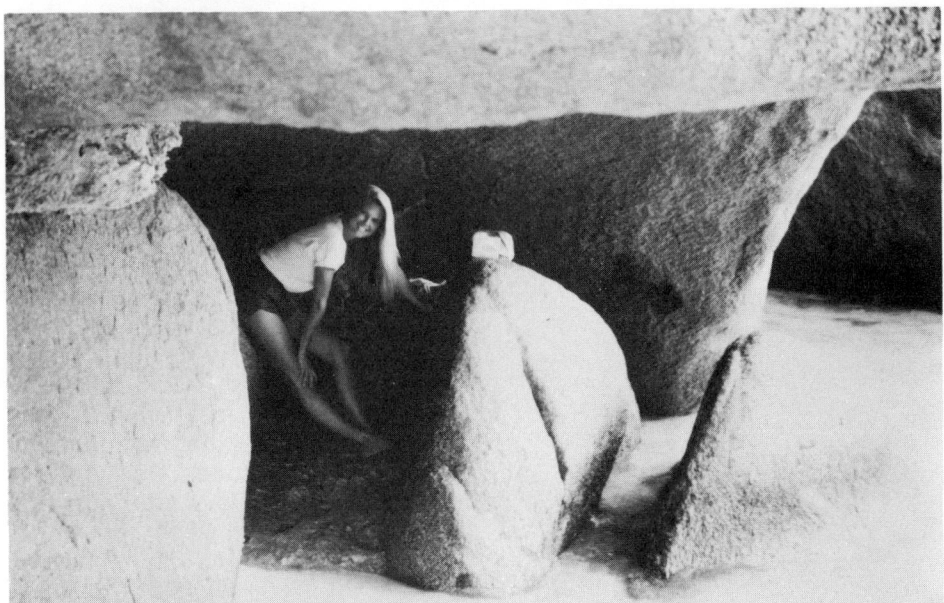

My "dressing room" in the Seychelles Islands

SAND EXERCISES

Sand exercises are another example of what I mean by exercise flexibility. How often have you sat in the sand watching the surf crash or listening to your radio? You could have been exercising! Sand makes a great environment for calisthenics, aerobics, yoga —really *all* exercising because it provides resistance. It's fun *and,* as an extra bonus, the sand itself acts as a natural pumice and helps to smooth your body as you work.

So you no longer have any reason to spend all day at the beach just lying on your towel. Exercise while you tan! You'll look and feel great!

P.S. Please remember that these are just a half dozen of my favorites. Try to come up with another half dozen of your own!

Backward Dig

This is a good one for the upper arms and the back. It's also so easy to do that it's really a pleasure. You can do it while you're lightening your hair with lemon juice or waiting for your hair to curl—like me!

Sit on the sand with your arms extended behind you, palms up. Dig a hole behind you by lifting handfuls of sand as high as you can. As the hole gets deeper, the angle of your digging changes and the muscles you work change as well. You can, by the way, use a shovel if you want to maintain your manicure.

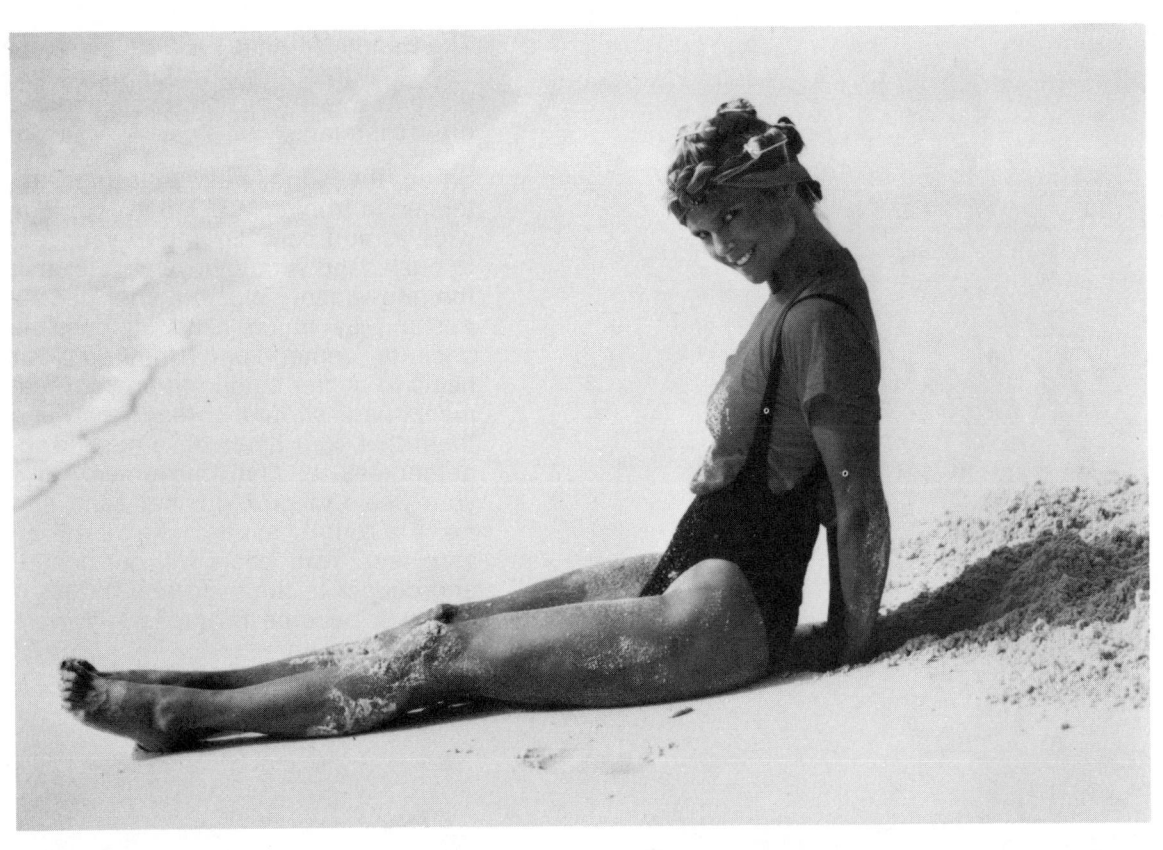

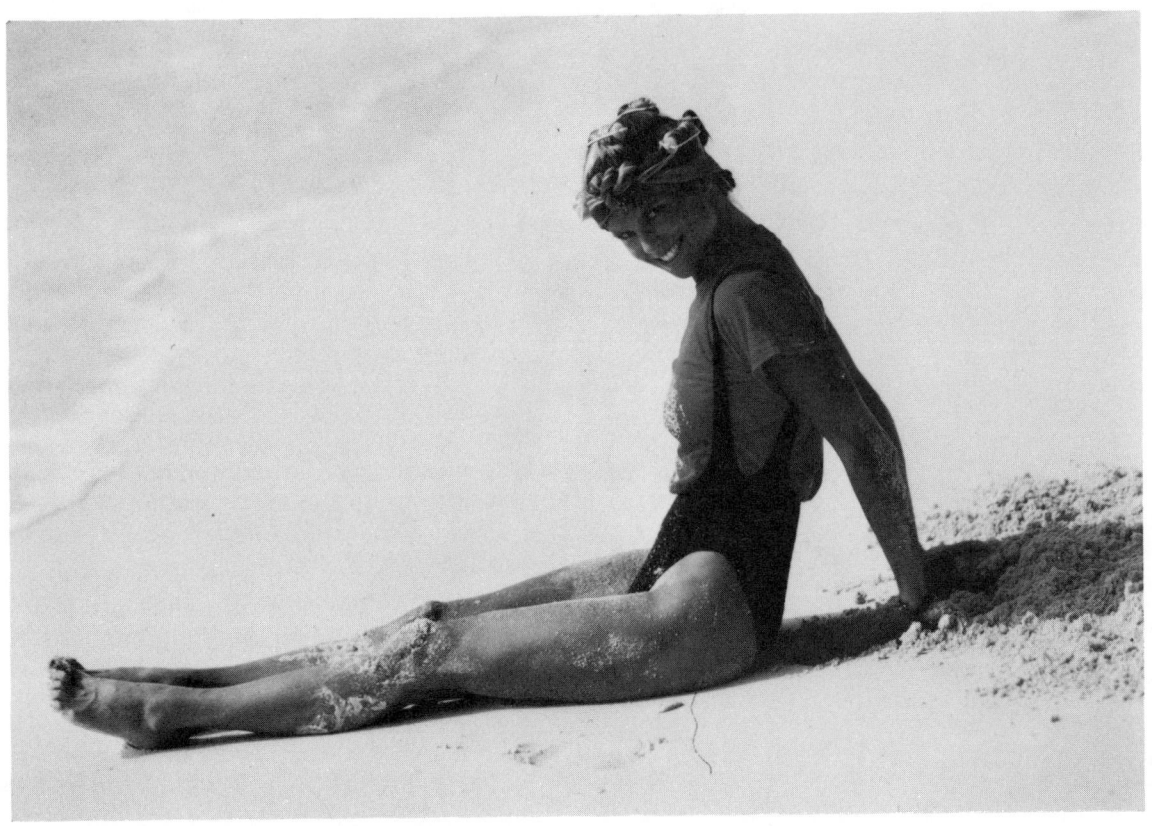

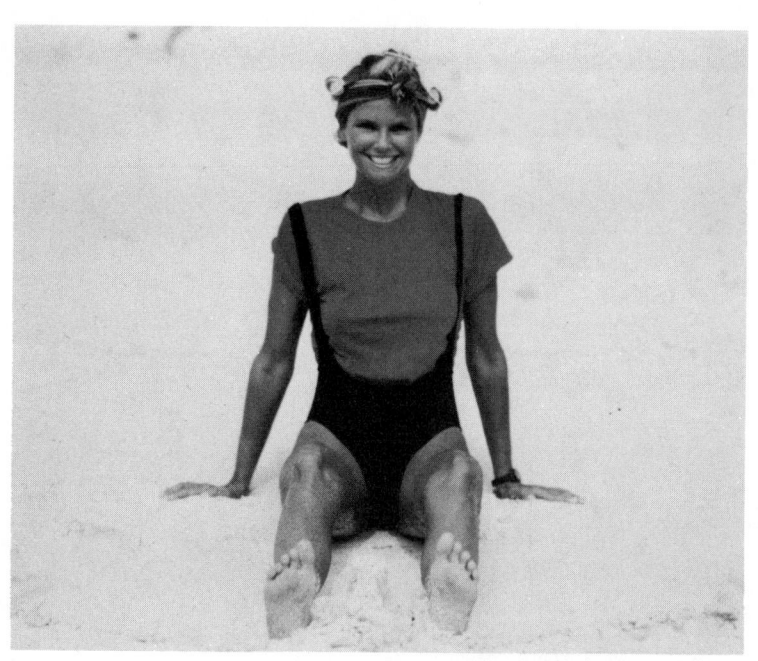

The Sandy Nautilus

This is a great exercise for your legs; it seems to work every muscle and is a great trimmer.

Sit in the sand with your legs extended in front of you. Open your legs wide as you can, digging in your feet to push sand with your heels. Reverse the movement, closing your legs—pushing as much sand as possible back to center—and bringing your heels to center again. When your feet meet there should be sand between them that your heels have pushed together—as a final movement, use your heels to pick up that sand and make a rough "sand castle" between your feet. Your heels will get deeper and deeper in the sand and the exercise will become progressively more difficult.

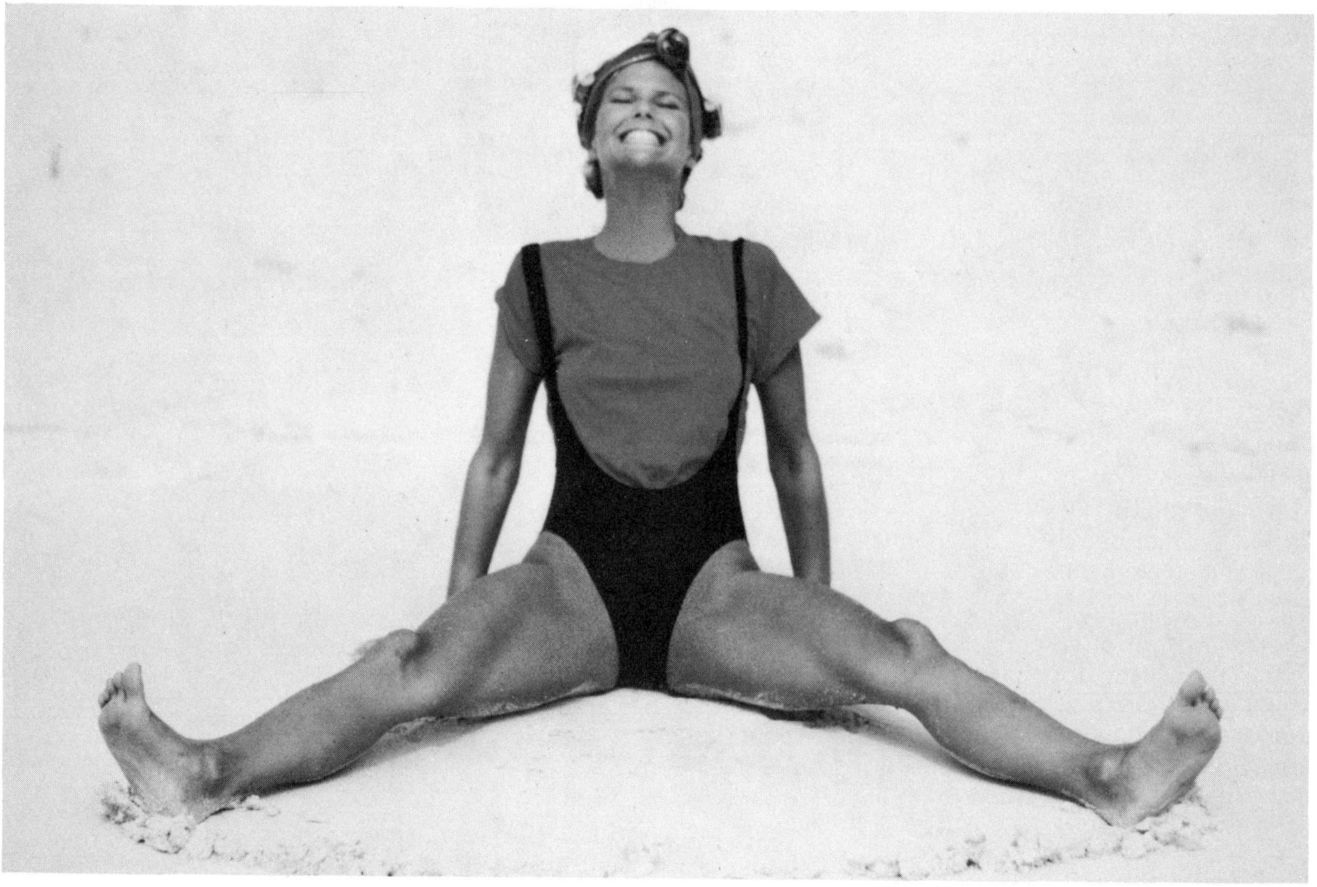

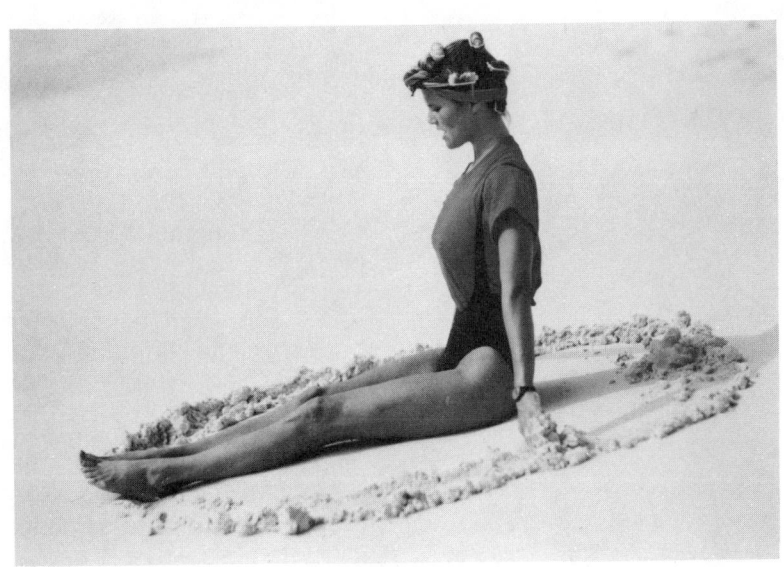

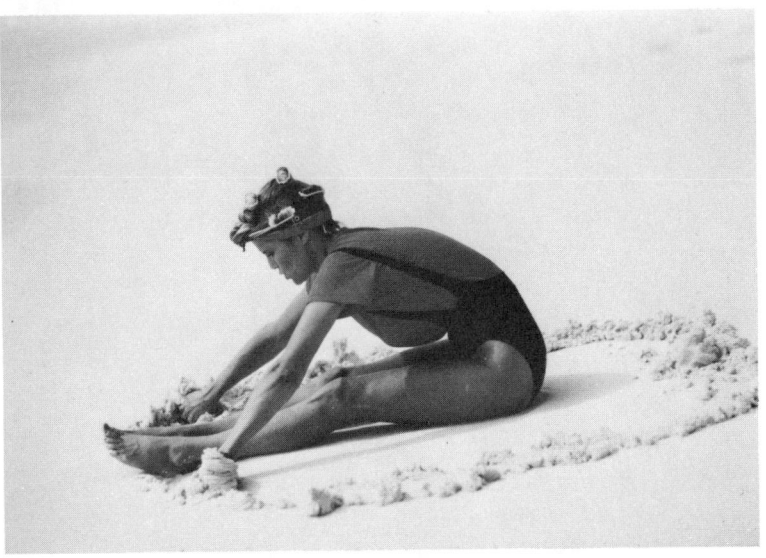

The Sand Circle
This is another one that's good for the arms. It also works the back and waist.

Sit in the sand with your legs extended in front of you and your arms outstretched and touching the sand. Make a big circle around yourself in the sand, bending forward as your arms approach your feet. Keep a straight back as your arms move behind you. The more sand you move, the greater the resistance and the better the workout.

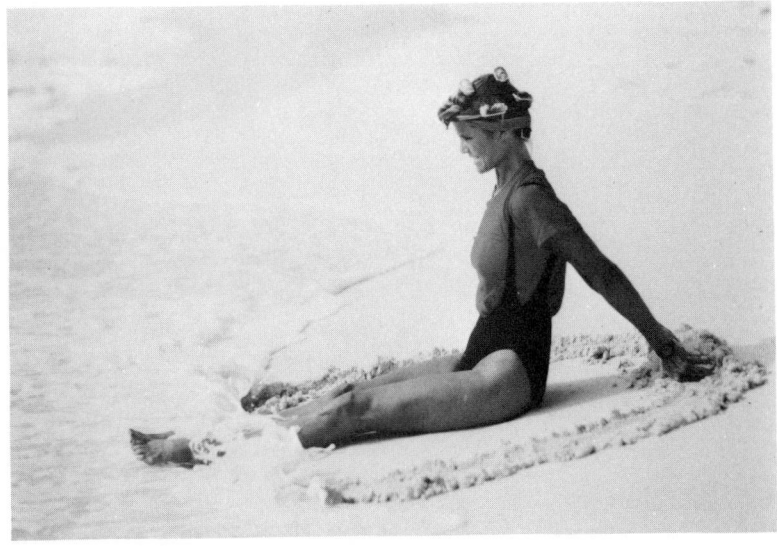

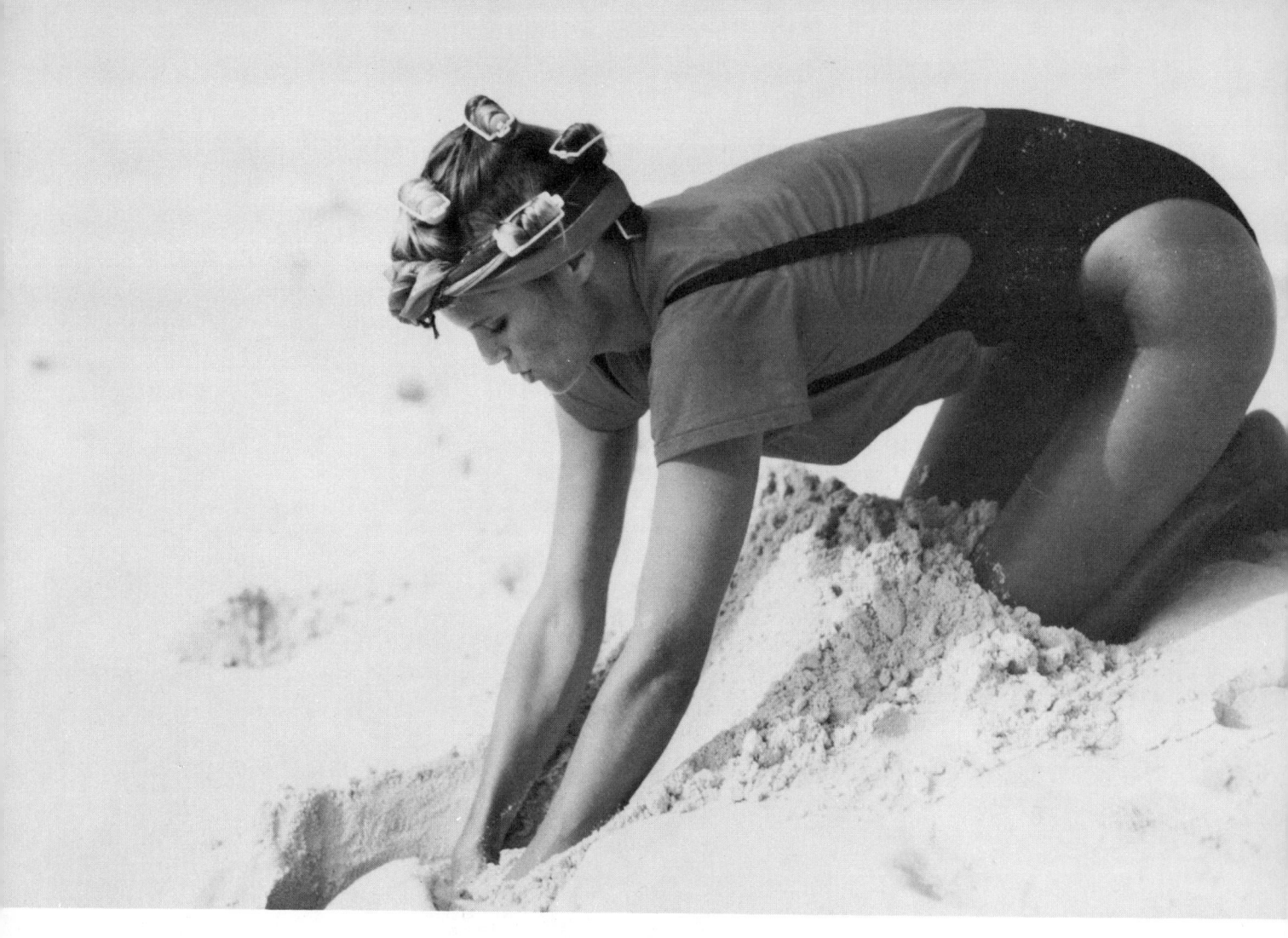

The Clam Digger

This is a good one for the stomach, but it also works the arms and back.

Get on your knees in the sand with your arms extended in front of you. Dig a hole by pulling the sand toward you. Make sure the hole isn't too close to you; the farther away, the more difficult the exercise. As the hole gets deeper, you'll be working those stomach muscles hard.

When the hole is as deep as you can make it, you're ready for the next exercise. . . .

Sand Sit-ups

Bury your feet in the hole you just dug. If the beach is on a slant, it's better to bury your feet so that you're facing the highest part of the beach. That way the beach can act as a slant board. Your feet should be buried and your legs, too, almost up to the knees. Now you're ready to do your sit-ups. By keeping your knees bent, you're making it easier on your back.

When you're finished with your sit-ups, you're ready for your next buried exercise. . . .

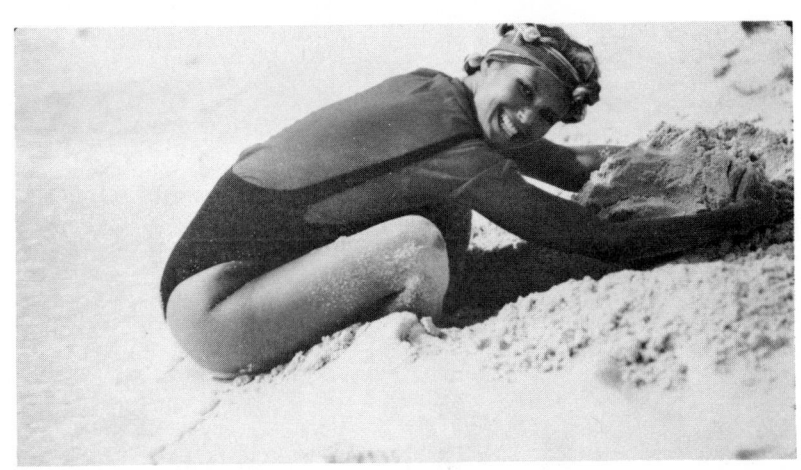

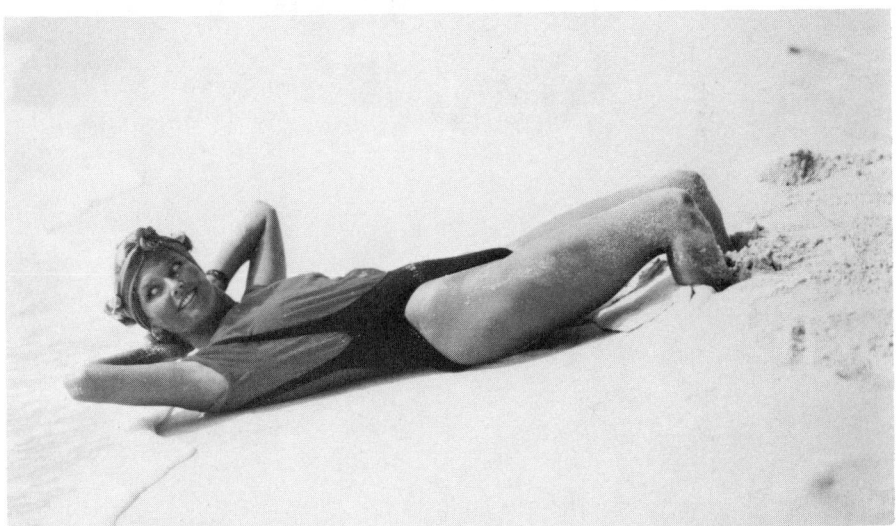

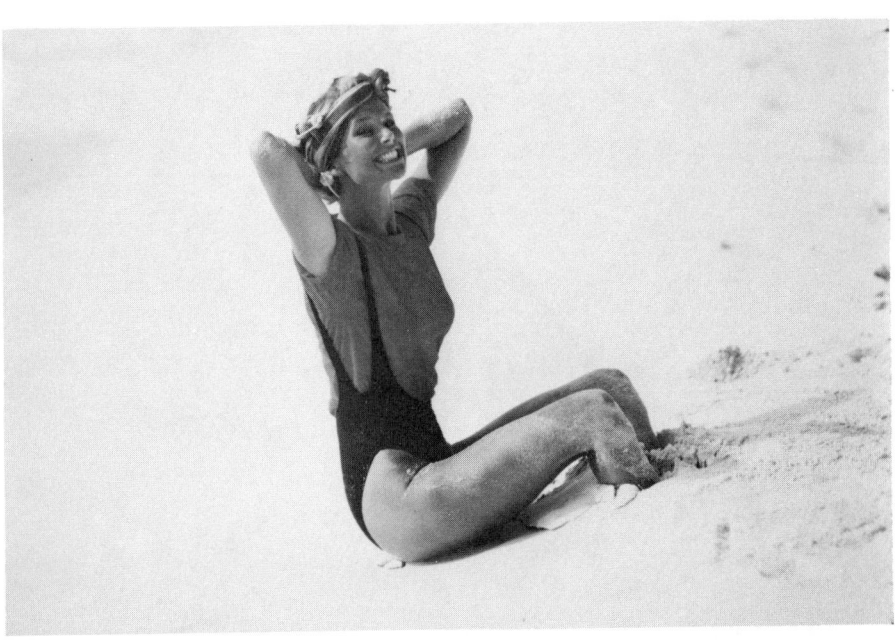

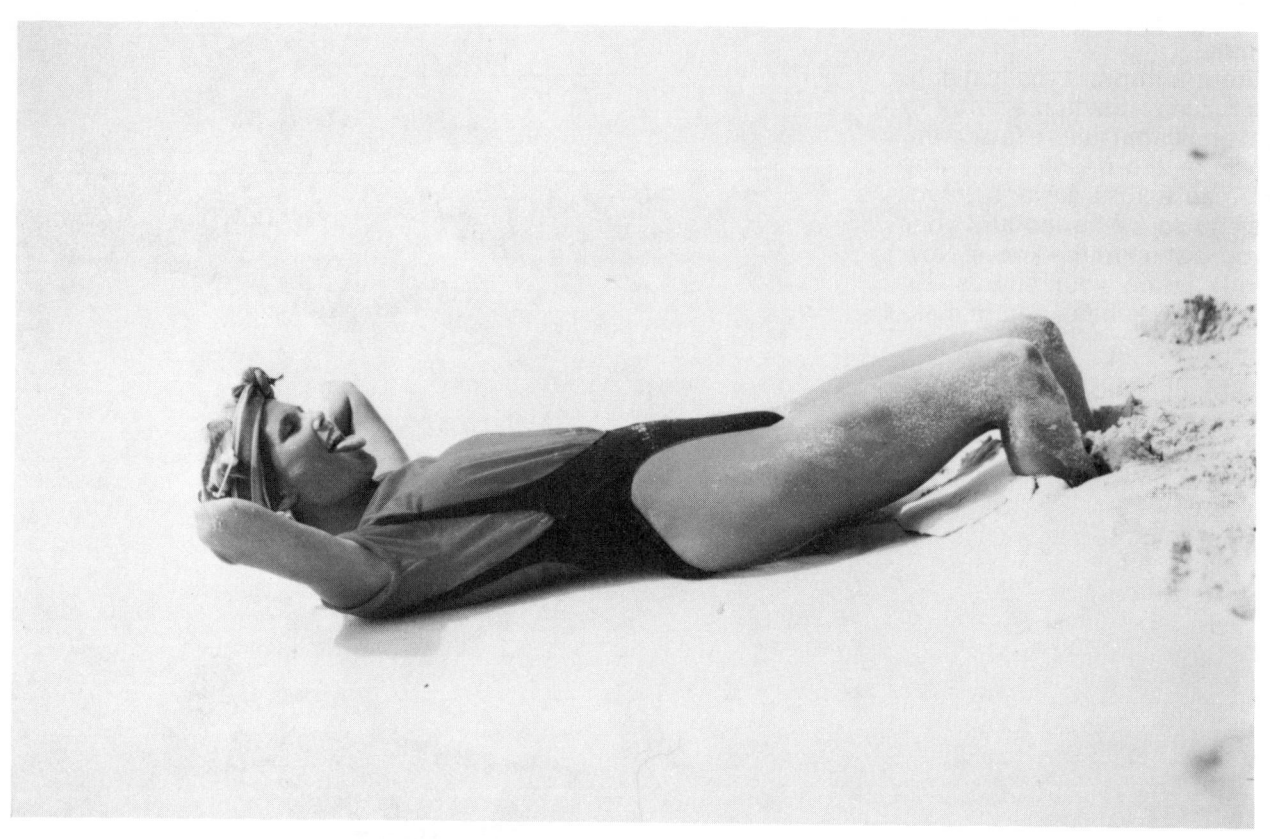

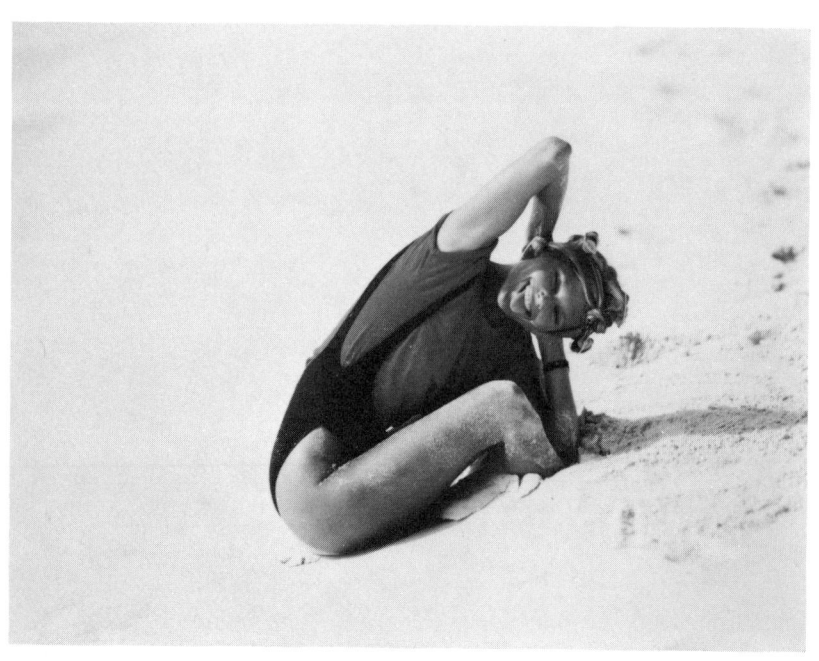

Elbow/Knee-Twist Sit-ups
This is a fine one for the waist as well as the stomach.

With your feet still buried in the ground, lie flat on your back, keeping your knees bent. Clasp your hands behind your head. Sit up, touching your knee with the opposite elbow, twisting your torso and trying to keep a flat back. Lie back slowly. Repeat with the other elbow touching the opposite knee.

Jump Rope

Bring your jump rope to the beach to liven up your jog. It's a great form of aerobic exercising. I like to do fancy jump-rope maneuvers I picked up from boxer Roberto Duran! Try to develop some of your own variations. Do it to music! Salsa's great!

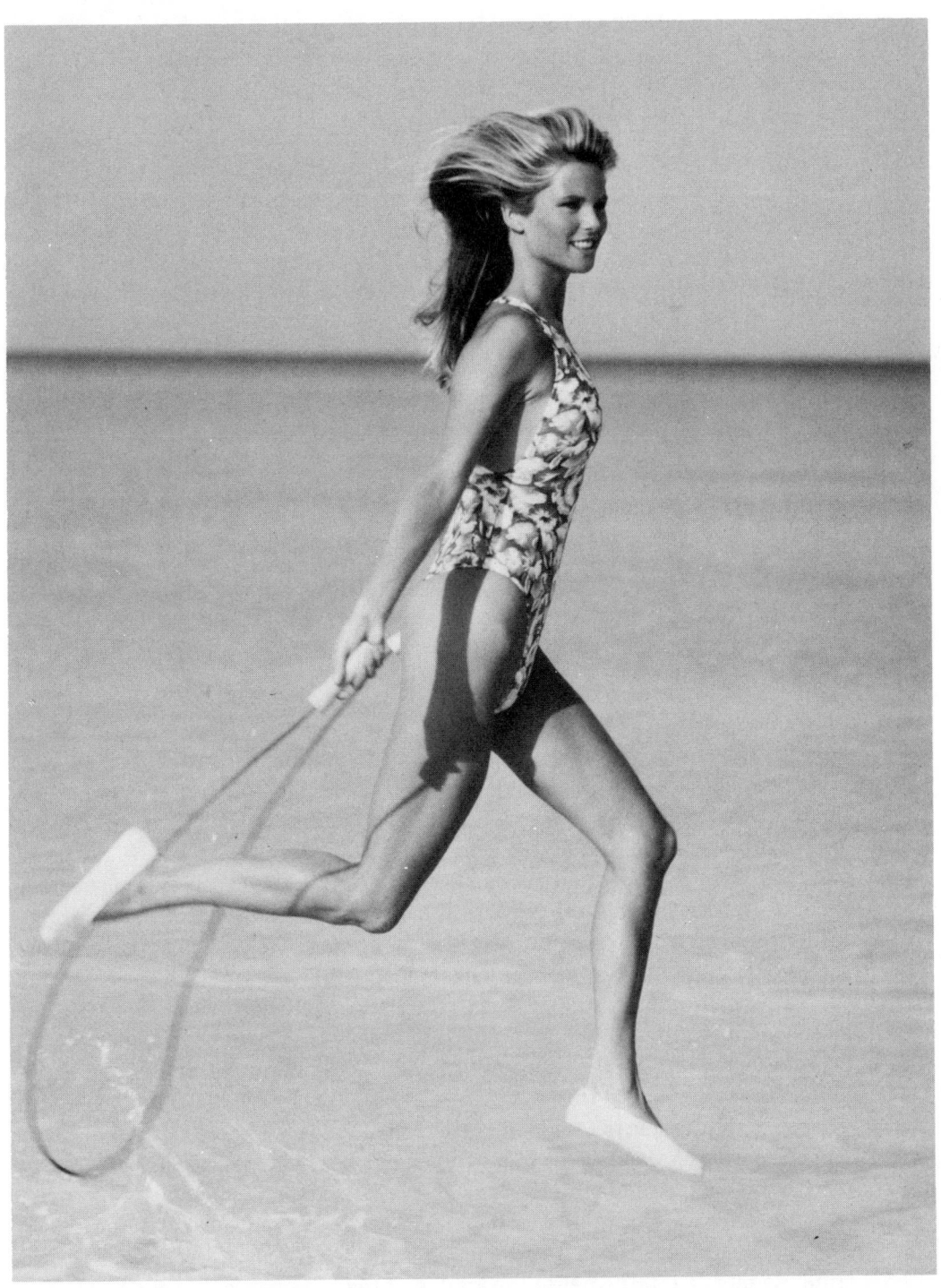

THE BEASTS OF SUMMER

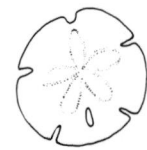

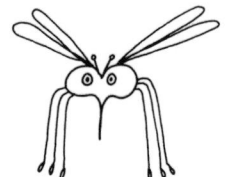

Bugs are tricky! *They* like to think they have a sly sense of humor, but it's *really* a mean streak! They certainly have pulled some fast ones on me. They know *exactly* what to do to send me screaming, itching, running, tearing at my clothes, leaping into water, onto chairs, and out of my skin! Some are more clever than others but *none* are to be trusted. I've compiled a list of tips and cautions, tried and true, to keep you one jump ahead of the bugs without all the leaping!

Calm down and don't eat sweets! It seems that people who are very emotional and people who eat a lot of sweets are the favorite victims of bugs. (Another great reason to give up sweets!) Because I try to avoid sweets, I know that in my case, the emotions are to blame!

Repellent. A good repellent is the first line of defense. I always carry two or three with me when I travel. I keep one in my beach bag, one on my bedside table, and one in my purse. I spray myself frequently wherever I'm exposed. I don't like to put repellent on my face but I do dab it behind my ears and along my hairline. (Why nobody has invented a suntan lotion with insect repellent is a mystery to me!)

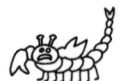

Avoid perfume. Bugs love perfume. It makes you smell like a delicious flower and they'll line up for a sample. So avoid it, even in the evenings, unless you're going to be indoors. Be sure that your body moisturizer and other beauty products are free of perfumes, too.

Bees love champagne almost as much as I do! So gulp it. (Just kidding!)

Bug-Bite Relief: Sooner or later you'll probably get bitten, so be sure you have some kind of cream or lotion on hand that stops the itching and stinging. There are lots of commercial preparations that will do the trick but you can always rely on a dab of witch hazel or rubbing alcohol to relieve the itch or sting.

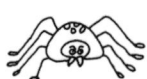

Mosquito netting. Yes, I know it sounds very *African Queen,* but it really works. On one trip to the Seychelles Islands I was plagued with bugs. I got my hands on some mosquito netting and sewed up my all-time best weapon in my bug battle: a net bag. It's just a giant net sleeping bag sewn on three sides with a drawstring on the fourth side, and it's wonderfully versatile. It's large enough to fit a pillow inside so I can actually sleep in it: step into it, slip under the covers, tuck in a pillow, and pull the string. One night on that trip a huge spider dropped from the ceiling right onto my face, but my net bag kept me safe. I only had to worry about my heart stopping!

I used it when I was on Bird Island because there were thousands of gnats and mosquitos, and if I were bitten, the photos would have looked awful. So when I wasn't posing I wore my net bag tied around me like a long skirt, ballerina style. I would throw it over my shoulders like a shawl and even slip my legs into it under the table at restaurants.

Even if you don't want to sew up a net bag, you can always find a big piece of netting to help protect yourself. I promise, you'll be glad you have it.

Another way to rig up a nighttime bug-safe canopy is to bring along two thumbtacks. Push your bed against the wall (not too close—remember those climbing bugs!), pin the net to the wall, and then drape it over your bed.

Me with my mosquito netting

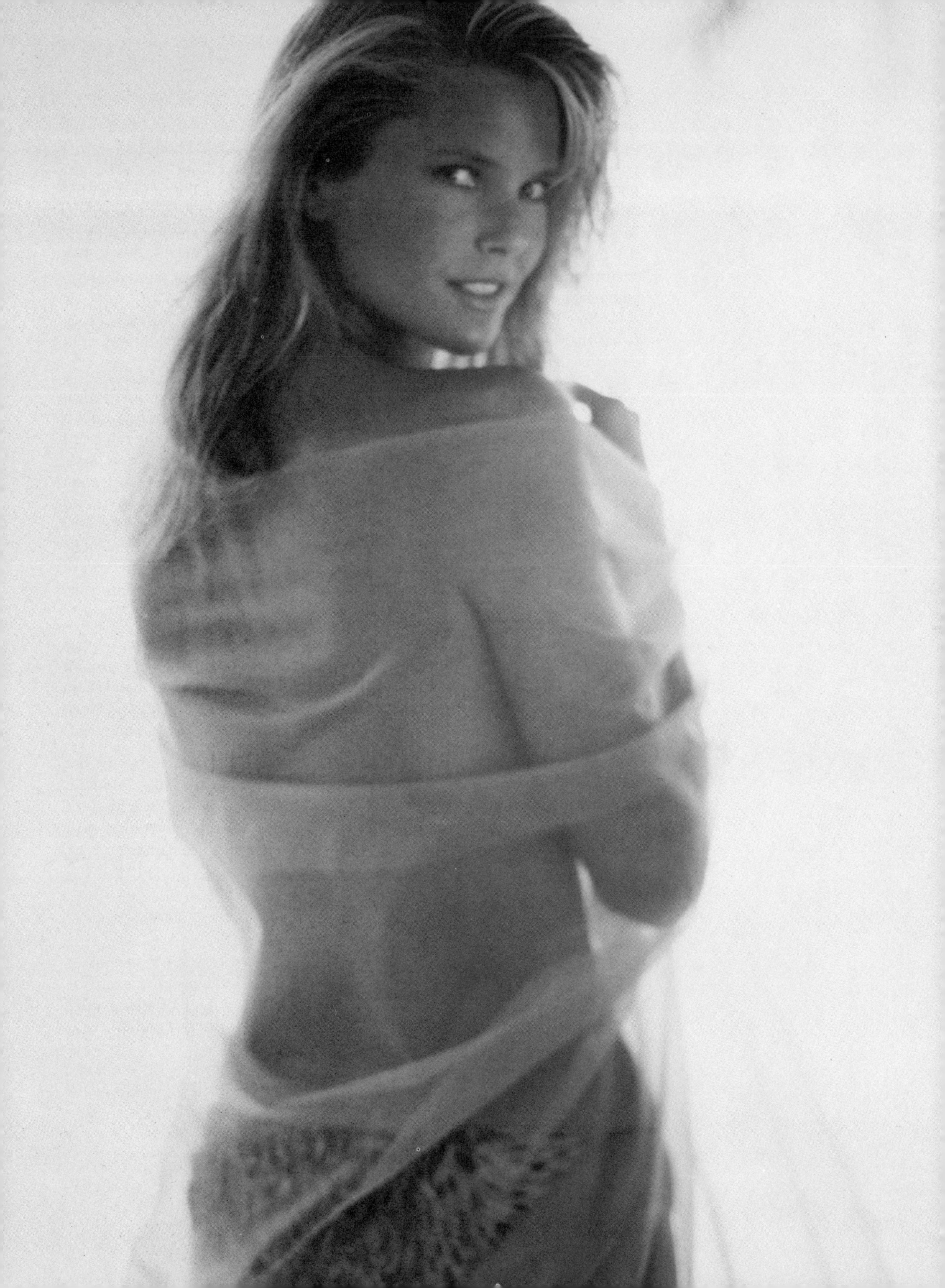

Look before you leap. Once I was in the Bahamas on a shooting. I had to get down on the sand on all fours for one particular shot. After I had been in that position for a few minutes I felt a terrible burning on my legs. I yelled but the photographer said he couldn't see anything. I held the pose but in another few minutes I was completely covered with sand-flea bites. Sand fleas, aptly named "noseeums" (no-see-ums), can do their damage while being almost invisible to the casual eye. My knees must have been in some sort of nest and they had swarmed all over me. I had so many bites that I became feverish and had to go home.

Now I never lie on an unfamiliar beach without a towel. I always check to see there are no bugs beneath my towel. And I spray insect repellent right on my beach towel.

Check your clothes and bedding. This is especially important in tropical places. When I work in a place that has scorpions, I'm always careful to put a pair of shoes next to my bed during the night or even on my bedside table. If I have to get up I never touch the floor barefoot and I never step into shoes without looking. I learned to do this when I lived in Mexico. Most everyone I knew who had been bitten by a scorpion had been attacked when they'd stepped out of bed in the middle of the night—right onto a scorpion! Of course you should always check your sheets before you climb into bed at night to be sure you'll sleep alone. And shake out your jeans, shorts, shirts—*anything*—before slipping into it. There's nothing worse than zipping a bug up into your pants!

Keep food under wraps. This is another lesson I learned the hard way. I was on a job in the tropics and because I'm a vegetarian, I'd packed some protein bars in case I didn't find anything to eat. When I came back to my hotel room the first night I reached into my suitcase for a nightgown and it was black with bugs. The moral is, if you don't want bugs in your room, don't bring food.

The Japanese have taken a giant leap for mankind! They have invented a machine that emits ultrasonic sound. We can't hear it but the bugs can and it drives them crazy. My mom has the plug-in model for kitchens (roach fighters, rejoice!) but there's also a battery-operated model in the form of a pin to wear on your lapel. I'm buying thousands of them. The perfect Christmas present, at last!

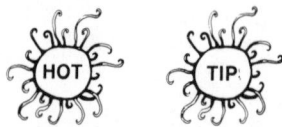

When you get a mosquito bite, don't scratch. Instead, make a little X on the bite with your fingernail and rub some Tiger Balm into the X. It's very soothing.

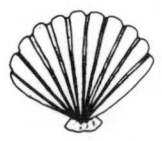

There are certain plants that would love to ruin our time at the beach. The most common ones are poison ivy, oak, and sumac. Some people have no reaction whatsoever to these plants but others are so allergic that they can wind up in the hospital. I once found a deserted beach in California at Big Sur and spent the afternoon nude enjoying the sea and the privacy. But that night I discovered all about plant allergies: I think I'd come into contact with every poisonous plant known to man. I didn't land in the hospital but I was miserable for a long time.

Poison ivy seems to be the most common pest plant found at a beach. By now you should know that it has three green, glossy leaves. Poison oak has three leaves but they're a little more ragged than poison ivy. Poison sumac has dark green leaves with light green backs.

If you do get stricken by any of the "poison" plants, I think you'd do well to avoid the lotions and ointments in the drugstore unless you've used them in the past without problems. Like sunburn medications, they are acting on the skin when it's damaged and they can cause allergic reactions. I think you're best off to go the old-fashioned route: Wash thoroughly with brown laundry soap and then apply a compress of skim milk diluted with water. (Make sure you wash the clothes you were wearing separately.) Of course, if you're swollen or in real pain, call your doctor.

In addition to the common plants, you've got to watch out for the exotics. Once I was in Hawaii and dressing up for a special dinner. As I left my hotel room I saw a beautiful plant with bright flowers. I picked one and tucked it behind my ear. I thought it looked wonderful but the next day I had a rash on my neck from oleander sap.

If you're in a strange place, be sure to ask the locals about any plants that could cause a reaction, and when in doubt, search out the tried and true flowers like bougainvillea or hibiscus.

THE PERILS OF PLANTS

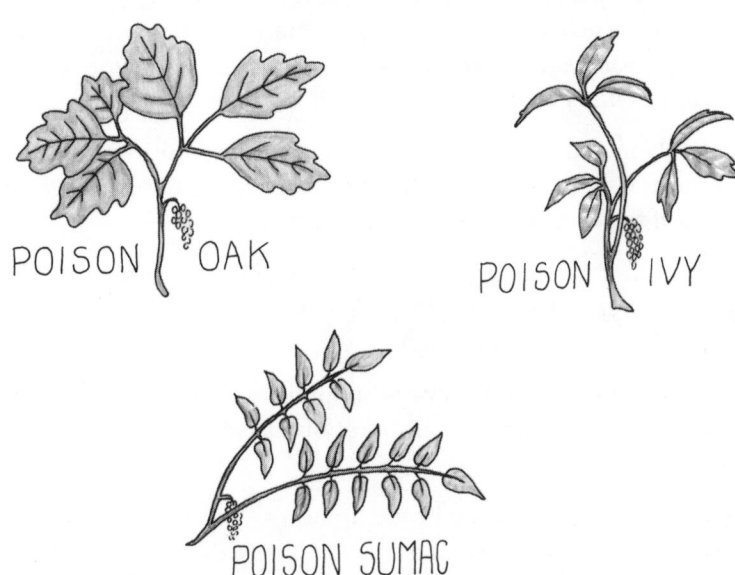

POISON OAK

POISON IVY

POISON SUMAC

Never, never run on a beach where the sand is anything but flat. If you run on a slanted beach you'll put an uneven stress on your muscles and you can hurt yourself badly.

If you're going to be at a beach that might have tar on it—which unfortunately includes many beaches today—tuck some nail-polish remover or strong household detergent in your beach bag for quick cleanups.

BEACH PHOTOS

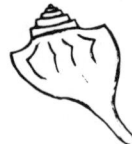

The beach is a super place to take photos. Next to photographing fights at ringside, it's one of my favorite locations. But there are some things you should know if you're bringing your camera to the beach:

Salt water is your camera's worst enemy. It corrodes parts and can cause serious damage. Keep your camera in a plastic bag to protect it from salt water. If it does get sprayed, wipe it immediately with a cloth that's wet with *fresh* water. If your camera goes overboard and gets soaked, don't despair. But do rush it to the nearest camera-repair store for immediate attention.

Sand is another enemy of your camera. It can scratch lenses and clog mechanisms. I always bring a can of pressurized air to the beach with me. I use it often to blow sand from camera parts. You can buy it at any camera-supply store.

Photographers' assistants make a point of carefully cleaning the cameras after a day of beach shooting. Know why? The salt air—the combination of moisture and salt—can eventually damage your camera. In addition to keeping your camera in a plastic bag, be sure to clean it when you get home from the beach. Use a soft cloth that's been dampened with fresh water.

Film can be damaged by excessive heat, so if you're taking film to the beach, be sure to keep it in the shade. You might even want to tuck it into the cooler with your food to be sure it stays cool and fresh.

Be extra careful when changing the film to guard against bright light. If there's no shady spot, use your body to make a shadow by putting your back to the sun and working in the shade.

I find it useful to keep all my camera supplies in a separate bag, reserved just for that purpose. That way I'm less likely to accidentally rub my lens with a wet, sandy beach towel.

If you're taking a photo in very bright light—at the beach or on a ski slope—set your camera one f-stop less than usual. This allows less light to reach the film, preventing overexposure.

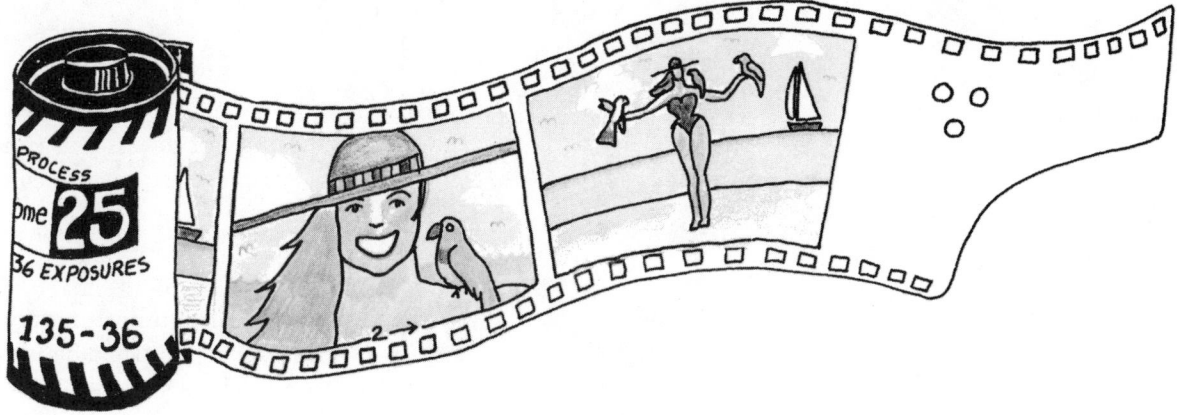

When photographing friends at the beach, remember that unless the sun is behind you, or your subject, it will distort your photo. The safest method is to be sure that the sun is coming from the side over one of your shoulders.

If you take lots of photos at the beach, or if you're planning a beach vacation (or need a gift idea for someone who is!), they now make relatively inexpensive sealed cameras that are sandproof and waterproof. These cameras even work under water and are a boon for scuba divers and snorkelers.

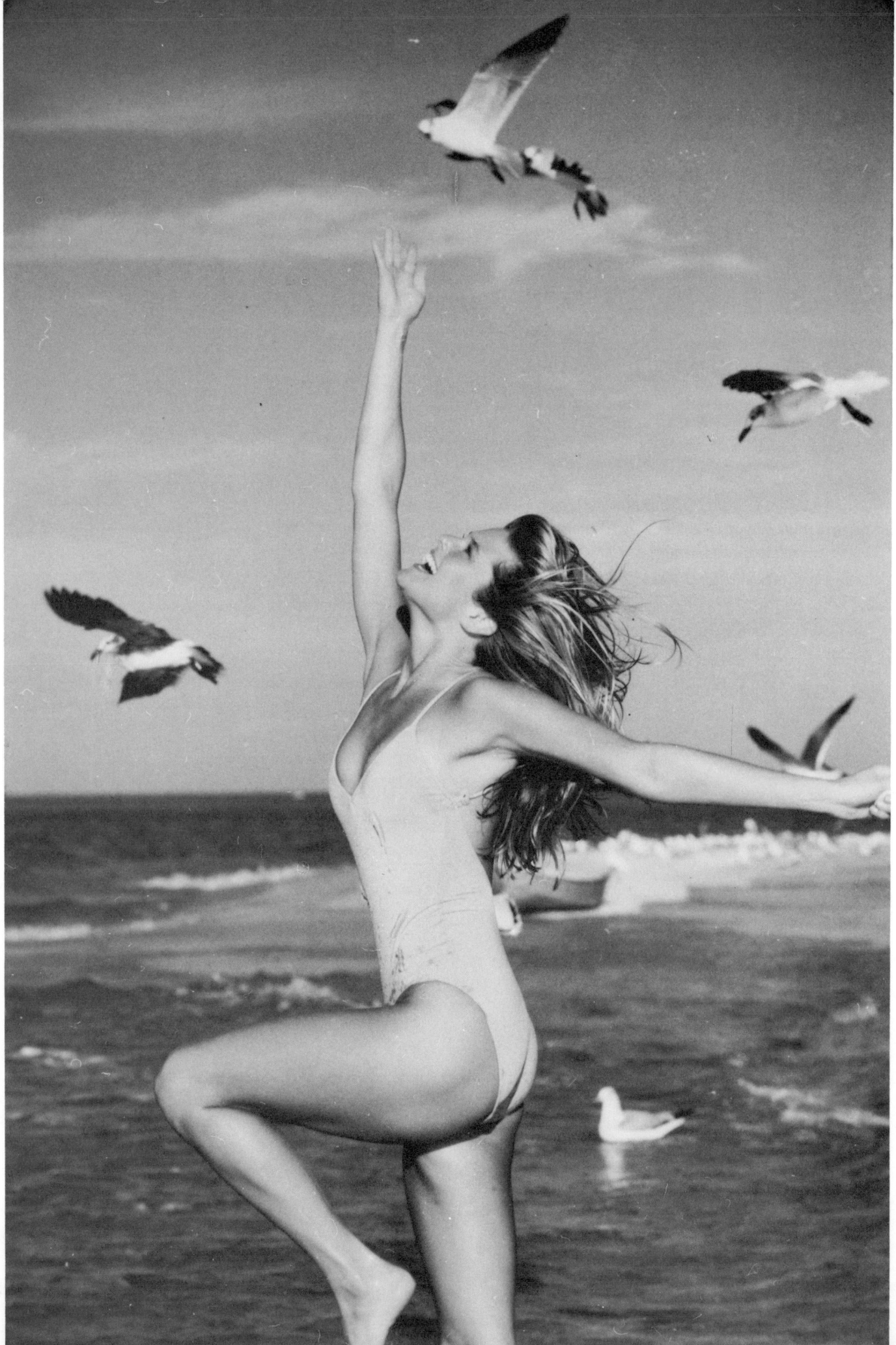

The beach and the ocean are my favorite places. They give me so much pleasure! But anyone who enjoys them has a responsibility to preserve them. I take that responsibility seriously. I'm an active member of both Greenpeace and the Cousteau Society. They both work to maintain and preserve the natural beauty of our oceans.

Maybe you should think about joining, too!
Write to them at:

The Cousteau Society
930 West 21st Street
Norfolk, VA 23517

Greenpeace U.S.A.
2007 R Street, N.W.
Washington, D.C. 20009

A SERIOUS NOTE

PHOTO
CREDITS